2438942779

A HISTORY OF INFECTIOUS DISEASES AND THE MICROBIAL WORLD

A HISTORY OF INFECTIOUS DISEASES AND THE MICROBIAL WORLD

LOIS N. MAGNER

Healing Society: Disease, Medicine, and History
John Parascandola, Series Editor

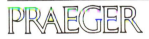

Westport, Connecticut
London

Library of Congress Cataloging-in-Publication Data

Magner, Lois N., 1943–
    A history of infectious diseases and the microbial world / Lois N. Magner.
        p. ; cm.—(Healing society—disease, medicine, and history; ISSN 1933–5938.)
    Includes bibliographical references and index.
    ISBN 978–0–275–99504–1 (alk. paper)
    1. Communicable diseases—History. 2. Microbiology—History. 3. Medical
microbiology—History. I. Title. II. Series: Healing society—disease, medicine,
and history.
    [DNLM: 1. Communicable Diseases—history. 2. Bioterrorism. 3. Communicable
Disease Control—history. 4. Disease Outbreaks—history. 5. Microbiology—history.
6. Virus Diseases—history. WC 11.1 M196h 2009]
    RA643.M32   2009
    362.196′9–dc22   2008051885

British Library Cataloguing in Publication Data is available.

Library of Congress Catalog Card Number: 2008051885
ISBN: 978–0–275–99504–1
ISSN: 1933-5938

First published in 2009

Praeger Publishers, 88 Post Road West, Westport, CT 06881
An imprint of Greenwood Publishing Group, Inc.
www.praeger.com

Printed in the United States of America

The paper used in this book complies with the
Permanent Paper Standard issued by the National
Information Standards Organization (Z39.48–1984).

10 9 8 7 6 5 4 3 2 1

To Ki-Han and Oliver, as always

CONTENTS

Series Foreword   ix

Acknowledgments   xi

Introduction: Welcome to the Microbial World   xiii

Abbreviations   xxiii

Chapter One: Disease and History: An Overview   1

Chapter Two: Miasma, Contagion, and the Germ Theory
of Disease   19

Chapter Three: Microbiology and the Foundations of Modern
Surgery and Therapy   49

Chapter Four: Viruses and Viral Diseases   73

Chapter Five: Sanitary Reform, Public Health, and the Battle
against Filth and Epidemic Diseases   95

Chapter Six: The Art and Science of Preventing and Controlling
Epidemic Diseases   111

Chapter Seven: Emerging Infectious Diseases   149

Contents

Chapter Eight: Biological Weapons and Bioterrorism   185

Chapter Nine: Infectious Agents and New Concepts: From Chronic
          Diseases to the Microbiome   195

Bibliography   209
Index   219

SERIES FOREWORD

The Praeger series *Healing Society: Disease, Medicine, and History* features individual volumes that explore the social impact of particular illnesses or medically related conditions or topics for a broad audience. The object is to publish books that offer reliable overviews of particular aspects of medical and social history, while incorporating the most up-to-date scholarly interpretations. The books in the series are designed to engage readers and educate them about important but often neglected aspects of the social history of medicine. Disease and disability have significantly influenced the course of human history, and the books in this series will examine various aspects of that influence.

Of the three previous books in the series, two examined the history of a particular disease, and the other focused on the role of a particular individual in American public health. *A History of Infectious Diseases and the Microbial World* has a broader scope than these books. As the title suggests, Lois Magner examines the history of infectious disease in general. Beginning with early attempts to understand the nature and cause of infectious diseases, she carries the story right up to the present, including current concerns about emerging infections and biological terrorism. Her analysis covers the social and cultural factors, as well as the scientific and technical factors that have influenced our understanding of infectious diseases and our efforts to combat them. She tells a fascinating tale that recounts the history of all of the major infectious diseases that have plagued humankind, including smallpox, cholera, malaria, tuberculosis, poliomyelitis, bubonic plague, and many others. The reader will learn about evolving theories of disease, the emergence of microbiology, and the development of drugs, vaccines, and public health measures against infectious diseases.

A History of Infectious Diseases and the Microbial World will be of interest not only to historians and health professionals, but also to any member of the general public curious about how infectious diseases have affected our world and how societies have tried to cope with them. In addition, Magner has written about the subject in a way that will provide the nonspecialist reader with a basic understanding of microorganisms and the mechanisms by which they cause disease. It is a book that will also be useful for students in courses in the history of medicine or public health.

John Parascandola

ACKNOWLEDGMENTS

I would like to express my deep appreciation to John Parascandola for his advice, criticism, and encouragement in the preparation of this book.

INTRODUCTION: WELCOME TO THE MICROBIAL WORLD

Modern societies no longer live under the constant threat of the deadly and incomprehensible plagues that terrified our ancestors. Much of the credit for this transformation belongs to the scientists who established the germ theory of disease and proved that microorganisms caused specific, infectious, epidemic diseases. Unlike toxins, poisons, and chemical agents that may be quite deadly, even in minute quantities, the very diverse agents that cause infectious diseases are able to multiply in the sick and spread from one person to another. As we shall see in this exploration of the relationship between infectious diseases and the microbial world, pathogenic (disease-causing) agents belong to categories as diverse as parasitic worms, protozoans, fungi, bacteria, viruses, prions, and viroids.

During the last twenty years of the nineteenth century, scientific germ theory revolutionized medical thought and the art of surgery. Understanding the relationship between pathogens—disease-causing microbes—and infectious disease did not, however, lead to immediate improvements in therapy. During the first half of the twentieth century, medical microbiology stimulated the development of drugs, antitoxins, antibiotics, and vaccines that made it possible to treat or prevent many major epidemic diseases. These efforts were so successful that many experts predicted the imminent conquest of infectious diseases. But by the 1980s, new infectious diseases had appeared, previously obscure diseases were invading new areas, and deadly pathogens were becoming resistant to once-powerful antibiotics. Specialists in infectious disease generally agree that emerging infectious diseases and drug-resistant pathogens have become major threats throughout the world.

According to the modern germ theory of disease, infectious diseases are caused by microbes that invade and damage the body of their host as they grow and multiply. Infectious diseases can be transmitted directly or indirectly from one living organism to another. Some diseases are highly contagious, which means that the sick can spread the disease to many new victims. In other cases, even though the sick may cough and vomit, they do not spread the disease to others. Some diseases can result in a carrier state, in which the individual seems healthy but is still capable of transmitting the disease to others. Thus, a major goal of microbiology is to identify the mechanisms by which specific microbes invade the body and spread to new hosts.

Understanding the properties and characteristics of the various disease agents is critical to understanding the development, transmission, and treatment of specific infectious diseases. Pathogenic microbes have evolved complicated strategies to evade the defense mechanisms of the host. If successful in evading the immune response, microbes can cause a persistent infection and chronic disease. Understanding how microorganisms evade the normal host defense mechanisms and the mechanisms employed in the evasion strategy will provide insight into those medical approaches that can be used to treat infection and prevent disease. Microorganisms cause diseases in a wide range of plants and animals as well as in human beings, but different groups of microorganisms are more likely to cause disease in particular kinds of hosts. For example, protozoa are almost unknown as pathogens in plants, but members of this group cause malaria and other major diseases in humans and other animals. Fungi cause the great majority of plant diseases, whereas bacteria cause many diseases in humans and other animals.

The microbial world encompasses the most ancient and prevalent forms of life on earth. Although our interest in microbes primarily grew out of the battle against infectious diseases, modern knowledge of microorganisms and their properties is providing insight into a world that remained invisible, unimaginable, and unexplored long after the invention of the microscope. New techniques, primarily derived from molecular biology, are making it possible to reevaluate the role of microbes in nature. Microbes are unavoidable—they are present in the air we breathe and on every surface we touch, and many hundreds of different species of bacteria colonize the human body, particularly the skin, mouth, and gastrointestinal tract. The normally harmless microbes that quietly live on or within the body have many important physiological functions, but they also seem to inhibit the growth of harmful bacteria. Thus, in addition to understanding the role of microbes as pathogens, it is important to think about the world of microbes in terms of the normal, inevitable, and generally harmless interactions that take place between microbes and the human body.

THE SCIENCE OF MICROBIOLOGY

Although a new world swarming with entities invisible to the naked eye was first described by the pioneers of microscopy in the seventeenth century, microbiology did not emerge as a scientific discipline until the nineteenth century. Historians as well as naturalists have often used the terms *bacteriology* and *microbiology* interchangeably, although microbiology is a broader term that encompasses an expanding list of subdisciplines: the study of bacteria (bacteriology), fungi (mycology), protozoa (protozoology), algae (phycology), and viruses (virology). Thus, in addition to the study of the minute organisms known to nineteenth-century scientists, microbiology now includes the study of microscopic entities that are not actually cells or organisms, in the traditional sense, although they are capable of multiplying, mutating, and causing disease. These noncellular transmissible agents include viruses and newly discovered infectious entities such as viroids and prions (see Chapter 4).

Bacteria are considered *prokaryotes*, that is, single-celled living entities that do not have a well-defined membrane-enclosed nucleus. Despite their apparent simplicity, bacterial species exhibit great diversity in terms of size, shape, nutritional requirements, and motility. Bacteria have adapted to a remarkably wide range of environments, including some that seem quite hostile to life. Many bacteria probably remain undetected because they cannot be grown with existing laboratory techniques. Recently, microbiologists have also become very interested in a group of prokaryotes known as the Archaea, which were originally discovered as inhabitants of extreme environments. Many of these microbes are known as extremophiles because of their adaptations to life in environments that are unusually hot or cold, acidic or basic. Classifying the prokaryotes has been a difficult and often controversial undertaking because microbes that look very similar under the microscope may be very different when examined in terms of genetic sequences and physiological properties.

During the 1970s, Carl R. Woese introduced the idea that the prokaryotes should be separated into two distinct groups, bacteria and the archaea, by using molecular sequences in their genetic material to deduce their genealogical relationships. The family trees derived from this approach, often referred to as molecular phylogenetics, were very different from traditional classifications primarily based on morphology. All living beings, according to Woese, should be divided into three domains: Eukaryota, Eubacteria, and Archaea. In general, although archaeans resemble bacteria under the microscope, these groups differ significantly in terms of genetic sequences and biochemical properties. Archaeans were originally found in extreme environments such as thermal vents in the deep sea, hot springs, alkaline or acid waters, extremely salty waters, underground petroleum deposits, and the digestive tracts of various animals, including cows and termites. Scientists have also discovered microbes living many miles above the surface of the earth in dust particles carried by clouds.

Newly discovered extremophiles continue to challenge previous assumptions about the environment in which life can evolve, exist, and flourish.

As methods of detecting microbes by identifying characteristic genetic signatures improved, archaeans were found in very diverse and even relatively pleasant environments, especially in the oceans. Recent work, therefore, provides strong evidence that the genetic diversity of the microbial world has been greatly underestimated and that many uncultured archaeal species exist in marine environments and in forest soils. Many archaean species are difficult or impossible to culture in the laboratory, but their ability to thrive in extreme environments is of interest in terms of the evolution of life on earth and the possibility that organisms similar to the archaea might exist in the extreme environments found on other planets.

In contrast to bacteria, fungi, algae, and protozoa have a well-defined, membrane-enclosed nucleus and therefore are called *eukaryotes*. The cells of all eukaryotes, whether they are single-celled microbes or multicellular plants and animals, contain a membrane-bound nucleus and organelles such as chloroplasts and mitochondria. The origin of eukaryotic cells is still unclear, although parasitic or symbiotic relationships between different prokaryotic ancestral cells were presumably involved in the evolution of the first eukaryotes. Indeed, subcellular organelles that are now essential components of plant and animal cells, such as mitochondria, chloroplasts, and the nucleus, might be the descendents of ancient bacteria and archaeans that colonized ancestral eukaryotic cells and became permanent residents.

Understanding the relationship between microbes and infectious diseases was one of the primary reasons for the study of microbiology, but pathogens—disease-causing microbes—constitute a very small part of the microbial world. Microorganisms play a critical, indispensable role in the recycling of chemical elements in the biosphere and in making atmospheric nitrogen available for use by plants. The decomposition of organic matter by microorganisms is the basis of sewage treatment. Long before microorganisms had been identified, human beings relied on microbial fermentation for the production of beer, wine, bread, cheese, yogurt, and other foods. As scientists learned to exploit the properties of microbes, microbial fermentation was used in the production of antibiotics, vitamins, enzymes, and various pharmaceutical products. Recognition of the ability of microbes to modify the environment has resulted in many practical, industrial applications. Microorganisms have been used as highly selective biological pesticides, as catalysts for reactions that are difficult or impossible to carry out using conventional chemical methods, and in the extraction of copper and gold from low-grade deposits and mine tailings. Biodegradable bacterial plastics have been used in surgical pins, sutures, and wound dressings; as components of time-release drugs, medicines, pesticides, or fertilizers; and as emulsifying agents and blood plasma substitutes. Microorganisms have been used to accelerate the breakdown of toxic wastes, pesticides, oil spills, and other pollutants, a process known as bioremediation.

Enzymes produced by the microbes known as extremophiles are valuable because of their stability under the conditions required for sophisticated laboratory processes and in rather mundane domestic products such as laundry detergents.

BACTERIOLOGY

Ancestors of modern bacteria were probably the first form of life on earth, making their appearance about three and a half billion years ago. Suggestive evidence of these first living entities has been detected in materials known as stromatolites, found in ancient sedimentary rocks. Researchers who tested samples of ice from Antarctica that were at least one hundred thousand years old discovered bacteria that were able to resume growth and reproduction under favorable conditions. These findings suggest that if Antarctic ice melts as the result of global warming, long-dormant bacteria might become part of the microbial population of the oceans. The introduction of ancient microbes into modern communities and the potential mixing of genes that have been isolated for millennia could transform the so-called genome of the ocean in unpredictable ways.

Because of their important place in the work of the founders of modern microbiology, the bacteria deserve special attention. The term *bacteriology* was first used in the early 1880s, when it primarily designated the new medical science devoted to the study of disease-causing germs. In keeping with the importance of the microscope in studies of the causative agents of disease, the term *bacterium*—from a Greek term meaning "little rod"—refers to the shape of many of the tiny entities revealed by that instrument. Bacteriology was crucial to the development of the germ theory of disease, a unifying theory that revolutionized medicine, surgery, and public health policy; that is, studies of bacteria made it possible to understand the causes of infectious diseases and postsurgical infections. When identifying bacteria, scientists and medical technicians still rely on criteria established during the nineteenth century: morphology, staining behavior, and physiological and serological properties. The Gram stain, introduced by Hans Christian Gram in 1884, separates most prokaryotes into two groups: Gram-positive and Gram-negative. Gram-positive and Gram-negative bacteria differ in the structure and chemical composition of their cell walls, which often determines their sensitivity to antibiotics.

Although the history of bacteriology is so closely linked to medical history, nineteenth-century scientists studied bacteria for many different reasons. From a very practical standpoint, understanding the role of bacteria in fermentation could improve and standardize the production of wine, beer, vinegar, cheese, and so forth. Bacteria were of interest in debates about spontaneous generation and the origin of life and the controversy surrounding Charles Darwin's theory of evolution. Agricultural and soil scientists were interested in the role bacteria played in nitrogen fixation and the breakdown of dead and decaying organic matter, processes that contribute to soil fertility. Naturalists were very interested in the complex task of classifying the bewildering array of microscopic creatures.

Scientists who are interested in understanding the diversity of all life-forms on earth suggest that there may be many hundreds of thousands, or even millions, of different species of bacteria. Bacteriologists have discovered and characterized only a small fraction of all the bacteria that exist today and have not yet fully explored the entire range of the properties of known species. Scientists originally organized bacteria in terms of their shapes and staining behaviors, but modern classification systems are generally based on molecular biology, rather than morphology; that is, scientists are increasingly using information obtained by sequencing bacterial nucleic acids as the fundamental principle of a new system of classification. In 1995, the first bacterial whole-genome sequence was published (*Haemophilus influenzae*). Ten years later, the sequences of at least 150 bacterial genomes had been completed and more than 250 were in progress. Despite the increasing sophistication and efficiency of the techniques for gathering and organizing sequence data from DNA and RNA, the classification of microorganisms remains a complex, confusing, and contentious field.

Robert Koch and other pioneers of microbiology devoted themselves to the problem of preparing pure cultures to prove that specific diseases were caused by specific bacteria. Medical microbiologists still rely on the isolation, purification, and characterization of individual species of bacteria to clarify the relationship between pathogens and diseases. The role of bacteria in disease remains a major focus of microbiology, but scientists are increasingly interested in basic questions about the intrinsic nature of bacteria—their physiology, metabolism, genetics, evolution, and place in nature. In general, microbiologists still work with pure cultures, but they are increasingly interested in understanding the behavior of microbes under more natural conditions. For example, the growth rates of bacteria in pure laboratory cultures can be very different from those in more natural environments and communities. *Escherichia coli* can double in about twenty minutes under optimal laboratory conditions, but its generation time in the intestinal tract is generally about twelve hours.

In natural environments, as opposed to laboratory cultures, bacterial cells may interact, communicate, and exchange genetic material with other microbial species. Instead of living as separate individuals, swimming or being tumbled about in a liquid medium, some microbes form large, complex communities known as biofilms that stick to solid surfaces, such as teeth, surgical instruments, and medical implants, much as barnacles stick to piers, docks, and boat bottoms. Pathogens in biofilms may be protected from disinfectants and antibiotics.

Attempts to understand how diverse microbial communities control or coordinate their responses to each other, their environment, and available resources led to surprising discoveries about bacterial communication, a process called *quorum sensing*.

Bacteria seem to use chemical signals to communicate with members of the same species and members of other species, primarily in response to population density. Chemicals that we know as toxins or antibiotics might have evolved as signals used in microbial conversations. An understanding of microbial communication may lead to novel therapeutic methods that could prevent the release of deadly microbial toxins or inhibit the progress of infectious diseases.

MYCOLOGY: THE STUDY OF FUNGI

Mycology is the branch of science that studies fungi, eukaryotic microorganisms that, like plants, have rigid cell walls, but, unlike plants, lack chlorophyll. Mycologists estimate that there may be more than one million species of fungi, a category that includes molds and yeasts. The fungi have been difficult to classify because they can assume many different forms. Molds typically live in complex networks of filaments called *hyphae*. In contrast, yeasts exist as separate, single cells. Some fungi alternate between mold and yeast forms, depending on environmental conditions. Fungal networks are often capable of penetrating and exploiting solid substrates that are impervious to bacteria. In popular usage as well as the medical literature, the terms *fungus* and *mold* are used interchangeably. Found in environments as different as arid deserts and tropical forests, fungi live primarily on dead, decaying organic material. Fungi play a vital role in the decomposition and recycling of organic matter, including the cellulose and lignin in plant debris and chitin and keratin from animal remains.

Fungi are generally harmless, but some produce hallucinogens and deadly toxins, and others cause serious diseases in plants, animals, and humans. Fungal plant diseases result in billions of dollars in damage to crops both before and after harvest. The American elm and the American sweet chestnut tree were brought to the verge of extinction by fungal pathogens. Dutch elm disease first appeared in Europe early in the twentieth century and was brought to the United States in the 1920s. Elm bark beetles originally acted as the vectors of the disease, but the fungus is also transmitted from the roots of infected trees to the roots of neighboring elms. Chestnut blight is caused by an airborne fungus that spread from imported Chinese chestnut trees, which are resistant to the disease.

Under certain conditions, normally innocuous fungi and their spores can cause respiratory diseases, allergies, skin infections, and life-threatening systemic infections. Indeed, early evidence for the germ theory of disease involved the relationship between molds and human skin diseases. Skin infections caused by fungi (dermatophytoses) include common nuisances, such as athlete's foot and ringworm (tinea), but severe illness can occur when fungi enter open wounds. Serious systemic diseases can occur when the lungs are attacked by fungi or spores contracted through inhalation. Histoplasmosis, caused by a mold commonly found in bird droppings, can range from asymptomatic to life threatening. *Coccidioides immitis* can cause a life-threatening disease known as coccidioidomycosis or desert fever, which is endemic in the southwestern United States. Paracoccidioidomycosis, generally found in Central and South America, can cause symptoms similar to tuberculosis. *Ochroconis gallopava*, a fungus that can infect the human brain and nervous system, has been isolated from hot springs that have been popular as spas. Systemic mycoses are among the opportunistic infections that occur in patients with impaired immune systems. *Pneumocystis carinii* is particularly well known as the cause of a rare form of pneumonia that led to the recognition of HIV/AIDS in the 1980s.

Molds and their spores have been blamed for a variety of conditions generally known as sick building syndrome. People who believe that they have suffered serious illnesses because of mold in their homes or workplaces argued that mold infestations had caused memory loss, brain seizures, breathing difficulties, violent chronic cough, stomach problems, and diarrhea. During the 1990s, *Stachybotrys chartarum*, a toxin-producing mold, was blamed for several deaths in contaminated houses. In many cases, however, evidence of a causal relationship between molds and illness was ambiguous. Nevertheless, reports of severe illnesses associated with mold infestations were widely circulated by the mass media, leading to lawsuits against building contractors filed by homeowners who claimed that water damage and mold infestations caused serious illnesses. In response to widespread fears that molds and their toxins were creating a public health threat, officials at the Centers for Disease Control and Prevention asked the Institute of Medicine to convene a panel of epidemiologists, toxicologists, and physicians to study the problem. In 2004, the Institute of Medicine released a study titled *Damp Indoor Spaces and Health*. The study concluded that anecdotal reports of health problems allegedly caused by toxic molds had generated a great deal of mass media attention but relatively little reliable, scientific evidence linking mold infestations to sick building syndrome. Given the widespread fear of toxic indoor mold, the panel recommended more rigorous research into the effects of indoor mold.

PARASITOLOGY

Parasites are creatures that live on or in another organism at the expense of the host. Although disease-causing microbes fit the definition, after the establishment of scientific germ theory, the term parasite was very rarely used in reference to bacteria, fungi, or viruses. Nineteenth-century evolutionary biologists often described parasites as degenerate life-forms, but parasites usually had complex life cycles and often could not be cultured in the laboratory by the methods developed for bacteria. Microbiology and parasitology gradually separated from each other as it became apparent that the infectious diseases of most concern to the wealthy, industrialized nations were caused by bacteria and viruses. European powers, however, were concerned with the parasitic diseases that affected people and animals in the colonies they controlled. Thus, parasitology was primarily associated with tropical medicine, colonial doctors, veterinarians, and entomologists and became peripheral to biomedical science. The major parasitic diseases are all but forgotten in much of the Western world, but parasitic diseases are still widespread, and some—such as Chagas' disease—are certainly capable of escaping from the areas where they are endemic.

By the end of the twentieth century, scientists were beginning to think seriously about the remarkable adaptations and properties that made disease-causing parasites so persistent and so successful. Techniques adopted from molecular biology and genomics made it possible to study previously intractable questions about the complex life cycle of major parasites and to explore new approaches to preventing and treating the devastating diseases they cause. Scientists are particularly interested in evidence that certain parasites, especially those with complex life cycles that require different host species, can alter the behavior of their hosts in ways that increase the probability that the parasite will be transmitted to a new host.

MICROBIAL ECOLOGY AND THE FUTURE OF MICROBIOLOGY

Since the 1990s, pioneers of a field known as microbial ecology have been exploring the complex microbial populations found in natural ecosystems. Microbiologists now know that disease-causing agents are only a very small component of the complex microbial world. They suspect, however, that the collective activities of these invisible, essentially unknown entities may have a profound impact on our environment and therefore on our health and well-being. Becoming familiar with the microbial world is therefore essential to understanding global patterns of disease and poverty, health and prosperity, and ultimately, to the quest for healing society.

ABBREVIATIONS

AHF	AIDS Healthcare Foundation
AIDS	acquired immune deficiency syndrome
ATCC	American Type Culture Collection
AZT	azidothymidine
BCG	Bacille Calmette-Guérin
BSE	bovine spongiform encephalopathy (commonly known as mad cow disease)
CDC	Centers for Disease Control and Prevention (an agency of the U.S. Public Health Service)
CJD	Creutzfeldt-Jakob disease
CMV	cytomegalovirus
CRS	congenital rubella syndrome
DDT	dichlorodiphenyltrichloroethane
DHF	dengue hemorrhagic fever
DNA	deoxyribonucleic acid
DPT	diphtheria, pertussis, and tetanus vaccine

DSS	dengue shock syndrome
EBV	Epstein-Barr virus
FBI	Federal Bureau of Investigation (an agency of the U.S. Department of Justice)
FDA	U.S. Food and Drug Administration
FMD	foot-and-mouth disease
HFRS	hemorrhagic fevers with renal syndrome
HIV	human immunodeficiency virus
HPV	human papilloma virus
HTLV	human T-lymphotropic virus
MDR-TB	multidrug-resistant tuberculosis
MDT	multidrug therapy
MMR	measles, mumps, and rubella vaccine
MRSA	methicillin-resistant *Staphylococcus aureus*
NAS	National Academy of Sciences
NIH	National Institutes of Health (an agency of the U.S. Department of Health and Human Services)
PCR	polymerase chain reaction
RNA	ribonucleic acid
RSV	Rous sarcoma virus
SARS	severe acute respiratory syndrome
SIDS	sudden infant death syndrome
SIV	simian immunodeficiency virus
STD	sexually transmitted disease
TMV	tobacco mosaic virus
Unaids	United Nations AIDS Program
USSR	Union of Soviet Socialist Republics
vCJD	variant Creutzfeldt-Jakob disease
VD	venereal disease
WHO	World Health Organization
XDR-TB	extremely drug-resistant tuberculosis

ONE

⤬⤬⤬

DISEASE AND HISTORY: AN OVERVIEW

Infectious diseases have affected human evolution and history in complex and subtle ways. Endemic and epidemic diseases may determine the density of populations, the dispersion of peoples, and the diffusion of genes as well as the success or failure of battles, invasions, migration, and colonization. Infectious diseases can be thought of as a reflection of evolution in progress, particularly if we focus on the mechanisms by which microbes adapted to new environments and exploited emerging opportunities to reach new hosts. In addition to illuminating the natural history of human disease, recent studies of microbes may provide insights into human evolution, early migration patterns, the domestication of plants and animals, and contemporary and future interactions between humans and microorganisms.

The microbes that cause infectious diseases flourished long before human life appeared, but the epidemic diseases that require dense human populations are relatively new. Many pathogens are species-specific, but some of the major epidemic diseases of human history, such as bubonic plague, malaria, yellow fever, and tuberculosis, can infect other animals. Wild or domesticated animals, which often live in quite dense groups, can serve as reservoirs for many diseases transmitted to humans directly or via insect vectors.

The survival of a pathogen that is species-specific depends on the pathogen's virulence, the size and population density of the host group, the immune response mounted by the host, and the pathogen's ability to find new victims. Certain pathogens can only be transmitted during the acute phase of a disease because the infectious agent disappears on recovery or death. When such an organism is introduced into a small population, virtually all individuals become infected and then recover or die. Such diseases could not establish permanent residence among small groups of people. Large herds of animals, however, carried many of the infectious agents that eventually adapted to human hosts. New disease patterns became part of the price paid for domesticating animals and creating densely populated, permanent villages, towns, and cities.

Pathogens that remain in the host during convalescence, persist in chronic lesions, or establish permanent residence in healthy carriers are likely to find new victims even among small bands of people. Some diseases are caused by commensal organisms—those that live harmlessly in or on their host until some disturbance triggers the onset of illness. Commensalism generally indicates a long period of mutual adaptation; thus, such diseases may be the most ancient. Mutated genes that produce variant forms of proteins, such as sickle cell hemoglobin, may reflect evolutionary adaptations in populations subjected to ancient scourges like malaria.

It is often assumed that modern and so-called primitive people differ in their susceptibility and resistance to disease. Comparisons of crude mortality rates for "moderns" and "primitives" are, however, likely to be very misleading. Mortality rates during an epidemic may reflect prior experience with the disease as well as the kind of care given to the sick. During an explosive epidemic in a small, isolated population, there may be no healthy adults left to feed children and care for the sick. Those who might have survived the disease may die because of the lack of food, water, and simple nursing care.

Changes in human behaviors and technologies provided new challenges and new opportunities for the microbial agents that cause disease; that is, hunting, foraging, cooking, the domestication of plants and animals, and the establishment of permanent villages, towns, and cities changed the relationship between humans and microbes over the course of many thousands of years. In more recent history, rapid and revolutionary changes in agriculture, animal husbandry, commerce, housing, travel, transportation, sexual mores, and medical techniques, such as the use of injections, blood transfusions, and tissue and organ transplants, have provided unprecedented opportunities for the transmission of infectious diseases.

Paleopathology, the study of the diseases that can be demonstrated in human and animal remains of ancient times, indicates that disease is older than the human race and was not uncommon among other species. Studies of ancient fossil remains, skeletons in museum collections, animals in zoos, and animals in the wild demonstrate the antiquity of disease. Paleopathology provides information about health, disease, death, environment, and culture in ancient populations. Because direct evidence of disease among ancient human beings is very limited, scientists must use indirect approaches to reach a tentative understanding of the prehistoric world. For example, studies of our closest relatives, the great apes and monkeys, indicate that wild primates suffer from many disorders, including arthritis, malaria, and parasitic worms. Scientists now think that the separation of the human line from that of the apes took place in Africa about five to eight million years ago. Our ancestors, the first "naked apes," presumably experienced disorders and diseases similar to those found among modern primates.

During the Paleolithic era, or Old Stone Age, human beings learned to make stone tools, build shelters, and create uniquely human social structures. Typically, they were opportunistic omnivores, living as scavengers and hunter-gatherers, traveling in small, mobile bands that probably included only a few dozen members. Contact with dead animals would have exposed hunters and scavengers to parasites, pathogens, and disease-carrying vectors. Until humans acquired mastery over fire and cooking, decaying flesh represented another source of life-threatening illness. Hunting, skinning, butchering, cooking, and eating wild animals brought humans into contact with many different pathogens and parasites.

Most of the evidence concerning disease in prehistoric humans comes from the study of skeletal remains. Bone is a dynamic living tissue constantly being modified in response to the stimulus of growth and to physiological and pathological stresses. Many factors, such as age, sex, nutrition, and illness, affect the bones, especially during growth. Starvation, severe malnutrition, and serious infectious diseases may leave diagnostic clues in bones and teeth. Severe episodes of diarrhea in infants, for example, can disrupt the development of teeth and bones. Most infectious diseases affect soft tissue, rather than bones, but some infectious diseases, such as tuberculosis, yaws, leprosy, syphilis, and fungal infections, leave diagnostic clues in the bones.

Where conditions favor the preservation of organic matter, coprolites (fossilized human feces) may be found in or near prehistoric campsites and dwellings, in cesspools, latrine pits, and refuse piles. Because certain parts of plants and animals are indigestible, information about diet, disease, and cooking techniques can be inferred from the analysis of pollen grains, charcoal, insect parts, and the eggs or cysts of parasitic worms in coprolites. In rare instances, the soft parts of prehistoric bodies have been preserved because of favorable burial conditions or the deliberate use of various mummification techniques. Mummified human remains provide evidence of infectious diseases and parasitic infestations. In the western hemisphere, natural mummification was more common than artificial methods, but the prehistoric people called the Basket-Makers deliberately dried cadavers and stuffed them into large baskets. Such mummies provide suggestive evidence for the existence of tuberculosis, hookworm, and other diseases in pre-Columbian America.

The transition from the Paleolithic way of life to new social patterns based on settled agriculture and animal husbandry is known as the Neolithic Revolution. Recent studies of the origins of agriculture suggest that it was almost universally adopted between ten thousand and two thousand years ago. The profound changes associated with the cultivation of crops, the domestication of animals, and the establishment of permanent settlements also led to major shifts in patterns of human disease. As their numbers and population density grew, human beings became suitable hosts for many disease agents previously found only in large herds of wild animals. Domesticating goats, sheep, pigs, and cattle improved the nutritional status of ancient people, but such animals harbored pathogens and parasites and attracted the vectors that transmit many infectious diseases. Some people adopted a nomadic or seminomadic existence, herding their animals between seasonal pasturelands or following their animals in search of water and pastureland. People and their domesticated animals often lived in very close proximity. Bringing people, dogs, sheep, goats, pigs, or cattle into close contact made it possible for infectious agents to attack new targets and to mix with other microbes. Germs could spread from animals to humans when they were licked, bitten, or touched, or through the air when animals coughed, and when animals were butchered and animals parts and products were used or eaten. Permanent dwellings, gardens, and fields provided convenient niches for insects, rodents, and other pests. Stored foods are likely to attract pests and become contaminated with excrement, insects, bacteria, molds, and their toxins. The basic food supply of early agricultural populations might have been more reliable than the food supply available to hunter-gatherers, but sedentary populations could be devastated by crop failures, starvation, and malnutrition, which would make them more vulnerable to infectious disease. Local famines could lead to attacks on neighboring or distant settlements, which could carry parasites and pathogens to new territories and populations.

Highly contagious diseases cannot be sustained by isolated bands of hunter-gatherers or farmers because the microbes that cause them generally cannot survive and multiply in the absence of fairly large numbers of susceptible hosts living in close proximity. Such microbes typically cause a disease of short duration that leads to immunity for those hosts that survive infection. To sustain a train of transmission, these microbes must continuously find susceptible individuals who will transmit the disease to other susceptible hosts. Settled, crowded populations offered many opportunities for the transmission of pathogens from person to person and from animals to humans. Villages, towns, and the networks that connected permanent settlements provided new opportunities for the transmission of infectious diseases. Networks of trade and travel, expanded by the use of horses and camels, wagons and ships, carried microbes to new environments, where they might find an array of susceptible hosts.

Some experts suggest that microbes that originally infected other animals cause the vast majority of human infectious diseases. The most likely source of the pathogens that infect humans would be domesticated dogs, sheep, goats, cattle, pigs, horses, and cats. But rodents, birds, marine mammals, and bats also transmit pathogens to humans and other primates. Microbes that colonized our hominid or primate ancestors are probably still with us, either as the common intestinal bacteria that help digest food or as pathogens such as the herpes and hepatitis viruses. Diseases of animals, known as *zoonoses*, may be relatively mild in their traditional hosts but can be very deadly when transferred to new host species. Although microbes are most likely to be transmitted to individuals of the same or closely related species, some pathogens are capable of jumping species barriers and attacking a broad range of hosts. Microbes may use different strategies of transmission to reach different host species. Many diseases can be carried by animals and transmitted to humans with the help of insect vectors so that direct contact with infected animals is unnecessary. For example, the protozoan that causes sleeping sickness (trypanosomiasis) is transmitted among horses as a venereal disease, but it is transmitted to rats and humans by means of fleas and flies.

Changing relationships between humans and animals continue to provide opportunities for pathogens to make the leap from their normal animal hosts to humans, or from humans to other animals. For example, directly or indirectly, humans have been responsible for the transmission of poliomyelitis, tuberculosis, malaria, influenza, and probably pneumonia, meningitis, and measles to other primates. Humans have also created conditions for the transmission of microbes from their domesticated animals to wild animals. When Europeans brought cattle carrying the rinderpest virus to Africa in the 1880s, the disease decimated African domestic cattle and quickly spread to wild animals, including buffaloes, wildebeests, giraffes, and antelopes.

CIVILIZATION AND DISEASE

Villages and towns that might have included several thousand people probably appeared about nine thousand years ago, but it is the development of large, densely populated cities that is generally considered a defining characteristic of the kind of culture or society known as a civilization. Complex civilizations began to develop between about 3500 and 1500 BCE in Mesopotamia, Egypt, the Indus River Valley, and northern China. In the Americas, unique civilizations arose significantly later. The cultural, historical, and environmental factors that led to the development of the first civilizations are still subject to considerable debate. No simple, definitive answer seems possible, but a variety of causes related to the probable advantages and challenges of geographic, climatic, and economic factors have been suggested. Under favorable conditions, the mastery of agricultural techniques led to food surpluses, increases in population, social stratification, specialized occupations, and the rise of powerful administrators, who governed and organized resources. An important accomplishment that is almost invariably associated with the development of early civilizations was the invention of writing and record keeping. Fragmentary evidence, preserved in the texts, artifacts, and human remains of ancient civilizations, provides some insights into the ways in which people thought about health and diseases. The infectious diseases and medical concepts of ancient Mesopotamia, Egypt, India, and China are particularly significant.

The belief that diseases are caused by supernatural agents, whether gods, demons, ghosts, or evil spirits, was essentially universal in prehistoric societies and in the remarkable civilizations that developed in the period between about 3500 BCE and 1500 BCE in Mesopotamia, Egypt, China, and India. In particular, the ancient texts reveal the development of distinct scholarly traditions in these early centers of civilization. Moreover, in India and China, the ancient texts still provide the philosophical basis of traditional medical practice.

Texts from ancient Mesopotamia reflect the belief that diseases and misfortunes were caused by demons, devils, and evil spirits. The texts also preserve evidence that physicians were familiar with a wide range of diseases, including schistosomiasis (also known as bilharzia or snail fever), dysentery, pneumonia, and various parasitic diseases. Medical texts from ancient Egypt include discussions of diseases associated with supernatural agents, but physicians also attributed disease to intestinal putrefaction, noxious winds, and insects as well as visible and invisible worms. Skeletons, portraits, and mummies provide ample evidence of the crushing burden of disease, including malaria, parasitic worms, and schistosomiasis. The incidence of schistosomiasis, a disease caused by tiny parasitic worms known as schistosomes, typically reflects agricultural and sanitary practices. Stagnant water, especially in irrigated fields, serves as a home for the snail that acts as the intermediate host for this parasitic worm, which has a complicated life cycle that involves humans and snails. When people enter contaminated bodies of water, the larval form of the parasite penetrates their skin, enters the capillaries and lymphatic vessels, and migrates to the internal organs. Severe infestations can result in damage to the lungs, liver, intestines, and urinary tract. Mature worms produce eggs throughout their three- to five-year life span. When eggs are discharged into freshwater in human urine or feces, they hatch to release a free-swimming form that must complete the next phase of its life cycle in a freshwater snail. Improving sanitary conditions and eliminating the snails that serve as intermediate hosts could eradicate the disease, but epidemiologists estimate that the disease still affects about two hundred million people in over seventy countries in Africa, Latin America, the Caribbean, and Southeast Asia.

The medical texts of ancient India alluded to at least one thousand diseases, but fever was considered the king of diseases. The emphasis on intermittent fevers, and the intervals between the febrile episodes, probably reflects experience with the patterns of malarial fevers. Hindu myths and legends depict a complex pantheon of gods and a vast array of demons capable of causing disease and pestilence. Legendary healers and gods wrestled with the demons that caused disease and pestilence. According to the scholarly traditions of Chinese medicine, disease was basically caused by factors that led to imbalance within the body; all therapies were directed toward restoring a state of harmony. Scholarly physicians, however, only cared for a tiny fraction of the population. Most people assumed that demons and spirits played a role in causing disease. Chinese records also provide clues about the development of trade networks with India, Rome, and Arabia that might have facilitated the spread of smallpox and other diseases.

THE FOUNDATIONS OF WESTERN MEDICINE

Western medicine traces its origins to the intellectual traditions established by Greek philosophers, naturalists, and physicians. The writings attributed to Hippocrates are considered the foundation of Western secular medicine, but even Hippocratic physicians traced their art back to Asclepius, the god of medicine. Nevertheless, Hippocratic medicine emphasized the search for natural explanations of disease based on careful observations of characteristic patterns of signs and symptoms. As in other medical traditions, the goal of healing was to restore balance and harmony to the body. Whatever success the Hippocratic physician may have had in caring for individual patients, his best advice when a city was struck by a major plague was to flee quickly, go as far as possible, and not return until the plague ended.

The plague that struck Athens in 431 BCE during the Peloponnesian War between Athens and Sparta demonstrated how little physicians could do when confronted with epidemic disease. The most vivid portrait of the plague was recorded not by a physician, but by the Greek historian Thucydides. Having survived his own battle with the disease, Thucydides left a detailed account of its symptoms and his observations of the effects of the plague on his fellow citizens. According to Thucydides, the disease began very suddenly, with headache, fever, and inflammation of the eyes, throat, and tongue. Sneezing, hoarseness, and painful coughing were followed by vomiting, violent spasms, pustules and ulcers of the skin, diarrhea, unquenchable thirst, exhaustion, depression, and severe mental confusion. Most victims died in seven to nine days. Only those who had survived an attack of the disease were willing to nurse the sick because those who recovered never contracted the disease again. By some estimates, the disease killed almost one-third of the Athenian population. Despite Thucydides' vivid description of the epidemic, and much speculation by modern historians and physicians, the specific cause of the epidemic remains uncertain. Among the diagnoses that have been offered are typhus, typhoid fever, scarlet fever, bubonic plague, smallpox, measles, anthrax, and influenza complicated by bacterial infections that triggered toxic shock syndrome. Whatever the plague of Athens may have been, it provides a striking example of the recurrent theme of social disintegration linked to war and epidemic disease.

Although Roman medical writers generally adopted Hippocratic theories, many of the practical achievements that characterize the Roman Empire are of particular interest in the history of medicine and public health. Centuries of warfare provided new opportunities for the movement of germs and pests throughout the Roman Empire, but Rome's unprecedented concern for sanitary engineering presumably played an important role in maintaining public health. Nevertheless, Rome itself could not totally avoid epidemic disease. The most influential medical writer of ancient Rome, the Greek physician Galen of Pergamum, left a description of a deadly epidemic that struck Rome in 165, apparently carried by soldiers returning from conflicts in Southeast Asia. According to Galen, who fled from the city, the symptoms of the disease included fever, diarrhea, inflammation of the pharynx, and dry or pustular skin eruptions. Physicians were unable to understand or cure the disease.

An admirable concern for the purity of water and the sanitary location of dwelling places is found in the text *On Architecture* (ca. 27 BCE) by the Roman architect and engineer Vitruvius. Also of interest is the suggestion by Marcus Terentius Varro that swampy places might be inhabited by extremely minute animals that could float in the air. According to Varro, these invisible entities could enter the body through the mouth and nose and cause serious illnesses. Diodorus of Sicily and Livy wrote about the dangers of allowing armies to camp close to swamps. Knowing that swamps were associated with debilitating fevers, generals attempted to force their opponents to camp near swamps or travel through marshy areas, a tactic that might be considered germ warfare. A more philosophical version of this concept was presented by Lucretius in his poem *On the Nature of Things.* Lucretius argued that the world was made up of many kinds of atoms. Some were essential to human life, but others caused deadly diseases. The mists associated with swampy areas were particularly likely to contain dangerous, disease-causing atoms that entered the body through the nostrils, mouth, or skin. The numerous references to fevers, and recognition of a relationship between swamps and intermittent fevers, apparently reflect the prevalence and importance of malaria in the Mediterranean region.

Malaria has been called the greatest killer in all of human history. When first introduced into a region, malaria may cause deadly epidemics, but in many areas, the disease becomes endemic, and almost all people are affected. Instead of immediately killing or immunizing its victims, malaria makes them more vulnerable to further attacks and to other diseases. Hippocratic physicians described malaria as a recurrent fever and paid very close attention to the time intervals between episodes of fever and chills. Fevers that appeared every third day were called benign tertian fevers. Those that struck every fourth day were known as quartan fevers. The most deadly form of the disease, malignant tertian fever, was common in North Africa and Asia Minor, but was almost unknown in Europe until the second century. After the protozoan parasite that causes malaria was discovered in the 1890s, the different patterns of malarial fevers were clarified by the identification of four different species of the parasites that cause human malaria.

PLAGUE AND LEPROSY

Leprosy and bubonic plague, the most feared of all pestilential diseases, have become inextricably, even if inappropriately, linked to the era known as the European Middle Ages. Indeed, epidemics of bubonic plague continued into the nineteenth century, and plague remains endemic or enzootic in parts of Africa, Asia, and the Americas. The plague pandemics that seem to provide an appropriate frame for the medical history of the Middle Ages—the Plague of Justinian in 541 and the Black Death of 1348—were separated by eight centuries.

The Justinian Plague was vividly described by the Byzantine historian Procopius in his history of the Persian Wars. In 540 Constantinople was attacked by a disease that probably began in Ethiopia or Egypt. At its peak, the disease killed thousands of people in the city of Constantinople each day. Contemporary accounts suggest that the disease spread by land and by sea throughout the world, but it is impossible to determine the exact magnitude of this first plague pandemic. The pandemic that struck Europe, Asia, and the Middle East in the middle of the fourteenth century is better documented, but many uncertainties remain. Contemporaries called it the *Great Dying*, but it is generally remembered as the Black Death. From 1346 to 1352, the Black Death probably killed 30 to 60 percent of the population of Europe. Survivors of the plague predicted that those who had not experienced the Great Dying would never be able to comprehend the magnitude of the disaster. Indeed, modern historians still dispute the mortality caused by the plague, its impact on medieval society, and even the generally accepted conclusion that the Black Death was bubonic plague (see Figure 1.1).

It was not until the end of the nineteenth century that scientists were able to explain the catastrophic web of relationships linking rats, fleas, bacteria, and people to bubonic plague. Not surprisingly, medieval attempts to limit the spread of the disease through prayers and quarantine regulations were quite ineffective. By the fifteenth century, several Italian cities had developed detailed public health measures. Unfortunately, because those who formulated quarantine rules did not understand the natural history of plague, some measures, such as deliberate massacres of dogs and cats, must have been counterproductive. Long periods of quarantine caused terrible hardships and promoted willful disobedience. Plague remained a threat in the eastern Mediterranean area well into the nineteenth century, although later outbreaks never achieved the prevalence or virulence of the Black Death.

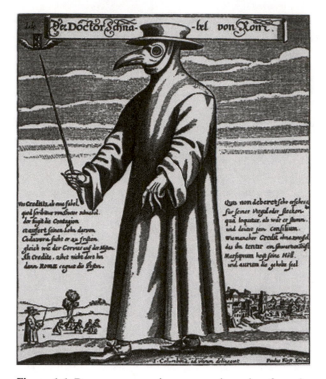

Figure 1.1 Doctors attempted to protect themselves from the plague by wearing a protective costume that included a long cloak, gloves, and a face mask. The long rod allowed the doctor to point at diagnostic lesions, instead of touching the patient. The long beak of the mask could be filled with strong-smelling herbs, exotic spices, and other substances that were thought to reduce the danger of inhaling tainted air. Engraving by Paul Fürst in 1656. Credit: Imagery from the History of Medicine.

During an outbreak in Hong Kong in the 1890s, bacteriologists Alexandre Yersin and Shibasaburo Kitasato independently isolated the plague bacillus from victims of the disease. Although Yersin and Kitasato discovered the causative agent, they were unable to clarify the means of transmission. In 1898, while investigating an outbreak of plague in India, Paul-Louis Simond discovered the bacillus that causes the disease in the stomach of fleas living on infected rats. Infected fleas transmit the plague from rat to rat and from rats to humans. The rat flea *Xenophylla cheopsis* is the most efficient vector of plague, but a few other species can transmit *Yersinia pestis*, the plague bacillus, to humans. Infected fleas also become victims of the plague bacillus because the rapidly multiplying bacteria form a plug that blocks the flea's stomach. When the flea bites a new victim, it regurgitates its blood meal along with many thousands of plague bacilli. Fleas are usually fairly loyal to their primary host species, which, for *Xenophylla cheopsis*, is the black rat, but rat fleas will attack human beings when their normal hosts die.

The plague bacillus was originally called *Pasteurella pestis* but was renamed *Yersinia pestis* in honor of Alexandre Yersin. *Yersinia pestis* provides an interesting example of the way in which a specific microbe can cause different clinical patterns of disease. In this case, the major forms of illness are known as *bubonic* and *pneumonic* plague. In rare cases, referred to as *septicemic* plague, *Yersinia pestis* invades the bloodstream, resulting in serious damage to major organs, hemorrhages, gangrene, delirium or coma, and death. If the plague bacillus enters the body through the bite of an infected flea, the disease follows the pattern known as bubonic because of the characteristic *buboes* (painful, inflamed swellings of the lymph nodes) that typically appear in the groin, armpit, and neck. When the bacteria spread to the lung, causing a condition known as secondary pneumonic plague, the victim can spread the disease to others through droplets of saliva expelled by coughing and sneezing. If the bacteria-laden droplets enter the respiratory system of a new host, the result is a deadly condition called primary pneumonic plague, which is highly contagious. In the absence of appropriate antibiotics, the mortality rate for bubonic plague may exceed 50 percent, but the pneumonic and septicemic forms of the disease are almost invariably fatal. Unfortunately, although several plague vaccines have been introduced since the end of the nineteenth century, these vaccines have not been very effective, especially against the pneumonic form.

At least three naturally occurring varieties of *Yersinia pestis* are known today. All three varieties cause virulent infections in humans and most mammals. Studies of *Yersinia pestis* suggest that it probably emerged as recently as twenty thousand years ago, when it became distinct from *Yersinia pseudotuberculosis*, which generally produces mild intestinal disease. *Yersinia pseudotuberculosis* apparently became a deadly pathogen by acquiring genes from other bacteria that allowed it to colonize a wider array of tissues and organs. The genome of *Yersinia pestis*, cultured from a victim of pneumonic plague, was sequenced in 2001. Genomic data can be used to identify the genes that determine the life cycle, evolutionary history, and virulence of *Yersinia pestis*. Eventually, these studies could lead to improved therapeutic drugs and more effective vaccines, but the same techniques could theoretically be used by bioterrorists to engineer more deadly forms of bacteria or strains of *Yersinia pestis* resistant to antibiotics. Less sophisticated terrorists could attempt to spread the plague by collecting infected rodents and their fleas from areas where the plague is still enzootic. According to military historians, this approach was actually used during World War II.

Ancient myths, legends, and chronicles associated mice with disasters, plagues, and pestilence, but they rarely distinguished between mice and rats. The black rat, *Rattus rattus*, is most closely associated with plague epidemics, but almost two hundred species of rodents have been identified as possible reservoirs of the plague bacillus. Plague is still enzootic among wild rodents found in Russia, the Middle East, Asia, Africa, and North and South America. After the plague pandemic of the 1890s reached San Francisco, California, plague bacilli spread to rodents throughout the western states. The prairie dog colonies of Colorado became the major plague reservoir in North America. Human cases are rare, but they have occurred in New Mexico, Colorado, Arizona, California, Oregon, and Nevada. Infected rodents have even transmitted plague to zoo animals.

Perhaps the most dangerous characteristic of *Yersinia pestis* today is its ability to camouflage itself as a so-called medieval plague of no possible significance to modern societies. However, the intrusion of human beings into previously undisturbed wild areas could bring them into contact with animals harboring plague bacilli. Changes in the ecology of a plague reservoir, caused by climate change or development, could expand the range of infected animals. Because human plague is rare and unexpected, sporadic cases may be misdiagnosed. Prompt treatment with antibiotics is usually effective, but the mortality rate for untreated plague remains as high as 50 to 90 percent, and since the 1990s, multidrug-resistant strains of *Yersinia pestis* have been detected. Much about the disappearance of plague from the ranks of major epidemic diseases is obscure, but in its animal reservoirs, the plague is still very much alive and presumably quite capable of taking advantage of any disaster that could alter relationships among rodents, fleas, and humans.

Some historians have expressed doubts about the identity of the disease that caused the pandemic now known as the Black Death. In place of bubonic plague, skeptics have suggested anthrax, typhus, influenza, a viral hemorrhagic fever, a microbe that no longer exists, or mass poisoning by mold toxins. Despite lingering uncertainties, most epidemiologists believe that *Yersinia pestis* was the cause of the epidemics historically known as bubonic plague. Many ambiguities in the descriptions of plague in different times and places might be a reflection of the different clinical forms of disease that can result from infection with *Yersinia pestis* and the tendency of witnesses to describe what they expect to see. Settling this dispute is difficult because modern societies are very different from those of the fourteenth, or even the nineteenth, centuries. Analysis of DNA recovered from the dental pulp of people buried in the fourteenth century in a mass grave in France provided evidence of *Yersinia pestis*. Researchers concluded that this proved that the Black Death was bubonic plague, but skeptics claim that this merely proved that some cases of plague occurred in fourteenth-century France.

More than any other disease, leprosy demonstrates the difference between the biological nature of illness and the attributes ascribed to the sick. Indeed, the word *leper* is still commonly used to mean one who is hated and shunned by society. Medieval attitudes toward the leper were based on biblical passages pertaining to "leprosy," a vague term that was applied to various chronic, progressive skin afflictions, from true leprosy to psoriasis (reddish, scaly patches), vitiligo (depigmented, white patches), and skin cancer. The leper, according to medieval interpretations of the Bible, was "unclean" and therefore a dangerous source of physical and moral pollution. Leprosy was probably endemic in the Middle East from at least 1500 BCE. Its presence in Europe in the Middle Ages has been confirmed by studies of skeletal remains that exhibit the deformities caused by the disease. Leprosy apparently became a major problem in Europe by the end of the twelfth century. After reaching its peak in the thirteenth century, leprosy all but disappeared from Europe. Changing patterns of commerce, warfare, and pilgrimages might have broken the chain of contagion by which leprosy reached Europe from areas where the disease remained, and still remains, endemic. Nevertheless, leprosy remained a significant public health problem in Norway well into the nineteenth century, when the new science of microbiology developed.

In 1873, Gerhard Hansen, physician and researcher at the leprosy hospital in Bergen, Norway, discovered *Mycobacterium leprae*, the bacillus that causes leprosy. To honor Hansen, and reduce the stigma associated with the term *leper*, the disease was renamed "Hansen's disease." Hansen's mentor and father-in-law, Daniel Cornelius Danielssen, coauthor with Carl Wilhelm Boeck, of *On Leprosy* (1847), a landmark treatise in the study of leprosy, had established Bergen as a major center of leprosy research. As part of his extensive research, Danielssen had injected bits of tissue taken from lepers into himself, members of his medical staff, and other volunteers. These experiments seemed to support his belief that leprosy was hereditary, rather than directly transmissible. After finding rodlike bacteria in leprous skin lesions, Hansen made numerous unsuccessful attempts to grow the bacillus on artificial media. Attempts to transfer the disease to rabbits and human volunteers were also failures, but the evidence indicated that Hansen's bacillus was the probable cause of the disease.

Recognition of the infectious nature of the disease led to the passage of laws that called for the mandatory isolation of lepers. Before 1875, admission to Norway's leprosy hospitals had been voluntary. Some of Hansen's experiments raised controversial questions about the use of human subjects. Hansen was tried for failing to obtain consent from a patient before conducting an experiment in which he inoculated her eyes with leprous material taken from a patient with a different form of the disease. In 1880, after his trial, Hansen lost his position as resident physician at the Bergen leprosy hospital, but he continued to serve as Norway's chief medical officer for leprosy. Although his colleagues and the Norwegian authorities generally believed that Hansen had performed human experimentation to answer important scientific questions that would lead to the advancement of medicine, he had violated Norway's laws and ethical standards.

Generally, Hansen's disease begins with skin lesions, followed by nerve damage, loss of sensation, and the progressive destruction of cartilage and bone that results in crippling deformities. What is most surprising about Hansen's disease is the fact that it is not very contagious; moreover, most people seem to be immune. Many people having extended and close contact with lepers, such as spouses, nurses, and doctors, do not contract the disease. Of course, this does not prove that leprosy was not more contagious in the past, but it does make it unlikely that the leper was ever as dangerous to others as was commonly assumed. Indeed, it could be said that leprosy and Hansen's disease stand for different concepts more than different diseases. Proving that the bacteria Hansen found in skin scrapings from leprosy patients actually caused the disease was very difficult. Indeed, some of Hansen's colleagues disputed his findings and insisted that leprosy was a hereditary disease. No animal model was available, and bacteriologists were unable to grow the leprosy bacillus on artificial media. Eventually. scientists discovered that *Mycobacterium leprae* can infect armadillos and certain monkeys, but there is no evidence that animals ever transmit the disease to humans.

Although the *Mycobacterium leprae* genome was sequenced in 2001, many aspects of the disease that it causes remain obscure. The bacteria seem to be transmitted primarily by means of nasal secretions, but most people are able to initiate an immune response that prevents the establishment of a chronic infection. In susceptible people, the microbe triggers an inflammatory response that damages the skin and peripheral nerves. Within the human body, these extremely slow-growing bacteria live within the white blood cells known as macrophages, which serve as scavengers, and in cells known as Schwann cells, which surround and protect peripheral nerves. After the appearance of the skin lesions that typically indicate the establishment of infection, damage to the peripheral nerves leads to the characteristic deformities historically associated with advanced leprosy. Infection can, however, lead to a very wide spectrum of clinical patterns, depending on the immunological response of the patient. Clinicians traditionally described two distinct forms, known as tuberculoid and lepromatous leprosy, and a series of intermediate types. The incubation period between infection and symptomatic leprosy varies widely, but the average is four years for tuberculoid and ten years for lepromatous leprosy. Tuberculoid leprosy, which occurs in patients capable of an immune response that limits the replication of the bacilli, results in minor nerve damage and skin lesions. Patients with the most severe form of the disease, lepromatous leprosy, experience severe skin and nerve damage that may lead to impaired vision or blindness, kidney damage, anemia, skin ulcers, loss of sensation, secondary infections of the skin and bone, and so forth. In some patients, changes in the immune response occur over time, resulting in changes in the clinical patterns. Epidemiologists had predicted that HIV/AIDS would be particularly deadly in patients previously infected with Hansen's disease. Surprisingly, although symptoms associated with Hansen's disease did not seem to worsen when patients developed AIDS, the drugs used to treat HIV/AIDS caused latent cases of Hansen's disease to become active.

Hansen's disease is now considered a tropical disease, but because of its long incubation period, an infected individual may develop symptoms years after migrating to another country. As a result of improved therapy and active control programs, during the last decades of the twentieth century, the numbers of registered leprosy patients undergoing therapy fell from some twelve million to about eight hundred thousand. Nevertheless, public health experts estimate that at least two to three million people still have permanent nerve impairment as a result of leprosy, and hundreds of thousands of new patients are discovered every year. As a result, leprosy is likely to remain a threat in endemic areas for many decades, and sporadic imported cases may appear in other areas.

Since the 1980s, the treatment of leprosy has been revolutionized by multidrug therapy (MDT), the simultaneous use of two or three drugs, a procedure that was instituted to counteract the emergence of drug-resistant bacteria. Aggressive treatment of patients with early leprosy is considered the key to interrupting the chain of transmission and eventually eradicating the disease. Treatment may be needed for six months to two years. According to World Health Organization reports, more than eight million patients have been successfully treated with MDT. Although this approach has transformed the lives of leprosy patients and reduced the prevalence of the disease, experts warn that the new case-detection rate in areas where the disease is most common has not fallen significantly. The long and variable incubation period, the continuing stigma, and attempts to hide the disease make it difficult to detect and treat. Many patients still think of leprosy as a curse, rather than a curable disease.

Public health experts believe that leprosy could be totally eradicated in the not too distant future if all victims of Hansen's disease were to receive appropriate therapy. Unlike bubonic plague, Hansen's disease does not seem to have a natural animal reservoir. Nevertheless, experts estimated that at the end of the twentieth century, about fifteen million people were still suffering from the disease, and only about 20 percent of those already infected were being treated. Estimating the number of people already infected is difficult because Hansen's disease is often misdiagnosed or unreported. Public health experts trying to control leprosy in impoverished areas point out that a medical solution will not cure what is basically a socioeconomic problem associated with poverty and overcrowding. However, Hansen's disease could be eradicated if sufficient resources were dedicated to this goal.

EUROPEAN DISEASES AND THE HISTORY OF THE AMERICAS

The history of infectious disease in the Americas was quite different from that of Europe, primarily because the Americas remained essentially isolated from the people, pathogens, and pests of Europe, Asia, and Africa until the fifteenth century. Epidemiologists suggest that the people of the New World did not experience the epidemic diseases found in Europe, at least in part, because of the absence of the domesticated herd animals that were the source of many of the pathogens that had adapted to humans.

Centuries before Europeans arrived in the western hemisphere, advanced cultures had developed in Guatemala, Mexico, and the Andean highlands. It is impossible to know what patterns their development might have assumed if the Americas had remained isolated from Europe. The consequences of contact between Europeans and the Aztec, Maya, and Inca civilizations were especially dramatic, primarily because Mexico and Peru had the highest population densities and the most extensive trade and transport networks in the Americas. Such factors provided ideal conditions for the spread of highly contagious European diseases such as smallpox, measles, and influenza.

The rapid, complete, and catastrophic conquest of the vast Aztec empire by a small band of Spanish explorers and soldiers is a major historical puzzle. Despite the superiority of European weapons, the Aztecs should have had the advantage in terms of numbers of warriors, knowledge of the environment, and access to supplies. Many possible factors have been suggested, but the devastating impact of smallpox, measles, and other infections diseases on Native Americans might account for the very different outcome of European intrusions into America, Asia, and Africa. Historians have estimated that early waves of smallpox may have killed 75 to 90 percent of the Native Americans who contracted the disease. Such high mortality rates have been observed in more recent so-called virgin soil epidemics—disease outbreaks among populations that have never previously encountered a particular pathogen. Estimates of the population of the Americas in 1492 and the magnitude of the demographic collapse that followed the European invasion remain controversial. The biological impact of the Spanish Conquest was so profound that it is difficult to ascertain whether particular diseases and pests were even present in pre-Columbian America. Recent studies of lice found in pre-Columbian mummies indicate, however, that the species of louse common throughout the world was present in the Americas before Europeans arrived. Lice are vectors of some deadly diseases, including typhus fever. Infectious diseases that were probably unique to the Americas before 1492 include Oroya fever, American leishmaniasis, Chagas' disease, and a skin disease known as pinta. Many sixteenth-century physicians thought that syphilis originated in the Americas, but this is still a matter of much dispute.

The European impact on the Americas sent ripples all around the world, affecting Africa as well as Europe. Because of the demographic catastrophe that overcame Native Americans and the demands of Spanish settlers for labor, the establishment of the slave trade brought vast numbers of Africans to the New World. Thus, the

Americas became the site of the mixing of the peoples and germs of previously separate continents. Yellow fever and malaria have been called the most important disease exports from Africa to the Americas, but other diseases that probably accompanied the slave trade include amebic dysentery, hookworms, roundworms, filariasis, Guinea worm, trachoma, leprosy, yaws, typhoid fever, and so forth.

TWO

❧❧❧

MIASMA, CONTAGION, AND THE GERM THEORY OF DISEASE

THE RENAISSANCE AND THE SCIENTIFIC REVOLUTION

In European history, the Renaissance has been thought of primarily in terms of the rebirth of the arts and sciences that accompanied the complex social, political, and intellectual transformations that took place between the fourteenth and seventeenth centuries. During this period, Europe experienced the disintegration of medieval economic and social patterns; the expansion of commerce, cities, and trade; and the growth of the modern state. The Renaissance coincided with a new age of exploration and discovery, but it was also a period in which old and apparently new epidemic diseases flourished. Just as the Renaissance transformed the arts, and the exploration of the Americas transformed the map of the known world, the Scientific Revolution transformed ideas about the nature of the universe and the nature of human beings as well as the relative authority of ancient texts, direct observation, and experimentation.

Anatomical and physiological investigations challenged many ancient doctrines, but new ideas about the human body coexisted with ancient assumptions about the cause and transmission of disease. Classical medical theory generally attributed epidemic diseases to poisonous vapors—known as miasmas—generated by putrid, decomposing materials that polluted the atmosphere. Dangerous miasmatic conditions were particularly associated with swamps and marshy areas. According to

Hippocratic doctrine, health and disease depended on interactions between environmental or atmospheric conditions and the four humors—blood, black bile, yellow bile, and phlegm—that made up the human body. In *Airs, Waters, Places,* one of the most important Hippocratic texts, disease was analyzed in terms of the relationship and interactions between individuals and their environment—including weather conditions and other local circumstances. This concept is generally known as the atmospheric-miasmatic theory of disease. Other medical writers speculated that the noxious particles in disease-causing miasmas might actually be living entities. These mysterious little animals, seeds, worms, or ferments might be disseminated through the air or transmitted directly from the sick to others by means of direct physical contact, that is, by *contagion.*

Ancient and primitive ideas about contagion dealt with the general notion of transfer through contact and should not be confused with the modern germ theory of disease. According to traditional concepts concerning contagion, just as heat and cold were transferred to neighboring bodies by direct contact, so, too, were putrefaction, uncleanliness, corruption, and disease. Epidemic diseases were frequently attributed to the appearance of comets, eclipses, floods, earthquakes, or major astrological disturbances that supposedly charged the air with poisonous vapors, but such concepts did not eclipse the assumption that some diseases, most notably leprosy, were highly contagious. Although it was possible to believe that disease was transmitted by both contagion and atmospheric conditions, until the acceptance of modern germ theory, the miasmatic theory of disease was generally more influential than any competing theory. The miasmatic theory of disease was vigorously defended by many of the great nineteenth-century public health reformers, who argued that poor sanitary conditions, filth, and noxious air caused the epidemic diseases that flourished in the rapidly growing industrial cities of Europe. In practice, sanitary reforms that helped remove the filth that allegedly generated noxious vapors or miasmas helped reduce the toll of epidemic diseases on cities and towns.

GIROLAMO FRACASTORO: ON CONTAGION, SYPHILIS, AND GERMS

Girolamo Fracastoro, poet, physician, and medical writer, has often been called the founder of the germ theory of disease, although his observations and conclusions were more ambiguous than this honorary title might imply. The kinds of evidence and speculation that Fracastoro invoked can be seen in his first significant book, *Syphilis, or the French Disease* (1530), in which he attempted to explain the origin, natural history, and treatment of the disease. In 1546, Fracastoro published *On Contagion, Contagious Diseases and Their Treatment,* a study that is considered a landmark in the evolution of the germ theory of disease. Reviewing and criticizing contemporary concepts of disease, Fracastoro analyzed the ways in which miasma and contagion theories explained, or failed to explain, the transmission of various infectious diseases. Fracastoro was intrigued by the fact that diseases could be specific to plants, animals, and humans. Even among humans, he noted, there were diseases that only affected the young or the old, while others affected women or men. Some diseases could attack all ages and both sexes, but some individuals remained unaffected in the midst of even the most widespread disease outbreaks.

Incorporating his own observations into a general analysis of existing theories of disease, Fracastoro speculated about the existence of living contagions or seeds of disease that were transmissible, specific for each disease, and capable of reproducing themselves. It was obvious that some diseases, such as syphilis and rabies, were only transmitted by direct contact with those who were already infected. Other diseases were transmitted by direct contact and by fomites, that is, inanimate articles, such as clothing and bedding that had been in contact with the sick. The seeds of some diseases, such as scabies, leprosy, tuberculosis, and pestilential fevers, seemed to be capable of hiding in appropriate fomites for months or even years, while retaining their ability to infect new victims. In addition to making use of direct contact and fomites, the seeds of some infectious diseases were apparently transmitted from the sick to new victims over significant distances in the absence of any known physical contact. These diseases included epidemic fevers, tuberculosis, certain eye diseases, and smallpox. The forces that allowed contagions to multiply and spread remained a mystery, although Fracastoro invoked interesting analogies between the transmission of human diseases and the transmission of putrefaction between fruits. It seemed to him that it was only logical to conclude that infection and putrefaction were ultimately the same phenomenon. Therefore, infection was essentially the same as the passage of putrefaction from one body to another. Struggling with the task of explaining what factors could account for both infection and putrefaction, Fracastoro could only imagine some interaction between the germs of putrefaction and particles of heat and moisture. Despite his intriguing hypotheses, Fracastoro's writings shared the confusion commonly found in the use of terms like *contagion* and *miasma*.

Thus, although the establishment of the germ theory of disease is often cast in terms of a conflict between contagion theory and miasma theory, until the late nineteenth century, these terms were not clearly differentiated. If the term *contagion* applied to harmful material that was transmitted directly or indirectly, it was compatible with miasma as disease-inducing noxious air. In any case, the concept that invisible germs or seeds might transmit diseases did not prove very useful in guiding medical practice and public health measures. Contagion theory suggested that quarantines, isolation, and disinfection could block the spread of epidemic diseases, but these methods had very limited success and imposed hardships that generated resentment and disobedience. Public health reformers generally believed that filth and poisoned air spread epidemic diseases. Removing the sources of noxious vapors often helped reduce epidemic diseases in crowded towns and cities that attempted to improve their general sanitary situation. By the end of the nineteenth century, bacteriologists were able to demonstrate that the filth and putrefaction associated with miasmas usually contained disease-causing germs. Understanding this principle made it possible to establish more effective public health measures.

In *Syphilis, or the French Disease*, Fracastoro provided a widely accepted name for an epidemic disease that many of his contemporaries thought had only recently appeared in Europe. At the time, syphilis was known by many names—the French called it the Neapolitan disease, the Italians called it the French disease, and the Portuguese called it the Castilian disease. In India and Japan, it was called the Portuguese disease, and the names Canton disease, great pox, and *lues venereum* were also used. Medical references to venereal diseases (VDs) are very old, but many sixteenth-century physicians thought that syphilis was a distinct, new disease. Other doctors argued that there was really only one venereal disease, but it could assume many different forms. Fracastoro, like most sixteenth-century physicians, believed that syphilis first appeared in Europe shortly after Christopher Columbus and his crew returned from their historic voyages to the New World. As Fracastoro explained, syphilis provided a good example of an epidemic disease that could be transmitted from person to person by very direct contagion. In *Syphilis, or the French Disease*, Fracastoro created the story of Syphilis, who had foolishly cursed the sun and was punished by becoming the first victim of a new disease (see Figure 2.1).

The term *venereal disease*, which refers to Venus, the Roman goddess of love, served as a euphemism for sexually transmitted disease (STD). Any disease that can be transmitted by sexual contact may be considered a venereal disease. For example, scabies and crab lice can be transmitted by direct contact, with or without sexual intercourse. A more restrictive definition includes only those diseases that are never, or almost never, transmitted by any mechanism other than intimate sexual contact. Until the emergence of AIDS, syphilis and gonorrhea were classified as the major venereal diseases, but diseases that were originally classified as minor venereal diseases—chancroid, lymphogranuloma venereum, and granuloma inguinale—can also lead to serious complications. Additional modern members of the STD category include genital herpes, trichomoniasis, nongonococcal urethritis, and so forth.

Syphilis has been called the great mimic because in the course of its development, it resembles many other diseases. Syphilitic lesions can be confused with those of leprosy, tuberculosis, scabies, fungal infections, and various skin cancers. Before the introduction of specific bacteriological and immunological tests, syphilis was such a diagnostic challenge that it was said that the physician who knew all of syphilis knew all of medicine. Typically, syphilis began with a small lesion known as a chancre

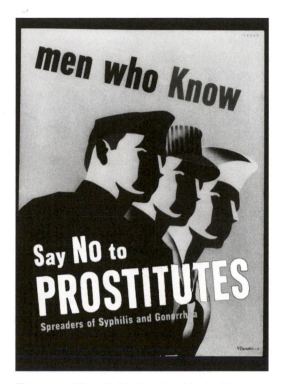

Figure 2.1 This World War II public health poster urged servicemen to avoid prostitutes because of the danger of contracting syphilis and gonorrhea. Credit: Public Health Image Library, Centers for Disease Control and Prevention, U.S. Department of Health and Human Services.

and progressed through a series of nonspecific symptoms that might include fever, headache, skin lesions, swollen lymph nodes, and deep aches in the bones and joints. Untreated syphilis could eventually damage the cardiovascular system as well as the nervous system, resulting in paralysis, dementia, and insanity. In addition, infected women could experience miscarriages and stillbirths, and infants that survived were likely to suffer from various defects.

The microbe that causes syphilis, *Treponema pallidum*, is a member of the *Treponema* group of corkscrew-shaped bacteria known as spirochetes. Syphilis is one of four clinically distinct human treponematoses; the others are known as pinta, yaws, and bejel. Only syphilis is classified as a sexually transmitted disease. In terms of microbiological and immunological tests, the causative organisms isolated from victims of these diseases are virtually identical. Some bacteriologists believe that the subspecies of bacteria that cause pinta, yaws, bejel, and syphilis are variants of an ancestral spirochete that adapted to different patterns of climate and human behavior. Pinta, which is endemic in Mexico and Central America, is characterized by mild to severe skin lesions. Yaws, a disease found in hot climates, leads to destruction of tissue, joints, and bone. Bejel, also known as nonvenereal endemic syphilis, is generally acquired in childhood among rural populations living in warm, arid regions.

Many Renaissance physicians were convinced that Columbus and his crew had imported syphilis from the New World to the Old World, but some scholars believe that syphilis might have been an old disease that had previously been misdiagnosed as leprosy. Recognition of the microbial agents that cause syphilis and yaws led to speculation that the slave trade could have brought Africans with yaws to the Americas. When changes in climate and clothing inhibited nonvenereal transmission of yaws, the spirochete adapted to this challenge and continued to find new victims by becoming a sexually transmitted disease. Although this hypothesis seems plausible and provides a fitting lesson about the evils of slavery, it seems to ignore the antiquity of interchanges between Europe and Africa.

Uncertainty about the origin of syphilis might be resolved by genetic studies of the modern treponematoses. Comparative analyses of genetic sequences of existing treponematoses seem to support the hypothesis that European explorers did indeed carry the microbe that causes syphilis from the Americas to Europe. However, an analysis of modern treponematoses does not rule out the possibility that the explosive epidemic of syphilis that began in Europe at the end of the fifteenth century might have been caused by a modified form of a microbe that caused nonvenereal disease in tropical parts of the Americas. Detailed genomic studies indicate that the spirochete that causes syphilis arose relatively recently and that it is closely related to a microbe found among children in Guyana that causes skin lesions, usually on the legs. Europeans could have carried the nonvenereal tropical disease back to Europe, where a modified microbe that was transmitted by sexual contact first appeared. Further studies of the genomes of the microbes that cause a broad range of treponemal diseases in Africa, Asia, South America, and so forth could provide detailed evolutionary trees.

The origins of venereal syphilis may still be in doubt, but some scientists believe that it is more appropriate to think of the treponemal family as very ancient and very adaptable organisms that can exploit different means of transmission and produce different effects; that is, the debate about origins may be overemphasizing the evolution of allegedly discrete subspecies of microbes that actually should be seen as members of a biological continuum. Ultimately, the genetic approach might provide more reliable evidence than studies of skeletons because the mildest forms of the disease would not produce bone lesions. Paleopathologists may have found evidence of treponemal infections in the New World dating back seven thousand years, but uncertainties remain concerning the age of these skeletal remains. Moreover, bone lesions cannot provide definitive conclusions about the microbes that caused them or the mode of transmission. Skeletal evidence concerning treponemal disease in Europe and Africa as well as America that clearly predates the voyages of Columbus remains controversial. Despite ambiguities and uncertainties, the history of syphilis does seem to provide an intriguing example of the early globalization of emerging diseases.

Fracastoro believed that syphilis could be cured by aggressive therapy with mercury, also known as quicksilver, in doses large enough to purge the disease from the body in a flood of sweat and saliva. Many doctors favored various forms of fever therapy and a remedy known as guaiac, or holy wood, from a tree indigenous to South America. The rationale for fever therapy is that high body temperature must be a natural defense mechanism and therefore a useful response to disease. Because of the unpredictable nature of syphilis, case histories could be found to prove the efficacy of every purported remedy, although most so-called remedies probably did more harm to the patient than to the spirochetes.

Some observers suggested that patients who received no treatment were better off than those who received conventional mercury therapy. Evaluating remedies for venereal diseases was complicated by widespread confusion between gonorrhea and syphilis. At the beginning of the twentieth century, the discovery of the microbe that causes syphilis and the introduction of a diagnostic blood test made it possible to diagnose the disease and follow its natural history. In 1905, Fritz Richard Schaudinn and Paul Erich Hoffmann identified the causal agent of syphilis, *Spirochaeta pallida*, which was later renamed *Treponema pallidum*. One year later, August von Wassermann discovered a specific blood test for syphilis. Hideyo Noguchi confirmed the identification of *Treponema pallidum* and proved that the spirochete was present in brain tissue taken from patients who had died of paralytic dementia, a condition that was then fairly common among patients confined to insane asylums. Hope for victims of syphilis, even those with advanced disease, appeared in 1910 when Paul Ehrlich demonstrated the effectiveness of a drug that was given the name "salvarsan." Despite the adverse effects often associated with this arsenic-containing drug, salvarsan remained the standard remedy for syphilis until it was replaced by penicillin after World War II. As a remedy for syphilis, penicillin was so safe and effective that public health officials optimistically predicted that the disease would disappear by the end of the twentieth century. Unfortunately, after decades of decline, the incidence of syphilis began to increase during the 1990s.

MICROBES AND MICROSCOPES

Both Marcus Terentius Varro and Girolamo Fracastoro speculated about tiny seeds or animals that might serve as the physical basis of contagion, but these hypothetical entities were invisible until the invention of the microscope. The art of grinding and polishing lenses for corrective eyeglasses was well established by the sixteenth century, when the first crude telescopes and microscopes were invented. Even with magnification no greater than five- to ten-fold, the first microscopes revealed remarkable details about insects and other creatures just barely visible to the naked eye. Improvements in the microscope created much greater magnification and led to the discovery of a whole new world of entities invisible to the naked eye. With simple magnifying lenses and compound microscopes, seventeenth-century scientists discovered a new world teeming with previously invisible entities, including protozoa, molds, yeasts, and bacteria. Antoni van Leeuwenhoek, the most ingenious microscopist of the seventeenth century, provided some of the earliest descriptions of the diverse forms of microorganisms. Indeed, he was apparently the first person to see bacteria under the microscope. A shopkeeper and businessman, rather than a scholar, Leeuwenhoek taught himself the art of making magnifying lenses to observe new worlds revealed by the microscope. Like his contemporaries, Leeuwenhoek studied plant and animal cells, insects, and so forth, but he was particularly intrigued by the "little animals" that could be found in sources as diverse as the human mouth, pond water, and the semen of men and other animals. Assuming that motility was characteristic of living beings, Leeuwenhoek concluded that the tiny moving things that he observed under his microscopes—including bacteria, protozoa, and rotifers—must be live animals. Some naturalists thought that the *infusoria*—a term that encompassed all types of microscopic creatures—could be tiny plants and animals spontaneously generated in pond water, broth, and other nutritive media, but Leeuwenhoek was quite sure that even the smallest creatures revealed by his microscopes must have descended from parents like themselves.

Eighteenth-century naturalists acknowledged the existence of Leeuwenhoek's little animals and the infusoria but found them very difficult to characterize and classify. The great eighteenth-century Swedish taxonomist Carl von Linnaeus placed all the infusoria in the category known as Vermes (worms). German naturalist Christian Gottfried Ehrenberg believed that the infusoria were complex creatures with internal organs, analogous to those of ordinary living beings. Like Leeuwenhoek, Ehrenberg opposed the idea that the infusoria were produced by spontaneous generation, but the crude staining methods in use at that time made it very difficult to characterize any individual species among the infusoria. In 1856, William Henry Perkin discovered the first of many aniline dyes while trying to synthesize quinine, a valuable remedy for malaria. By the 1860s, many different aniline dyes were being used as biological stains, supplementing or replacing natural dyes such as indigo, carmine, and blueberry juice.

With improved microscopes and staining techniques, nineteenth-century scientists attempted to characterize and classify the confusing world of microbial life. The German botanist Ferdinand Cohn, the first prominent scientist to take a special interest in bacteriological research, suggested that bacteria should be considered microscopic plants. Many scientists, however, thought that bacteria were too primitive to fit into traditional botanical or zoological categories. Even the boundary between bacteria and inanimate matter was ill defined. Some naturalists objected to systems that characterized bacteria in terms of morphology, as if they were actually distinct species of plants or animals. Species names should not be applied to various forms of bacteria, they argued, because these minute entities appeared to change form as they grew in various media or arose by means of spontaneous generation. Despite unresolved debates about the nature of infusoria, Cohn's work essentially defined the domain of bacteriology in the 1870s and the possibility that bacteria could be arranged and classified according to shape and motility.

Improvements in the design of microscopes in the nineteenth century as well as new methods of sample preparation and staining made it possible to distinguish various forms of microbial life. Further studies of the microbial world, however, required even higher magnification and better resolving power than could be obtained with ordinary microscopes, which cannot distinguish details smaller than the wavelength of light. The first primitive electron microscopes were produced in the 1930s. Microscopes that used electron beams instead of ordinary light made it possible to investigate smaller and smaller entities, including the fine structure of bacteria and other microorganisms as well as the entities once known as invisible-filterable viruses. The 1986 Nobel Prize in Physics was awarded to Ernst Ruska, for his contributions to the design of the electron microscope, and to Gerd Binnig and Heinrich Rohrer, for their design of the scanning tunneling microscope.

LIVING ENTITIES AS CONTAGION

Experimental evidence that contagious human diseases could be transmitted by tiny parasites was established in the seventeenth century through Giovanni Cosimo Bonomo's studies of the so-called itch mite (*Sarcoptes scabiei*). This tiny insect, barely visible to the naked eye, causes scabies, a skin disease commonly known as the itch. The itch mite can be transferred directly from person to person or by means of bedding and clothing used by infested people. Physicians debated the alleged causal association between mites and scabies until the 1840s, but affected people traditionally treated the itch by searching for tiny insects under the skin and removing them with sharp pins or needles. Even after physicians carried out careful experiments that seemed to prove the causal relationship between mites and scabies, skeptics continued to argue that disease-causing material on the skin of people with incipient scabies might have attracted the little insects.

During the 1830s and 1840s, several other discoveries helped to establish the relationship between minute parasites and diseases of humans and other animals. A particularly influential example occurred in 1834 when Agostino Bassi demonstrated that a deadly silkworm disease known as muscardine was caused by a parasitic fungus, which was later named *Botrytis bassiana*. The disease-causing fungus could be transmitted by direct contact between silkworms and indirectly by contaminated food. Bassi predicted that similar living agents might cause other contagious diseases. His prediction was confirmed by the discovery of a fungus that causes the scalp disease known as favus, a tiny worm that causes trichinosis in pigs and people, and the parasitic roundworms that cause hookworm. During the eighteenth century, naturalists described hundreds of different molds, but the best-studied fungi were related to plant diseases. Fungal diseases of potatoes, wheat, coffee, cereals, grapes and grapevines, the American sweet chestnut, the American elm, and so forth have resulted in starvation, human disease, and economic crises. Although observations of the devastation caused by fungal diseases of plants are probably as ancient as agriculture itself, the fungi were particularly difficult to classify because they can assume many different forms.

THE NEW GERM THEORY OF DISEASE

Like Girolamo Fracastoro, the German pathologist Jacob Henle attempted to analyze and clarify prevailing theories about the transmission of infectious diseases. Their work was, however, very different, despite the fact that Jacob Henle's *On Miasmata and Contagia* (1840) is also generally considered a landmark in the history of the germ theory of disease. Henle analyzed the old concepts of contagion and miasma in the context of nineteenth-century science. Reviewing evidence about patterns of disease transmission, Henle provided a critical analysis of contagious, miasmatic, and miasmatic-contagious diseases. Observations of various diseases suggested that malaria was a purely miasmatic disease, whereas smallpox, measles, typhus, influenza, dysentery, plague, and so forth were both miasmatic and contagious. Diseases such as syphilis, gonorrhea, and rabies were acquired only through contagion. In addition to discussions of patterns of disease transmission, Henle's analysis incorporated evidence from microscopy, cell theory, pathology, and studies of the relationship between minute parasites and specific diseases.

According to Henle's hypothesis, *contagia animata* (living organisms) caused contagious diseases because whatever the morbid matter of disease might be, it obviously had the power to increase in the afflicted individual. By 1840 physicians were very familiar with inoculation and vaccination, medical interventions that had been widely accepted as ways of minimizing, or even eliminating, the threat of smallpox. In both procedures, doctors took a minute amount of pus from a smallpox or cowpox pustule and transmitted the infectious material to large numbers of people. The process could be repeated many times, using material from the pustules that developed in inoculated or vaccinated people to continue an essentially endless chain of inoculations. The same kind of argument could be made for other infectious, epidemic diseases because the medical literature confirmed the fact that one affected individual could initiate an outbreak of disease in a previously unaffected community. Therefore, Henle concluded, contagion must be an animate entity that multiplied within the body of affected individuals. Obviously, smallpox could not be caused by some unidentified chemical in miasmatic vapors because poisons, toxins, or any other chemical substances do not have the ability to increase in amount; only living things have the power of multiplying themselves. Poisons and toxins were often extremely powerful, even deadly, at very small doses, but they always remain fixed in amount and incapable of initiating epidemics. Miasma was traditionally defined as something that mixed with and poisoned the air, but this failed to explain the transmission of disease, Henle argued, because the existence of miasma had never been scientifically demonstrated. Miasma was only assumed to exist because no other causative agent of disease could be demonstrated.

Based on all available evidence, it was logical to explain the pattern of infectious epidemic diseases by assuming that a living parasitic agent was the cause. When the parasites had sufficiently increased in number, they might leave their victim through the lungs by means of coughs and sneezes. By traveling through the air like dust particles, the parasites could reach new victims even if they did not have direct contact with those who were sick. If the parasite was excreted by the intestines, it would enter sewers and wells. Water from such wells would allow the parasite to reach many new victims. After reviewing recent studies of the relationship between minute parasites and specific diseases, Henle discussed the nature of the proofs that would be required to establish a causal relationship between microbial germs and disease. Finding some microorganism in the sick did not prove that it had a causal role. The agent must be isolated and cultured so that it was free from any toxins or traces of diseased tissue. At the time, obtaining pure cultures of microbes was virtually impossible. Acknowledging the lack of rigorous evidence for the germ theory of disease, Henle argued that science could not wait for unequivocal proofs because scientists could only conduct meaningful research when they were guided by a reasonable theory. Until the last decades of the nineteenth century, however, scientists were unable to explain the many ways in which disease-causing germs were transmitted. Although Henle's theory was generally ignored by his contemporaries, since the establishment of microbiology, his essay on contagion has been honored as a classic contribution to the history of medicine.

In addition to analyzing patterns of disease transmission, both Fracastoro and Henle suggested another way of understanding the characteristics of the seeds or germs that allegedly caused infectious diseases. Both noted that direct studies of the germs that caused human disease might be difficult or impossible, but the processes involved in putrefaction, fermentation, and infectious disease seemed to share fundamental traits. Therefore, proof that fermentation and putrefaction were caused by microscopic living agents would support the hypothesis that microbes caused disease. Fermenting agents had, of course, been used for thousands of years to produce beer, wine, bread, yogurt, and so forth, but Fracastoro could only speculate about the existence of living agents of fermentation and putrefaction. When Henle argued that living entities caused infectious diseases, scientists were in the midst of a debate about whether the microscopic entities observed in fermenting liquids were the cause or the product of fermentation. During the 1830s, several scientists had suggested that the growth of yeast cells might be the cause of fermentation. Theodor Schwann, best remembered as one of the founders of Cell Theory, argued that because yeasts were independent living cells, fermentation provided a useful model system for investigating the fundamental activities of all plant and animal cells. In a series of experiments on fermentation, Schwann challenged the theory of spontaneous generation and suggested that microorganisms cause the chemical changes involved in putrefaction and fermentation. Schwann's hypothesis was ridiculed by many of the most famous chemists of the nineteenth century. Justus von Liebig insisted that fermentation was a purely chemical process and that microbes were the product, rather than the cause, of fermentation. The debate essentially ended when Louis Pasteur attacked Liebig's position and proved that microorganisms cause specific fermentations as well as putrefaction and infectious disease.

MEDICAL MICROBIOLOGY

In terms of fundamental concepts, microbiology is closely linked to the ancient doctrine of contagion, the germ theory of disease, and debates about the infusoria discovered by seventeenth-century microscopists. As a scientific discipline, however, microbiology emerged in the second half of the nineteenth century. By the 1880s, the foundations of microbiology and bacteriology were established, primarily through the work of the French chemist Louis Pasteur and the German physician Robert Koch. In France, where Pasteur's influence was dominant, the study of bacteria was considered part of the larger discipline of microbiology. Koch preferred the term *bacteriology* to describe his work, which was appropriate given the fact that his greatest successes involved the identification of the agents that cause several major bacterial diseases, including anthrax, tuberculosis, and cholera. Bitter and disruptive disputes between the French and German pioneers of microbiology were not uncommon and, at least in part, reflected the hostilities between their countries.

The early techniques of microbiology were fairly crude, which made the identification of pure strains extremely difficult and tedious. Pasteur, Koch, and others had to find media and experimental animals in which different bacteria would grow. Most important, they had to convince their contemporaries that diseases had specific causes and that the diseases they chose to study—diseases of wine and beer, silkworms and sheep, dogs and humans—were caused by microbes, which were organized, living, reproducing organisms. By growing pure strains of bacteria in laboratory cultures, examining their characteristics, and transmitting them to experimental animals, Pasteur, Koch, and their disciples clarified the relationship between specific germs and specific diseases. Through their research and publications, Pasteur and Koch established the theoretical, methodological, and ideological foundations of the new science of microbiology. However, their lives, their work, and their conflicts reflected the interplay between scientific research, basic and applied science, and the political and social environments within which scientists are embedded.

Despite their conflicts and differences in approach to research, Pasteur and Koch were champions of what has been called the *etiological principle*; that is, they shared the conviction that diseases could be understood and controlled if scientists discovered their specific causes. For infectious diseases, that meant rigorous proof that a specific microbial agent caused a particular disease. Based on this evidence, scientists could say with certainty that the disease would not occur without that microbe and that every case of the disease was caused by the microbe under investigation. The etiological principle, primarily associated with microbiology, has dominated medical thought since the end of the nineteenth century. It has guided attempts to understand, control, and cure new and old diseases. However, the founders of scientific germ theory also realized that the ability of a microbe to cause disease involved many interrelated factors such as the characteristics of the microbe, the susceptibility of the individuals exposed to the microbe, and the environment that allowed microbes to survive and find new victims.

LOUIS PASTEUR

Louis Pasteur was not the first to argue that germs caused infectious diseases, but his work was of paramount importance in demonstrating the relevance of germ theory to infectious disease, surgery, hospital management, agriculture, and industry. Generally involved in several major lines of research at the same time, Pasteur made major contributions to the study of fermentation; spontaneous generation; the diseases of wine, beer, silkworms, farm animals, and humans; the development of protective vaccines; and virology. In terms of human health and welfare, Pasteur's work on vaccines as well as the development of techniques for sterilizing growth media and medical instruments and the process now known as pasteurization have saved more lives than any specific therapeutic intervention. In addition to his genius for selecting challenging, but feasible, research problems, Pasteur had a genius for self-promotion and was more than willing to publicly debate his critics. These debates helped bring scientific germ theory to the attention of a broad audience (see Figure 2.2).

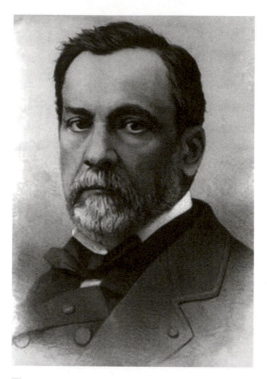

Figure 2.2 Louis Pasteur. Credit: Library of Congress Prints and Photographs Division. Washington, D.C.

When he began his research career, Pasteur expected to devote himself to chemistry and physics, but his innate curiosity, and requests for his help in solving problems plaguing French agriculture and industries, led to his work on fermentation and medical microbiology. As Professor of Chemistry and Dean of Sciences at the University of Lille, Pasteur was expected to demonstrate that science could be applied to improving local industries. While investigating problems involved in the fermentation of beet juice, Pasteur became interested in the relationship between microorganisms and fermentation, especially when the process was unsuccessful. Various ferments were traditionally used to produce beer, wine, vinegar, yogurt, bread, and so forth, but the nature of the fermentation process was mysterious. Ferments were vaguely defined as active substances that could transform substances capable of fermentation, the way a small amount of yogurt causes the transformation of a much larger amount of milk into yogurt. Experiments on a variety of fermentations—including those that produced wine, beer, and vinegar—led Pasteur to the conclusion that fermentation is always dependent on living germs that served as specific, organized ferments. Through his studies of fermentation, Pasteur discovered that changes in the population of microorganisms were associated with healthy fermentations that produced desirable outcomes, such as wine and beer, and spoiled fermentations that could be thought of as putrefactions, or the diseases of wine and beer. Previous speculations about the role of living yeast cells in fermentation had been ridiculed by the most illustrious organic chemists of the period. According to Justus von Liebig and his associates, fermentation was a purely chemical process, and microorganisms were the product, rather than the cause, of fermentation. Experiments on a variety of fermentations led Pasteur to the conclusion that all fermentations are caused by specific organized ferments, which could be referred to as germs or microbes. The hypothesis that fermentation, putrefaction, and infectious disease were closely related phenomena had been suggested by Fracastoro, Schwann, and Henle. Thus, the possibility that ferments were related to the germs that caused disease was not a new idea, but it was Pasteur's experiments and arguments that forced his contemporaries to consider the role of germs in fermentation, putrefaction, and disease.

Studies of fermentation led Pasteur to a declaration of war on the ancient doctrine of spontaneous generation. Friends warned him against being drawn into a contest that could not be won, for one cannot prove a universal negative; that is, one cannot actually prove that spontaneous generation never occurred, never occurs, or never will occur. An experimental attack on this question was essential, Pasteur insisted, because microbiology, medicine, and surgery could only progress when scientists and physicians abandoned the doctrine of spontaneous generation. According to ancient folklore and classical natural philosophy, living creatures, such as insects, frogs, and mice, could originate from nonliving matter. The Greek philosopher Aristotle accepted the doctrine of spontaneous generation, as did most seventeenth-century natural philosophers, until Francesco Redi initiated an experimental study of the generation of insects. Redi's work did not destroy the doctrine of spontaneous generation, but it helped move the debate away from insects and mice to the "little animals" revealed by the microscope. Eighteenth-century naturalists carried out various experiments to determine whether microbial life was spontaneously generated in nutrient broths, but the results of these tests were inconsistent.

During the nineteenth century, the design of experiments for and against spontaneous generation became increasingly sophisticated. For all practical purposes, however, Pasteur won the debate by proving that the existence of germs in the air was the critical issue in formulating experimental tests of the doctrine of spontaneous generation. Building on an experimental approach that can be traced back to Francesco Redi, Pasteur set out to prove that under present conditions, microbes only arise from preexisting microbes; that is, microbial life does not spontaneously arise in sterile media, if germs in the air are rigorously excluded. Therefore, according to Pasteur, all the so-called evidence that his opponents had presented to support spontaneous generation was the result of careless technique and experimental artifacts.

Without resolving fundamental philosophical questions about the origin of life, Pasteur's attack on the doctrine of spontaneous generation led to the pragmatic conclusion that fermentation, putrefaction, infection, and epidemic diseases were caused by microorganisms found in the air and on virtually all surfaces, including medical instruments, bandages, sponges, and the hands of physicians, surgeons, and nurses. Therefore, the rigorous practice of sterile technique was essential to microbiology, medicine, and surgery. The debates about the possibility of spontaneous generation were also of great importance in developing the process now known as pasteurization, or partial sterilization, which is used to destroy potentially harmful microorganisms in foods and beverages.

Food scientists consider milk pasteurization one of the most successful public health achievements of the twentieth century. Unpasteurized milk was responsible for a large share of all food-borne illness, especially among infants and children, because of the high risk of contracting tuberculosis, undulant fever (brucellosis), dysentery, and other infectious diseases. More than a century after the general adoption of pasteurization, the kinds of bacteria most commonly found in raw milk are somewhat different from those that threatened nineteenth-century children. Bovine tuberculosis and brucellosis may be very rare, but even milk obtained from cows that are certified as healthy may contain campylobacteria, salmonella, listeria, *Escherichia coli*, or other harmful bacteria. Although public health officials warn that unpasteurized milk, juice, and other products may harbor deadly bacteria, like Pasteur's nineteenth-century opponents, many people still believe that pasteurization destroys mysterious natural principles. Public health authorities estimate that hundreds of thousands of people in the United States ignore state laws banning the sale of raw milk for human consumption.

Although most physicians rejected the idea that Pasteur's studies of the relationship between microorganisms and healthy fermentations were related to human disease, his work was recognized for its value to important French industries such as the production of wine and beer. Another significant demonstration of the potential benefits of applying the science of microbiology to practical problems occurred when Pasteur accepted a request from the French Minister of Agriculture to investigate an epidemic disease that was threatening the country's silk industry. In addition to demonstrating the existence of two distinct microbial diseases in silkworms, Pasteur discovered that the epidemic was triggered and sustained by a complex web of factors that included environmental and nutritional deficiencies as well as microorganisms.

During the years spent on his studies of fermentation and the diseases of silkworms, Pasteur established the ideas and methods that led to his best known work, that is, the discovery of the microbial agents that cause various diseases of higher animals and the establishment of vaccines for anthrax and rabies. While investigating a disease known as chicken cholera, Pasteur isolated a microbe from infected birds and, almost by accident, discovered that laboratory cultures of the microbe could be used as a protective vaccine; that is, Pasteur realized that he had created a weakened, but still viable chicken cholera microbe that acted as a preventive vaccine. At the time, the only known vaccine was Edward Jenner's cowpox vaccine, which was used to prevent smallpox, a deadly viral disease that will be discussed in detail in Chapter 6.

As the causative agents of infectious diseases were discovered, Pasteur and others attempted to create protective vaccines by deliberately attenuating (weakening) these pathogens in the laboratory. The development of a protective vaccine for rabies, a rare but fatal disease, provided Pasteur's most famous triumph and most difficult challenge. The decision to study a disease as rare and dangerous as rabies, when Pasteur could have chosen from more common diseases that might have been easier to work with, seems puzzling. Although Pasteur referred to memories of the howls of a rabid wolf that had terrorized the village in the countryside where he grew up, the challenge posed by rabies certainly allowed Pasteur to indulge his flair for the dramatic. Moreover, because rabies was invariably fatal in humans, no experimental intervention could make the outcome any worse for a victim of the disease. The first step in all of Pasteur's previous work on specific infectious diseases had been to find the microbe and establish a laboratory culture. All efforts to identify the "virus of rabies" proved futile. At the time, the term *virus* was used in a general sense for agents of disease, especially those that were difficult or impossible to identify by existing methods. It was impossible to grow the rabies virus in laboratory cultures, but it was possible to transmit the disease to a series of experimental animals—dogs or rabbits—using spinal cord preparations from rabid animals. Pasteur discovered that the invisible rabies pathogen could be progressively weakened by suspending the spinal cords of infected animals in a drying chamber for longer and longer periods of time. By inoculating dogs with a series of increasingly virulent preparations, Pasteur could prevent the development of rabies in dogs that had been bitten by rabid animals or inoculated with virulent laboratory preparations.

As soon as Pasteur was sure that he could reliably protect dogs from rabies, he had to consider the greater challenge of protecting human beings from the threat of rabies. Clearly a rabies vaccine, even if it were safe and effective, was not a candidate for mass immunizations because human rabies was too rare a condition to justify a series of potentially dangerous injections. Immunizing all the dogs in France was impossible and would not provide sufficient protection for people because wild animals served as a reservoir of disease. Thus, the only logical approach was to use the vaccine in humans when the threat of rabies was imminent and death was presumably inevitable. In 1885, Pasteur's vaccine was administered to a nine year-old boy who had been severely bitten by a mad dog. Given the nature of the injuries, physicians who examined the boy were sure that he would die of rabies. Despite the painful series of rabies injections, the boy made a complete recovery. Pasteur's account of this case was presented to the Academy of Science of Paris in October 1885; an English translation was published in *Popular Science Monthly* in January 1886. When news of the rabies vaccine became public, it generated both bitter criticism and excessive optimism. Although many reports called the rabies vaccine the greatest achievement of medical science, Pasteur's adversaries—antivaccinators, antivivisectionists, conservative physicians, and veterinarians—emphasized the crudeness of the vaccine, the dangers of the procedure, the immorality of human experimentation, and the problem of diagnosing rabies in humans. Nevertheless, popular accounts of the successful use of the rabies vaccine were published throughout the world, enhancing Pasteur's reputation and leading to the establishment of the Pasteur Institute. The media sensation triggered by the rabies vaccine also heightened interest in the germ theory of disease and led the public to expect miraculous benefits from medical research.

Inevitably, the rabies vaccine produced tragic failures as well as successes. Unlike the smallpox vaccine, the rabies vaccine was only administered after an individual had been bitten by an animal that was thought to be rabid. Successful immunization depended on how soon the inoculations began and the individual's reaction to the vaccine. Critics contended that success measured only by the failure of patients to die of rabies was meaningless. Indeed, it is true that the difficulty of predicting the outcome of dog bites is a complicating factor in assessing Pasteur's rabies vaccine; that is, rabies was invariably fatal if contracted, but not all encounters with mad dogs result in human rabies, and not all so-called mad dogs are actually rabid. Thus, many people who were not actually infected by the rabies virus might undergo an unnecessary series of painful and dangerous inoculations. However, when victims of dog bites faced the possibility of dying of rabies, many thousands decided that they preferred to accept the risks inherent in the Pasteur vaccine.

Rabies-related human deaths in wealthy nations are very rare today because of routine vaccination of pet dogs and safer vaccines for people bitten by rabid or possibly rabid animals. About forty thousand people in the United States are treated for rabies exposure every year, primarily because of contact with wild animals, usually raccoons, bats, or coyotes. Ironically, in a few highly publicized cases, the rabies virus has been transmitted to organ transplant recipients because the organ donors had been infected but not yet diagnosed. Although rabies-related deaths caused by donated organs are extremely rare, several cases have occurred in people who received kidneys, livers, lungs, and corneas from infected donors. Transplant experts acknowledge that transplanted organs and tissues can transmit various diseases but warn that testing for all potential infectious diseases is virtually impossible given the scarcity of organs, time constraints, and lack of resources.

Almost all human rabies deaths today occur in developing countries in Africa and Asia, but the threat of rabies is still a significant problem in many parts of the world. Each year, rabies kills about fifty-five thousand people, and millions undergo preventive inoculations after being bitten by a rabid animal. Effective rabies control strategies depend on understanding the distribution and incidence of rabies in all possible host species. Rabies is primarily found in domestic and stray dogs in Africa, Asia, India, and Latin America. In North America, southern Africa, parts of the Caribbean, and Europe, wild carnivores are the major mammalian reservoir of the virus. In Africa, rabies has been found in foxes, jackals, bats, cats, shrews, mongooses, genets, cattle, antelopes, and various rodents. In 2006, the Alliance for Rabies Control initiated plans for World Rabies Day to raise support for the prevention of human rabies and the control of rabies in animals. The First World Rabies Day was held on September 8, 2007, as a means of calling attention to this much dreaded but preventable disease.

ROBERT KOCH

Very different from Louis Pasteur in training, temperament, and his approach to medical science, Robert Koch was most successful at formulating the principles and techniques of modern bacteriology. Koch lacked Pasteur's flair for the dramatic, but his simple and ingenious laboratory techniques were fundamental to the establishment of modern microbiology. While still a practicing rural physician, Koch conducted his first successful research project and proved that anthrax, a disease that primarily attacked sheep and cattle, was caused by a specific bacillus. Anthrax was a threat to people who worked with infected animals or came in contact with contaminated animal products. Depending on the way in which the bacteria were acquired, the disease could assume different clinical patterns, which are known as cutaneous, gastric, or inhalation anthrax. The most common form of the disease in humans, cutaneous anthrax, is characterized by severe, localized skin ulcers known as malignant pustules. Gastric anthrax, contracted by eating undercooked meat from infected animals, and inhalation anthrax, a virulent pneumonia once known as wool-sorter's disease, were almost always fatal. By 1860, several scientists had observed rather large, rod-shaped bacteria in the blood of anthrax victims, but their evidence for an association between these bacteria and the disease was largely circumstantial. Thus, although Koch was not the first scientist to find the causative agent, *Bacillus anthracis*, in the blood of animals dying of anthrax, he was the first to provide rigorous proof that anthrax was caused by a specific microbe.

Using blood from infected animals, Koch successfully transmitted the disease to rabbits and mice. He was then able to continue passing the disease through a series of experimental animals. To provide further proof that the disease was caused by *Bacillus anthracis* itself, rather than some poison in the blood of sick animals, Koch grew the bacteria in a series of laboratory cultures and demonstrated that even after ten to twenty transfers, his bacterial cultures could cause anthrax in experimental animals. These experiments ruled out the possibility that the disease was caused by some poison from the original animal. Obviously, only an entity capable of multiplying in animals and in laboratory cultures could create such a chain of infection.

While observing the growth of anthrax bacilli on microscope slides, Koch noticed that as the medium evaporated, the threadlike chains of anthrax bacteria were transformed into beadlike spores. By adding fresh medium, he could reverse this transformation. The existence of two forms of *Bacillus anthracis* and the durability of its spores explained many of the mysteries surrounding the transmission of the disease. The spores formed by *Bacillus anthracis* could remain dormant, but potentially viable, under harsh conditions for long periods of time. The spores served as a reservoir of disease in contaminated pastures and were able to revive and infect animals that consumed contaminated vegetation. Spores were the most general means of disseminating the disease among animals, but people who slaughtered, butchered, or skinned infected animals were exposed to active bacilli. People who worked with wool or hides from infected animals could be exposed to anthrax spores. Thus, an understanding of the natural history of anthrax immediately suggested a general strategy for controlling the disease, beginning with specific measures for disposing of animals that had died of anthrax. If carcasses were incinerated or buried in deep, dry trenches, spore formation could not occur. Surveys of disease patterns in sheep, cattle, and horses suggested that sheep were the normal reservoir for anthrax. Simply separating other animals from sheep interrupted the chain of infection.

In 1876, when Koch was convinced that he had isolated the microbe that caused anthrax, established its life cycle, and explained the natural history of the disease, he contacted Ferdinand Cohn for advice and criticism. Primarily a botanist, Cohn was the first prominent German scientist to take a special interest in bacteria. After examining the nature of Koch's experimental findings, Cohn arranged for the publication of Koch's paper, "The Etiology of Anthrax Based on the Developmental Cycle of *Bacillus anthracis*," in the journal *Contributions to Plant Biology*. Even after the publication of Koch's classic work on anthrax, critics of the germ theory of disease continued to argue that the disease was caused by toxic material in the blood, rather than the so-called anthrax bacillus. These attacks on the validity of germ theory drew Pasteur into the battle. Carrying out a series of one hundred transfers from culture to culture, Pasteur purified the bacteria in media composed of broth or urine. Only a living organism capable of multiplying in the course of these transfers could be the virulent agent; that is, the dilution factor for this painstaking procedure was so great that no trace of even the most potent poison that might have been present in the original sample could possibly remain. Pasteur noted that some skeptics had taken their specimens from animals long after death occurred. In such cases, he concluded, their experiments involved the germs of putrefaction, rather than the specific anthrax germ. Another peculiarity of the anthrax bacillus was discovered in connection with a dispute as to whether chickens could be affected. Under normal conditions, chickens are not susceptible to anthrax, but Pasteur proved that it was possible to transmit the disease to chickens. These experiments drew attention to the complex phenomenon of differential susceptibility to specific pathogens among various species.

Although it was Koch who provided unequivocal proof that *Bacillus anthracis* caused anthrax, it was Pasteur who developed a preventive vaccine and worked out an explanation for the role played by spores and earthworms in perpetuating and propagating the disease. To create a preventive vaccine, Pasteur grew *Bacillus anthracis* under controlled laboratory conditions to select an attenuated strain that did not produce the disease. In the case of the anthrax bacillus, maintaining a specific temperature range was critical to prevent spore formation or the death of the vegetative form. With the cooperation of the Agricultural Society of Melun, a public demonstration of Pasteur's anthrax vaccine was held in 1881 at Pouilly-le-Fort. At the time of the well-publicized demonstration, Pasteur was still trying to produce a safe and effective vaccine from live attenuated bacteria. Although Pasteur and his associates did not reveal the extent of this problem, his research notebooks indicate that he actually used a chemically treated dead anthrax vaccine developed by his associates Charles Chamberland and Émile Roux. Nevertheless, the public demonstration was a great success. Even after being inoculated with a highly virulent strain of the anthrax bacillus, the vaccinated sheep and cows remained healthy. The control group of unvaccinated sheep and cows contracted anthrax. By 1894, millions of sheep and cattle had been vaccinated against anthrax.

In addition to the threat that anthrax-contaminated soils pose to domesticated animals, the disease can infect wild herbivores, and even the carnivores that prey on them. In Africa, naturalists have reported deaths from anthrax in many different species, including elephant, lion, cheetah, zebra, buffalo, giraffe, antelope, hippopotamus, and rhinoceros. Deer and elephants have died of anthrax in game parks in India. In Canada, outbreaks of anthrax among bison have been recorded since the 1960s. Animal hides from infected animals can carry anthrax spores. Cutaneous and inhalation anthrax cases have been traced to untanned animal hides that were used to make drums. Textile workers have also contracted the disease from goat pelts. The transmission of anthrax from infected animals to humans who handle their hides or eat undercooked meat is not uncommon in many developing countries, especially in much of sub-Saharan Africa; but in the United States, since the terrorist attacks of September 11, 2001, a diagnosis of anthrax immediately raises fears of bioterrorism. Cutaneous anthrax, historically the most common form of human anthrax, can now be treated with antibiotics, but even with aggressive treatment, inhalation anthrax is still considered a life-threatening condition.

After establishing the causative relationship between one specific microbe, *Bacillus anthracis*, and one specific disease, Koch turned to the general problem of wound infection. Many investigators had observed bacteria in the deadly infections that often followed surgery or traumatic injuries, but they could not determine whether microbes were the cause of the disease, or if the disease was the product of pathological processes or nonspecific entities. In part, Koch's work on wound infection in laboratory mice was meant to support the concept that bacteria are distinct, fixed species. If bacteria did not exist as separate species, it made no sense to say that a specific microbe—such as *Bacillus anthracis*—caused a specific disease. Unfortunately, the significance of these experiments on wound infections in mice was not generally appreciated when Koch presented his results, presumably because Koch could not demonstrate their relevance to human disease.

Critics of the germ theory continued to argue that microbes were nonspecific and easily transformed into different types. The apparent generation of new forms in the laboratory, Koch contended, was not proof of transformation of type, but evidence of poor technique and contamination by microbes in the environment. Essentially, this was the same argument Pasteur had made concerning the doctrine of spontaneous generation. Supporters of germ theory realized that it would be impossible to convince skeptics that specific germs caused specific diseases if they could not prove that microbes existed as distinct species. In particular, Koch argued that advocates of the germ theory of disease needed simple, reliable methods of establishing pure cultures. The animal body might well be the optimum cultivation apparatus for pathogenic bacteria, but bacteriologists had to cultivate pure strains outside the animal body to establish the role of bacteria in causing disease. To obtain pure strains of bacteria, Koch developed techniques that transformed nutrient broths into solidified media to capture individual bacteria and allow them to grow into separate colonies, like little islands on a sea of jelly. Medium solidified by the addition of gelatin was useful for cultivating many different organisms, but gelatin can be liquefied at body temperature and can be digested by some bacteria. Agar, a product used in Asian cooking and adopted by some Europeans as a thickening agent for jellies, produced gels that could be added to hot soup without melting. Moreover, gels made with agar, a polysaccharide derived from red algae, are inert to bacterial digestion. A simple but very effective device for culturing microbes on agar gels was introduced by Koch's associate Richard Julius Petri. Although the use of solid media was initially called *Koch's plate technique*, thanks to the universal adoption of the petri dish, today, Petri's name is probably more familiar to students of microbiology than Koch's.

Another technical problem addressed by Koch and his associates was a reexamination of various public health measures such as the use of agents called *disinfectants* and *antiseptics*, which were thought to reduce the threat of putrefaction and infection. Typically, antiseptics were applied to external wounds, and disinfectants were used on inanimate objects and surfaces. Microbiology made it possible to understand the difference between disinfection, killing vegetative cells, but not necessarily all spores, and sterilization, completely killing both spores and vegetative cells. In testing the activity of reputed antiseptics, Koch discovered that many traditional antiseptics and disinfectants did not really kill or inhibit the growth of bacteria.

In contrast to Pasteur, who had taken rabies, one of the most dramatic but relatively rare threats to human life, as his greatest challenge, Koch chose to investigate tuberculosis and prove that a specific microbial agent, *Mycobacterium tuberculosis*, was the cause of the disease in all its diverse clinical forms—phthisis, consumption, scrofula, miliary tuberculosis, Pott's disease, and so forth. After decades of controversy as to the nature of tuberculosis, Koch proved that the various forms of the disease occurred because *Mycobacterium tuberculosis* could attack, colonize, and damage virtually all tissues of the human body. In 1882, when Koch reported that he had discovered the tubercle bacillus, accounts of his work and speculation about a possible cure for one of the major killers of the nineteenth century appeared in newspapers throughout the world. To understand the excitement generated by Koch's research on tuberculosis, it is essential to appreciate the way in which this dreaded disease permeated the whole fabric of nineteenth-century life. When Koch began his work, epidemiologists estimated that tuberculosis was the cause of death for one in every seven people. The impact of the disease on society was amplified by the fact that it was particularly likely to sicken or kill young adults. Even in the 1940s, pathologists commonly found evidence of tuberculosis when performing postmortem examinations on people who had not displayed symptoms of the disease during their lives.

Not unlike AIDS in the 1980s, tuberculosis seemed to claim the lives of a disproportionate number of young artists, writers, composers, and musicians, leading to the myth that the fever of tuberculosis was linked to the fires of creative genius. Koch's discovery dispelled this myth with proof that *Mycobacterium tuberculosis* was most often found in the impoverished residents of filthy, dark, crowded dwellings in city slums. As in the case of AIDS, the alleged connection between creativity and tuberculosis was the accidental result of the prevalence of the disease. The association between the disease and poverty, however, was indicative of fundamental inequities in society. Another blow to romantic myths about tuberculosis was the discovery that the tubercle bacillus was very similar in size, shape, and staining properties to the microbe associated with leprosy, a disease universally considered loathsome, rather than romantic. Sentimental visions of tragic young victims of tuberculosis discreetly coughing up bloodstained sputum into dainty handkerchiefs were replaced with the realization that infected individuals were filling the air around them with clouds of bacteria with their coughing and spitting. Looking at the history of tuberculosis and leprosy in terms of social context and literary allusions is probably the best demonstration of the fact that the pattern of human suffering associated with a particular disease cannot be reduced to a description of its microbial agent. Although all forms of tuberculosis are caused by a specific pathogen, controlling the disease required thinking in terms of a complex web of causation. Pulmonary tuberculosis, the most common form of the disease in humans, provided the most efficient means of transmission because its victims coughed up and spit out germ-laden sputum. In poorly ventilated, windowless, dirty, dusty tenement rooms, tubercle germs could remain viable for days, or even months. With this knowledge, public health reformers called for systematic campaigns to isolate the sick and break the chain of transmission, which was only the first step toward dealing with fundamental social problems related to poverty, housing, crowding, and unsanitary conditions.

Many other pathogens, Koch noted, had been relatively easy to isolate and characterize, but the tubercle bacillus presented special difficulties. It was much smaller than the anthrax bacillus, and its growth rate was surprisingly slow, even under optimal laboratory conditions. The persistence of the tubercle bacillus in the body was puzzling, but bacteriologists eventually discovered that *Mycobacterium tuberculosis* is able to use macrophages, white blood cells that usually engulf and destroy microorganisms, as its primary host. Many animals, including cattle, horses, monkeys, rabbits, and guinea pigs, contract tuberculosis, but not all strains of the tubercle bacillus can grow in every species. The bacillus that causes tuberculosis in cattle, goats, and sheep, *Mycobacterium bovis*, is closely related to *Mycobacterium tuberculosis*. Humans presumably acquired tuberculosis when they domesticated goats and cattle. Many bacteriologists assumed that milk from cows with bovine tuberculosis was a danger to children, but Koch mistakenly claimed that humans could not be infected with the bovine tubercle germ. Apparently, Koch underestimated the danger posed by milk from tuberculous cows because of his emphasis on the role of sputum in spreading pulmonary tuberculosis. Despite Koch's influence, scientists recognized the danger posed by milk from infected cows, and public health reformers called for testing dairy cattle and pasteurizing milk sold for human consumption. Opponents of pasteurization were encouraged by Koch's conclusion, but recognition of bovine tuberculosis as a public health threat, especially for young children, was an important factor in the battle to control tuberculosis.

Clinicians and critics of the germ theory of disease were not convinced that Koch's work on the tubercle bacillus proved that a single pathogen could be responsible for an illness as complex as tuberculosis, or that conditions as different as phthisis (tuberculosis of the lungs) and scrofula (tuberculosis of the lymphatic system that caused swelling of the neck) were different forms of the same disease. Based on autopsy findings, pathologists generally concluded that pulmonary tuberculosis and miliary tuberculosis must be different diseases. Many physicians rejected the idea that tuberculosis was a contagious disease. Instead, they argued that tuberculosis was an inherited disorder, as demonstrated by families in which many members, generation after generation, were affected by the disease. Critics of germ theory also argued that if the tubercle bacillus was as widespread as Koch asserted, given the fact that not all people contracted tuberculosis, the bacillus could not be the true cause of the disease. Advocates of the germ theory of disease responded that such an argument was like saying that bullets do not kill because not every soldier on the battlefield is killed by a barrage of bullets. Rather than dispute Koch's arguments about the transmission of tuberculosis, some critics attempted to trivialize his work by claiming that he had not discovered anything new because others, such as the English epidemiologist William Budd and the French physician Jean Antoine Villemin, had previously claimed that tuberculosis was contagious. Moreover, Villemin had demonstrated that tuberculosis could be transmitted from humans to rabbits by means of sputum, blood, and bronchial secretions.

During his studies of wound infections and tuberculosis, Koch formulated the criteria that must be satisfied to prove that a specific microbial agent causes a specific disease. Similar principles had been suggested previously by Jacob Henle and others, but Koch provided a more rigorous approach to establishing the relationship between specific germs and specific diseases. Thus, these criteria are now known as Koch's postulates. A thorough study of the relationship of the microbe to the natural history of the disease provided valuable, but still circumstantial evidence. Skeptics could argue that even if the microorganism appeared in association with the disease, it might not be the cause of the disease. Rigorous proof of a causal relationship required complete separation of the microbe from the diseased animal, tissue fragments, body fluids, and all possible contaminants. As a first step, according to the classical version of Koch's postulates, researchers must prove that a specific microorganism is found in victims of the disease and not in the tissues of healthy individuals or in those suffering from other diseases. The microbe should then be isolated and cultivated in the laboratory to separate it from contaminating tissue, possible toxins, and other microbes. After the microbe thought to cause the disease had been grown as a pure laboratory culture, it should be introduced into healthy animals. If experimental animals inoculated with pure laboratory cultures of the microbe contracted the disease, with all its typical symptoms and properties, and the microbe could be isolated from those animals, the investigator could reasonably conclude that the microbe in question was in fact the cause of the disease. Although Koch thought that researchers should carry out all of these steps, if at all possible, before making claims about the etiology of infectious diseases, not all human diseases could be transmitted to experimental animals, and some microbes could not be cultivated in the laboratory. Research on some human diseases, such as typhoid fever, leprosy, and cholera, was inhibited by the lack of animal models, but Koch was confident that progress in bacteriology would ultimately lead to the control of epidemic diseases. His attempt to find a cure for tuberculosis was, however, a great failure, bordering on scandal.

Whether a microbe or a hereditary weakness caused tuberculosis, in the absence of a therapeutic agent, victims of the disease were generally condemned to a long, lingering decline that inevitably terminated in death. For those who accepted the relationship between the tubercle bacillus and the disease, Koch's discovery stimulated hope that his work would make it possible to identify infected individuals in the early stages of the disease to break the chain of transmission. On the other hand, the ability of physicians to detect asymptomatic infections would inflate estimates of the prevalence of the disease and increase public anxiety about the threat posed by people with tuberculosis. Unless Koch's identification of the tubercle bacillus culminated in the discovery of a therapeutic agent or preventive vaccine, his work would lack the triumphant aspects of Pasteur's work on anthrax and rabies.

When Koch announced in 1890 that he had found a substance that inhibited the growth of the tubercle bacillus in laboratory cultures and in guinea pigs, the media and the public were eager to assume that a cure for tuberculosis was imminent. Newspapers quickly disseminated stories about the mysterious agent that Koch called tuberculin, leading to the widespread belief that a cure for tuberculosis had been discovered. Although Koch realized that his preliminary findings might not be applicable to tuberculosis in humans, he did attempt to conceal the identity of tuberculin (a crude extract of tubercle bacilli) from other scientists and physicians. Nevertheless, hordes of desperate and hopeful patients, physicians, and scientists came to Germany seeking access to tuberculin treatment.

Unfortunately, Koch's claims for the usefulness of tuberculin as a therapeutic agent were tragically wrong. He was right, however, in predicting that tuberculin would become a valuable diagnostic tool for detecting early and asymptomatic cases of tuberculosis. Tuberculin did not cure the sick, but it did discriminate between uninfected and infected people. Whereas a healthy person had almost no reaction to the agent, those who had been infected experienced severe reactions, including vomiting, fever, and chills. Indeed, some patients died because of their reaction to tuberculin. Immunologists later identified the tuberculin response as part of the complex immunological phenomenon called *delayed-type hypersensitivity*. When it became apparent that tuberculin was not a miraculous cure for tuberculosis, and that it sometimes accelerated the disease process, public opinion rapidly turned against Koch. Up to the end of his life, however, he continued to hope that some improved form of tuberculin would provide a cure or a preventive vaccine. Although the tuberculin episode seriously damaged his reputation, in 1905, Koch was awarded the fifth Nobel Prize for Physiology or Medicine in recognition of his pioneering work on tuberculosis.

Recognition of the role played by the tubercle bacillus proved that tuberculosis was a contagious, preventable disease, rather than a constitutional or hereditary defect in the patient. Sensitive tuberculin skin tests and X-ray examinations made it possible to diagnose infectious individuals and break the chain of transmission. Despite the widespread distribution of the tubercle bacillus in the early twentieth century, the incidence of tuberculosis as well as the mortality rate declined as living standards improved. No specific cure for tuberculosis became available until the 1940s, when Selman A. Waksman and coworkers discovered streptomycin.

When marked variations in the virulence of different varieties of tubercle bacilli were discovered, scientists hoped that a particularly weak strain could be used as a preventive vaccine. But developing and evaluating tuberculosis vaccines that can be useful in areas where almost everyone has been exposed to the bacillus and many have had a primary infection proved to be very difficult. The most commonly used tuberculosis vaccine is a live, attenuated strain of *Mycobacterium bovis* developed by Albert Calmette and Jean-Marie Camille Guérin in the 1920s. Bacille Calmette-Guérin (BCG) has been widely used as a vaccine against childhood tuberculosis, but American physicians generally rejected BCG because it made the tuberculin skin test useless as a diagnostic tool. Despite recurring questions about the safety and efficacy of BCG, preventive vaccination remains the basis of antituberculosis campaigns in many developing nations, especially in areas confronted by the increasing prevalence of antibiotic-resistant strains of *Mycobacterium tuberculosis*.

The bacillus that causes tuberculosis is a member of the *Mycobacterium tuberculosis complex*. Historically, the mycobacteria that cause tuberculosis and leprosy are the most important members of this group, but other mycobacteria can cause life-threatening respiratory diseases in humans, especially in those whose immune systems have been compromised. A disease known as Buruli ulcer is caused by *Mycobacterium ulcerans*. This progressive, crippling disease is classified by the World Health Organization as a neglected tropical disease. Since the 1990s, illnesses caused by mycobateria have increasingly appeared in people with normal immune function.

GERM THEORY, HYGIENE, AND HEALTH REFORM

By the end of the nineteenth century, the germ theory of disease had transformed human understanding of infectious diseases. The list of infectious diseases associated with specific germs included anthrax, bubonic plague, cholera, diphtheria, gonorrhea, leprosy, pneumonia, scarlet fever, tetanus, tuberculosis, and typhoid fever. Microbiologists were optimistic about the possibility of discovering the specific germs for many other diseases. The germ theory of disease also succeeded in becoming so well known and widely popularized that historians have referred to the popular version of the theory as the "gospel of germs." Indeed, American magazines often adopted and promoted ideas about bacteriology and germ theory before medical journals acknowledged the importance of these concepts. Interest in the germ theory of disease was widespread among the middle and upper classes, especially among health reformers, who explained bacteriology in terms of its applicability to domestic hygiene and sanitation. Although germ theory influenced social reforms and social norms in complex ways, popularizers generally emphasized the threat of invisible germs to human health and life. More optimistic popularizers predicted that the science of bacteriology would lead to the conquest of epidemic disease in the not too distant future.

Bacteriology provided a new rationale for sanitary and hygienic measures in homes, hospitals, cities, and towns. The germ theory of disease was invoked in the development and marketing of items now considered modern necessities such as indoor plumbing, vacuum cleaners, germicides, disinfectants, and antibacterial soaps. Damp cellars, dusty drapes and carpets, sinks, drains, and toilets were seen as the breeding grounds of the so-called house diseases attributed to microbes. Eventually, the standard goals of domestic hygiene and sanitary reform were incorporated into city codes and enforced by inspections so that all new buildings had to meet sanitary codes and incorporate proper plumbing and drainage.

Germ theory had important implications for the way in which people cleaned their homes and prepared foods, and even influenced the length of women's skirts. Well-known American health reformers like Ellen G. White, the spiritual leader and prophetess of the Seventh Day Adventist Church, and John Harvey Kellogg, physician-in-chief of the Adventist's highly successful Battle Creek Sanitarium, incorporated the germ theory of disease into their gospel of wellness. Stressing the importance of the new science of bacteriology in his popular health lectures, Kellogg preached the gospel of vegetarianism and shocked his audiences with horror shows that featured terrifying germs found in meats. In her writings, Ellen White advised her followers to avoid disease by following the laws of hygiene and maintaining the highest possible standards of cleanliness of home, body, and clothing. Uncleanliness allowed the growth of germs, poisoned the air, and led to death and disease. In justifying her command that Adventists adopt a vegetarian diet, White cited both biblical passages and scientific reports that allegedly proved that the tissues of domesticated animals were swarming with parasites and disease germs. White warned against drinking milk unless it had been pasteurized to kill bacteria or eating bread unless it had been thoroughly baked to kill yeast germs.

By the end of the nineteenth century, the public had learned the importance of fighting the invisible hordes of germs that surrounded them and attempted to invade their homes. Fear of filth and bacteria stimulated changes in housekeeping and fashion. Housewives were warned about the germs that hid in heavy drapes, carpets, ornate textured wallpaper, upholstered furniture, and dusty knickknacks. Wealthy people removed many of the traditional components of their Victorian-style homes and adopted cleaner, more streamlined styles. Fear of bringing the germ-laden dust and filth of city streets into their homes motivated women to replace floor-length dresses with skirts that ended above the ankle. Many men shaved off the beards, mustaches, and sideburns that were said to provide a sanctuary for germs. Although the germ theory may have overshadowed arguments about the social, economic, and political roots of disease, there were many affinities between public health campaigns based on miasmatic theories of disease and public health reforms based on germ theory. Sanitary reformers, who had relied on the miasmatic theory of disease transmission, could simply add germs to the list of dangers found in the environment, along with noxious air, sewer gases, contaminated water, filth, and putrefaction.

THREE

❧ ❧

MICROBIOLOGY AND THE FOUNDATIONS OF MODERN SURGERY AND THERAPY

CONTAGION AND CHILDBED FEVER

Historical studies suggest that different professional communities—surgeons, physicians, sanitarians, and veterinarians—developed somewhat different ways of thinking about the germ theory of disease and its practical implications. It is clear, however, that germ theory had a profound impact on the practice of surgery, preventive medicine, and public health policy long before it led to effective therapies for wound infections and infectious diseases. By the beginning of the twentieth century, microbiologists were able to identify the cause and means of transmission of many infectious diseases. Thus, microbiology allowed public health experts to focus on the pathogens that caused epidemic diseases, determine how they were able to spread, and propose measures that would protect the public. The germ theory of disease also explained the ways in which physicians, surgeons, and obstetricians transmitted deadly microbes to their patients.

Childbed fever (also known as puerperal fever) provides a classic example of the way in which a once rare disease could be transformed into a devastating epidemic condition by changes in medical practice. In the case of childbed fever, the major historical factors were a change in birth attendants from midwives to medical men and a change in the location of childbirth from the home to the hospital. Puerperal fever is a life-threatening illness, marked by high fever, infection of the uterus, painful abscesses in the chest and abdominal cavity, and septicemia (blood poisoning) that occurs shortly after childbirth. Case histories in the Hippocratic texts indicate that puerperal infection was rare but not unknown in ancient Greece. By the nineteenth century, a sporadic event had been transformed into a well-known and much feared epidemic disease. During the second half of the eighteenth century, a period generally remembered as the Age of Enlightenment, male doctors first began to displace the female midwives who had traditionally assisted women during childbirth. This was also the period in which childbed fever became a significant threat, especially in the maternity wards that accommodated impoverished women in cities and towns throughout Europe. Hospital maternity wards provided a new niche in which infectious agents could be transported from one victim to the next. The battle against puerperal fever could be seen as part of the story of the development of antiseptic surgery because puerperal fever is essentially equivalent to wound infection, but the first physicians to realize that puerperal fever was a contagious and largely preventable disease did so before the establishment of the modern germ theory of disease. In terms of their education and clinical experience, the American poet and physician Oliver Wendell Holmes and the Hungarian obstetrician Ignaz Philipp Semmelweis were very different, but they reasoned their way to the same conclusion: puerperal fever was a contagious disease carried to patients on the hands of their doctors.

In 1843, Oliver Wendell Holmes read a paper to the Boston Society for Medical Improvement titled "The Contagiousness of Puerperal Fever." Although the paper generated little interest at the time, it has become a classic in the history of medicine. Holmes became interested in childbed fever when he heard about a physician who had died of pathologist's pyemia—now known as septicemia, or blood poisoning—about a week after he conducted the autopsy of a victim of the disease. During the week before his death, the physician attended several women in labor; all of these patients contracted puerperal fever. The most reasonable explanation for this pattern of cases, Holmes concluded, was that puerperal fever was caused by a contagion transmitted from one patient to another by the attending physician.

Many physicians believed that puerperal fever was an epidemic disease associated with seasonal miasmas, but unlike influenza, the epidemics in various towns, villages, and hospitals did not seem to correlate with a particular time of year. Other doctors accepted the idea that puerperal fever might be a contagious disease peculiar to pregnant women but insisted that the contagion was not carried by physicians. A review of puerperal fever cases, however, revealed that the disease almost always attacked only the patients of specific physicians, notably, those who conducted autopsies before delivering babies. Therefore, Holmes argued, the logical conclusion was that specific physicians must have transmitted the contagion. If this was true, society should condemn a series of puerperal fever cases associated with a particular physician as a criminal offense, rather than dismissing such a cluster of cases as an unfortunate coincidence. To prevent the transmission of puerperal fever, Holmes insisted that obstetricians should not participate in postmortems. A doctor who considered it necessary to be present at an autopsy as an observer should wash thoroughly, change his clothing, and allow twenty-four hours to pass before attending women in labor. Although Holmes presented a logical case for the contagiousness of puerperal fever and a practical approach to breaking the chain of transmission, he could not explain the specific cause of the infection. His contemporaries continued to believe that the disease might become contagious in some cases, but that it was almost always the result of epidemic influences in the atmosphere or spontaneous infections peculiar to particular women.

Holmes, who had studied law before he decided to become a doctor, presented a logical argument, but his case was not firmly grounded on direct observation or large numbers of cases. His examples of the serial transmission of childbed fever cases were generally dismissed by his colleagues as merely anecdotal, rather than compelling. In contrast to Holmes, Ignaz Philipp Semmelweis, who had observed large numbers of patients with puerperal fever, and had conducted autopsies on many of them, presented a strong statistical argument for the contagiousness of the disease. Nevertheless, even though he proposed a theory of causation and a practical approach to preventing transmission of the disease, he, too, failed to influence the medical community. Indeed, Semmelweis was all but forgotten by the time the doctrine of antisepsis became associated with the modern germ theory of disease. The foundation of what Semmelweis called his "doctrine" was the statistical and empirical evidence he collected while working at the First Obstetrical Clinic at the Vienna General Hospital. In the 1840s, the Vienna Hospital provided obstetrical services for impoverished women in return for their use as "teaching material." Doctors, medical students, and researchers could anticipate seeing thousands of childbirth cases and hundreds of autopsies annually. Medical students had the opportunity to participate in examinations, deliveries, and autopsies. The maternity wards were divided into two separate divisions: one was supervised by midwives training midwifery students; in the other division, medical students conducted examinations and deliveries under the supervision of physicians. Women in labor were sometimes examined by several doctors and medical students. Conscientious doctors and students moved freely between the maternity ward and the adjoining dissection room.

In general, the maternal mortality rate at the Viennese maternity clinic was not unusually high for a nineteenth-century charitable hospital. What was striking was the difference between the mortality rate in the division served by midwives and the medical division. Whereas the mortality rate in the midwives' division was about 2 to 3 percent, the mortality rate in the medical division, which Semmelweis supervised, was usually about 7 to 10 percent. Unable to explain this discrepancy, Semmelweis conscientiously examined patients in labor and examined the bodies of puerperal fever victims, but the mortality rate for puerperal fever surged as high as 18 percent. According to prevailing medical theory, childbed fever was caused by putrid atmospheric conditions or an "epidemic constitution." Patients in the maternity wards might be particularly susceptible to the noxious atmosphere because of abnormalities in the body induced by pregnancy, childbirth, and lactation. Even wealthy private patients who gave birth at home might succumb to noxious atmospheric influences, but many nonspecific complicating factors—overcrowding, fear, anxiety, malnutrition, and so forth—might increase the incidence of puerperal fever in the maternity wards that served the poor.

Rejecting these widely accepted theories, Semmelweis formulated his doctrine: puerperal fever was identical to wound infection and was caused by the introduction of "cadaveric matter" (decaying organic material) into the body. The doctrine was based on a flash of insight he had experienced after the death of his friend and colleague Jakob Kolletschka in 1847. According to the autopsy report, Kolletschka died of pathologist's pyemia, a deadly infection induced by a small wound caused by a dissection knife. The fatal infection, Semmelweis reasoned, must have been caused by a small amount of cadaveric matter introduced into Kolletschka's body by means of the dissection knife. Reading the autopsy report, Semmelweis realized that the devastating effects of pyemia were strikingly similar to those seen in victims of puerperal fever. It was obvious that after childbirth, women were particularly susceptible to fatal infections because the trauma of birth, particularly, the separation of the placenta from the wall of the uterus, creates a large internal wound. Therefore, Semmelweis concluded, cadaveric matter must be the cause of both pyemia and puerperal fever. Just as the dissecting knife was capable of introducing cadaveric matter into the anatomist's bloodstream, the contaminated hand of the physician who had performed an autopsy was capable of carrying cadaveric matter to his patients when they were most vulnerable to infection.

When doctors and medical students followed Semmelweis's order to scrub their hands with a strong disinfectant until all traces of cadaveric material were removed, the mortality rate in the medical division of the maternity wards dropped below 3 percent. Semmelweis attributed the remaining cases to the decomposition of residual fetal or placental tissue that remained in the uterus of a small percentage of maternity patients. When this trapped organic material decayed, it became essentially equivalent to cadaveric matter. Thus, the doctrine explained all cases of puerperal fever—the sporadic cases that occurred among private patients and the all too common cases in maternity hospitals—because the primary cause was always decaying organic matter. Miasma, epidemic influences, or unknown spontaneous factors were excluded by the doctrine. Unfortunately, Semmelweis's doctrine was generally misunderstood as a simplistic attempt to link childbed fever to cadaveric matter. Many doctors were willing to accept rigorous washing to eliminate cadaveric material on their hands, but they generally rejected the idea that puerperal fever was the product of a specific contagion transmitted by doctors. Nor did they realize that hand washing alone would not eliminate the transmission of infections in hospitals or private practice because instruments, dressings, bedding, and clothing could also carry unknown, invisible sources of infection.

For Semmelweis, the discovery of the cause and prevention of puerperal fever was complete in 1847, but he did not fully explain his findings until 1861, when *The Etiology, Concept, and Prophylaxis of Childbed Fever* was published. Four years later, Semmelweis died in a mental asylum, probably from an infected wound. In retrospect, it seems obvious that if Semmelweis and Holmes could have persuaded the medical community to adopt their approach to preventing puerperal fever, the burden of postsurgical infections could have been reduced as well, but their ideas were generally ignored. In 1879, Louis Pasteur discovered a pathogen, now known as a hemolytic streptococcus, that seemed to be the cause of puerperal fever. Eventually, streptococci were identified as the causative agents of scarlet fever, septic sore throat, rheumatic fever, erysipelas, and necrotizing fasciitis.

Shortly after Semmelweis died, Joseph Lister began to publish a series of papers describing the antiseptic system that revolutionized surgery and hospital management. When asked whether Semmelweis had influenced his work, Lister explained that he knew nothing about Semmelweis when he began a series of clinical experiments inspired by Pasteur's papers on the germ theory of fermentation, putrefaction, and disease. Although Semmelweis had discovered his doctrine in 1847, Lister did not learn about his work on puerperal fever until 1893, when he received a biographical tribute to Semmelweis by Theodore Duka, a Hungarian physician practicing in London. Even though Semmelweis had not been aware of the microbial agents that caused puerperal fever and did not understand the broader implications of his work, Lister graciously acknowledged Semmelweis as a "clinical precursor" who was finally beginning to receive justifiable posthumous honors. By 1880, as part of the Listerian system, antisepsis was generally incorporated into obstetrical practice throughout Europe. Nevertheless, even in the early twentieth century, when mortality rates for other infectious diseases were falling, death rates for puerperal fever remained quite high. Indeed, in the Western world, puerperal fever remained the most common cause of death associated with childbirth until World War II.

JOSEPH LISTER AND ANTISEPTIC SURGERY

Surgery has undergone a remarkable transformation from one of the least respectable branches of medicine into one of the most successful and powerful areas of specialization. Although surgeons had performed difficult and challenging operations for hundreds of years, it was only during the nineteenth century that surgery was radically changed by incorporating reliable methods for dealing with pain and infection. The introduction of general anesthesia in the 1840s and antisepsis in the 1870s made it possible for the great majority of patients to endure and survive major operations. Anesthetics made it possible for surgeons to perform more complicated operations than their predecessors, but even minor operations could lead to life-threatening infections.

Throughout history, healers had adopted various substances for their supposed infection-fighting properties, but, as Robert Koch demonstrated, most of these so-called antiseptics and disinfectants were ineffective, and some were more destructive to human tissues than to microbes. As Florence Nightingale, pioneer of modern nursing and sanitary reform, often said, most of these agents were useless, except when their odor was so noxious that it forced people to open windows and bring fresh air into the sickroom. Thus, Joseph Lister's demonstration of the value of a rigorous system of antisepsis, dedicated to killing the germs that might come into contact with a surgical wound, was a key factor in the evolution of modern surgery and the establishment of the hospital as the proper place for surgery and childbirth.

Until hospitals adopted Lister's antiseptic practices, these charitable institutions were dangerous places, almost invariably associated with bad air, filth, poverty, and high rates of infection. In 1811, Benjamin Rush, eminent American physician and statesman, complained that although hospitals were established for the relief and cure of diseases, they seemed to breed infections and life-threatening hospital fevers. Moreover, hospitalized patients often died of diseases that were rarely, if ever, fatal among private patients who were cared for at home. The same problems were still common in many charity hospitals in the 1870s, where patients often died after minor operations or childbirth. Lister encountered these abominable conditions when he began his career as a surgeon. Like most of his colleagues, Lister initially assumed that infection was caused by the entry of noxious air into a wound. During his search for ways of preventing wound infection, he became interested in the implications of germ theory for surgery and hospital infections. After reading about Louis Pasteur's work on the relationship between microbes and fermentation, Lister began a study of wound infection in various animal models. Insights gained through these experiments and in hospital wards provided the theoretical and practical basis for the Listerian antiseptic system.

When Lister began his work on the antiseptic system, infection often killed more than 60 percent of the patients brought to hospitals with compound, or open, fractures (a fracture in which the broken ends of the bone protrude through the skin). In contrast, patients who experienced simple fracture (a fracture in which the skin remains unbroken) usually recovered without serious complications. The prognosis for compound fracture was so poor that many surgeons recommended immediate amputation above the site of the wound. Lister was convinced that patients with compound fractures could be saved if the open wound could be properly disinfected and kept free of infection. Having tested many disinfectants, Lister selected carbolic acid (also known as phenol) as the most powerful germicide that could be used to prevent wound infection without causing excessive damage to normal tissue. In addition to serving as a general disinfectant for cesspools, outhouses, stables, and drains, carbolic acid was said to overcome noxious odors. Although carbolic acid is a valuable disinfectant, at full strength, it is highly corrosive, and it is toxic when ingested or inhaled. Undiluted carbolic acid was too caustic to use in general surgery, but Lister demonstrated that its adverse effects on skin were acceptable in dealing with potentially fatal compound fractures. Moreover, carbolic acid has a local anesthetic effect when it comes in contact with human skin, and it does not cause blistering. Nevertheless, undiluted carbolic acid was too caustic for use in general surgery or for the treatment of abscesses and incised wounds. To diminish the adverse effects of carbolic acid, while maintaining the highest possible antiseptic activity, Lister spent many years testing various ways of diluting it or mixing it with other fluids.

By 1865, Lister was successfully managing compound fractures and applying his system to surgical operations by disinfecting the surgeon's hands, all surgical instruments, and the patient's skin at the site of the operation. Based on Pasteur's studies of the distribution of germs on surfaces and in the air, Lister insisted on incorporating the antiseptic system into all aspects of hospital care. To reduce the danger posed by air-borne germs in the operating room, Lister adopted various devices that enveloped the patient and the surgeons in a fine mist of dilute carbolic acid. Eventually, Lister realized that he could obtain equally good results without the irritating spray. By 1880, experience and experiments convinced him that some of the very harsh aspects of the antiseptic system—the attempt to create an antiseptic atmosphere in the operating room and washing deep wounds with strong carbolic acid—were unnecessary, as long as the surgeon and his assistants rigorously enforced all the essential components of the system, before, during, and after the operation.

For many years, the medical community ignored Lister's antiseptic system, but by the end of the century, his methods had largely transformed surgical practice and the hospital environment. Surgeons found that following Listerian techniques during surgery and in postsurgical care prevented postsurgical infections, greatly improving patient survival even after complex operations. Scientists and surgeons became interested in new techniques for killing microbes and explored the relative merits of heat versus chemical sterilization and antiseptic versus aseptic methods. The goal of *antisepsis* is to kill the germs in and around a wound by means of germ-killing agents. The goal of *asepsis* is to prevent the introduction of germs into the surgical site. Attention to both goals proved essential because almost all wounds contain some microbes, and antiseptics alone cannot guarantee uncomplicated healing. Louis Pasteur and his colleague Charles Chamberland demonstrated that heat sterilization was superior to chemical disinfection of surgical instruments. Chamberland's work led to the development of the autoclave, a device that provides sterilization by means of steam heat under pressure.

Improvements in methods of sterilization and the surgical routine were enthusiastically adopted by Lister's disciples, but the rigorous adoption of antisepsis and asepsis was not rapid or universal, nor were all hospitals capable of providing the supportive staff and resources that made success possible. Some of the improved techniques were more difficult for surgeons to adjust to than others. In particular, the antiseptic solutions that surgeons and nurses used to wash and scrub their hands before surgery were extremely harsh and unpleasant. William Stewart Halsted, a pioneer in the development of local anesthesia and aseptic surgery, realized that the human hand could not be sterilized, despite rigorous washing. Therefore, he experimented with the use of flexible rubber gloves that could be sterilized before surgery by subjecting them to harsh disinfectants. Despite complaints that gloves would reduce sensitivity and make surgery more difficult, the use of rubber gloves generally became part of the surgical ritual in the 1890s. Eventually, the full aseptic ritual included special surgical gowns, caps, masks, and gloves and the banishment of spectators from the operating room. Some hospitals installed special mirrors or glass domes so that observers could watch without contaminating the operating room. Bringing the antiseptic system to hospital wards as well as the operating room was a major challenge. For example, hospital bandages were generally made of rags that could carry dangerous microbes. No matter how skillful the surgeon, no matter how clean the operating room might be, patients washed with filthy sponges, bandaged with contaminated dressings, and covered with soiled bedding were likely to contract life-threatening infections.

SERUM THERAPY, SALVARSAN, SULFA DRUGS, AND ANTIBIOTICS

Microbiology and the germ theory of disease stimulated the development of new approaches to understanding and preventing infectious diseases, but identifying specific pathogens did not immediately lead to improvements in therapy. The germ theory of disease allowed scientists to demonstrate that the virulence of infectious diseases varied with many factors, including the means and duration of exposure, the way in which germs entered the body, and the physiological status of the host. Microbiology also made it possible to develop protective vaccines that took advantage of the body's own defense mechanisms. As Pasteur had so dramatically demonstrated in his work on rabies, it was even possible to attenuate invisible pathogens that could be used as protective vaccines.

Microbiologists had demonstrated that germs were widely distributed, but even during the most deadly epidemics, some people escaped infection and others recovered without complications. The fact that people who survived one attack of a disease were usually unaffected during later epidemics suggested that the human body was able to recognize and fight off microbial invaders; that is, survivors seemed to acquire immunity. The Latin term *immunity* originally referred to an exemption in the legal sense, but in medical usage, the term refers to resistance to infection by pathogenic microbes. In the late nineteenth century, scientists showed that immunity was at least partially due to noncellular factors in blood serum. The magic bullets or so-called natural disinfectants in the blood were called *antibodies*, and the viruses, bacteria, and toxins that induced them were called *antigens* (antibody generators). The fact that scientists could induce immunity to specific pathogens by creating protective vaccines suggested that it might be possible to develop other approaches to mobilizing and amplifying the body's innate defenses. By the end of the century, bacteriologists had established a new approach to treatment that was called *serum therapy*. The potential benefits of this approach were first demonstrated in the treatment of diphtheria and tetanus.

Diphtheria is an often deadly infectious disease caused by *Corynebacterium diphtheriae*, a bacillus discovered in 1883 by Theodor Klebs and Friedrich Loeffler, who were investigating reports of unusually frequent outbreaks of a condition variously referred to as malignant sore throat, croup, throat distemper, malignant angina, and diphtheritis. Although diphtheria seemed to kill young children by suffocation, autopsies revealed widespread damage to the internal organs, especially the heart, kidneys, and nervous system. The appearance of a thick, leathery gray membrane in the throat is the most characteristic symptom of diphtheria. Doctors sometimes performed a tracheotomy to prevent death by asphyxiation, but the operation generally produced only temporary relief and seemed to amplify other symptoms. Intrigued by the fact that *Corynebacterium diphtheriae* seemed to remain localized in the throat, even though the disease caused systemic damage, Pasteur's associates Émile Roux and Alexandre Yersin demonstrated that the bacteria released toxins into the bloodstream. The discovery of the toxin in the bloodstream helped explain why tracheotomies and attempts to disrupt the membrane often failed. Temporary improvements in respiration could not reverse the effects of the toxins already in the circulation. In the laboratory, researchers were able to separate the toxin from the bacteria by filtering growth medium. Bacteria-free filtrates of growth medium injected into experimental animals produced symptoms of the disease. Bacterial toxins were also found in other diseases, including tetanus, anthrax, cholera, gas gangrene, whooping cough, scarlet fever, food poisoning, and toxic shock syndrome.

During the late nineteenth century, diphtheria was one of the most common killers of children between two and fourteen years of age, but the disease also killed older adults. Diphtheria is usually acquired by inhaling bacteria released into the air by coughing and sneezing, but the severity of the illness may depend on whether the infection was contracted through the nose, skin, or throat. Individuals who contract chronic, asymptomatic nasal diphtheria are a serious threat to others. Diphtheria bacteria that enter the body through small cuts or abrasions can cause skin ulcers and wounds that heal very slowly. Infections of the throat, acquired by inhaling the bacillus, are most likely to cause severe illness. The case fatality rate for diphtheria was usually estimated at about 5 to 10 percent, but especially virulent outbreaks seemed to claim 30 to 50 percent of those affected. Determining the case fatality rate was difficult because many people acquired immunity after a mild, undiagnosed illness.

Through their work on diphtheria and tetanus, Emil von Behring and Shibasaburo Kitasato established a new form of treatment known as serum therapy. Diphtheria antitoxin was the first innovative and successful therapy directly based on germ theory to reach large numbers of patients and convince physicians that germ theory was relevant to medical practice. The rabies vaccine had gotten much publicity and generated great excitement, but human rabies is a very rare condition. Moreover, the first vaccine, Edward Jenner's smallpox vaccine, was introduced in 1798, long before the development of the germ theory of disease. Koch's discovery of the tubercle bacillus and tuberculin had generated widespread hope, but ended with great disappointment. Serum therapy, in contrast, was considered a great innovation and a major addition to therapeutic medicine, as indicated in 1901, when Emil von Behring was awarded the first Nobel Prize for Physiology or Medicine. Although diphtheria is essentially a forgotten disease in the United States, diphtheria antitoxin has become part of Alaskan folklore. The Iditarod dog sled race is held annually to commemorate the route taken in 1925 to bring diphtheria antitoxin from Nenana to Nome, Alaska, a journey of some eleven hundred miles, during an outbreak of diphtheria.

Like Lister and Koch, Behring was interested in chemicals that could kill germs and initially hoped to find compounds that could act within the body as internal disinfectants. Although chemical agents that were deadly to microbes in the test tube were generally too toxic for human use, some chemicals that were too weak to kill bacteria seemed to neutralize bacterial toxins. Behring's colleague Shibasaburo Kitasato had isolated *Clostridium tetani*, the bacillus that causes tetanus. Spores of *Clostridium tetani* are widely dispersed in dirt and soil. Like the diphtheria bacillus, *Clostridium tetani* produced a toxin that caused tetanus when injected into experimental animals. Behring and Kitasato inoculated experimental animals with increasing, sublethal doses of tetanus toxin and demonstrated that blood from the animals that survived contained *antitoxins* (substances that neutralized the bacterial toxins). In these experiments, Behring and Kitasato separated serum, the clear liquid portion of the blood, from the solid, cellular components. Blood serum containing antitoxins could be used to protect other animals from *Clostridium tetani* and its toxin.

Serum therapy seemed to offer a means of using the so-called natural disinfectants produced by the immune system to kill or neutralize bacteria and their toxins. Unlike the immunity produced by bacterial infection, the protection provided by serum therapy was short-lived because it was based on antibodies produced by immunized animals. Another approach to generating immunity was made possible when scientists discovered that formaldehyde could be used to inactivate the diphtheria toxin. Chemically modified toxins, which were called toxoids, could be used to induce long-lasting immunity. Diphtheria toxoid became part of the widely used childhood vaccine known as DPT (for diphtheria, pertussis, and tetanus). With diphtheria antitoxin to treat the sick and the Schick test, developed by Béla Schick, to determine whether people were susceptible to diphtheria, doctors discovered that the vast majority of adults were immune because of prior infection and that many apparently healthy people were carriers of *Corynebacterium diphtheriae*.

Since the discovery of serum therapy and the adoption of preventive immunization, diphtheria has been essentially removed from the list of once common childhood diseases. Diphtheria is the prime example of a major bacterial disease that has been successfully managed by preventive immunizations. Nevertheless, because diphtheria is still endemic in some areas and can be transmitted by healthy carriers, the disease is still a serious threat to children and adults who are not fully immunized. Where immunizations rates have fallen, either because of the breakdown of the public health sector or fear of vaccines, diphtheria outbreaks have returned. During the 1990s, the collapse of the former Soviet Union was followed by a precipitous decrease in routine immunizations and a resurgence of diphtheria. Epidemiological evidence that diphtheria was being transported to other areas led to a 1995 declaration by the World Health Organization (WHO) that the disease had become an international public health threat.

In 1902, when Behring gave his Nobel Prize lecture, he predicted that serum therapy would lead to a complete triumph over infectious diseases. Theoretically, serum therapy should make it possible to induce life-saving immunity to all infectious diseases. In practice, however, serum therapy proved impractical or ineffective for most infectious diseases, and the optimism triggered by Behring's discovery quickly faded. Nevertheless, when no preventive vaccines or drugs are available for deadly diseases, such as viral hemorrhagic fevers, doctors have attempted to save lives by collecting serum from survivors of the disease. Immune serum has been used to treat victims of Lassa fever and Ebola fever, but human convalescent serum is extremely rare because so few patients have survived these diseases. Lassa fever virus sickens thousands of people and causes many deaths in Sierra Leone, Liberia, and elsewhere in West Africa. Other arenaviruses cause Argentine, Brazilian, Bolivian, and Venezuelan hemorrhagic fevers. In the absence of effective vaccines, researchers hope that a broad-spectrum arenavirus antiserum could be used to save many lives. However, developing and testing antiserum or vaccines for hemorrhagic fever viruses would be very difficult and prohibitively expensive because of the need for biosafety level 4 animal containment facilities.

The toxins produced by bacteria have found an important place in biomedical research as well as in clinical medicine. By the end of the twentieth century, molecular biologists were taking advantage of the remarkable properties of various bacterial toxins. The use of botulinum toxin for cosmetic purposes is probably the best-known example. Previously, *Clostridium botulinum* toxin was universally feared as the cause of paralysis following the ingestion of improperly preserved foods. A more significant medical application for bacterial toxins was the creation of hybrid molecules, created by linking toxins to specific antibodies. These monoclonal antibodies have been referred to as "poisoned arrows" or "smart bombs" that can deliver modified toxins to specific targets such as tumor cells.

Serum therapy, also referred to as immunotherapy, stimulated attempts to understand the body's natural immunological defenses to find ways to stimulate and supplement them. Antibodies are remarkably powerful and specific components of the immune response to infectious agents, but it is obvious that many people are unable to produce effective antibodies quickly enough to meet life-threatening microbial challenges. Attempts to supplement the natural immune response led to the search for drugs that could mimic the effect of antibodies.

Salvarsan, an arsenical drug specifically aimed at the pathogen that causes syphilis, provided an effective demonstration of Paul Ehrlich's conviction that infectious diseases could be cured by synthetic drugs that killed microbial invaders without harming their human hosts. Like Pasteur, Ehrlich's theoretical interests were closely linked to practical problems; that is, he wanted to understand the body's natural immunological defenses and transform experimental pharmacology into the search for therapeutic agents. Modifications of drugs that could kill microbes in the test tube could lead to the synthesis of so-called magic bullets, that is, therapeutic agents that could help destroy infectious agents without damaging normal human cells. An effective chemotherapeutic agent would be a toxic substance that had a greater affinity for receptors in the pathogenic agent than for those in human cells. Beginning with dyes, and later expanding his studies to include arsenic compounds, Ehrlich modified the chemical structure of countless chemicals in an effort to produce effective drugs against disease-causing microorganisms. In 1908, Ehrlich was awarded the Nobel Prize in Physiology or Medicine for his contributions to immunology, toxicology, pharmacology, and therapeutics. Ehrlich's achievements include the development of salvarsan and other drugs, clarification of the distinction between active and passive immunity, recognition of the latent period in the development of active immunity, and an ingenious conceptual model for antibody production and antigen-antibody recognition.

Ehrlich's first targets were the trypanosomes, the causative agents of African sleeping sickness, Gambia fever, and nagana. Searching for chemicals that might be particularly toxic to these parasitic protozoans, Ehrlich began a series of experiments with an arsenical drug called *atoxyl*, which had been used for certain skin conditions. Atoxyl was quite effective against trypanosomes in the test tube but was not suitable for internal use because it caused nerve damage and blindness. After proving that it was possible to create many derivatives of atoxyl, Ehrlich and his colleagues systematically tested hundreds of modifications, hoping to find derivatives that would be safe and effective in experimental animals. Because spirochetes were thought to be similar to trypanosomes, Ehrlich's group also conducted tests on these corkscrew-shaped bacteria. Working in Ehrlich's laboratory, Sahachiro Hata tested arsenical compounds on the spirochetes that cause syphilis, chicken spirillosis, and relapsing fever. After hundreds of derivatives were tested, Hata identified one that cured chicken spirillosis in birds, relapsing fever in rats, and syphilis in rabbits. By 1910, Ehrlich had evidence that this compound, known as Preparation 606, was deadly to the spirochetes that cause syphilis but relatively safe for people. Preparation 606, an organic arsenic compound also known as arsphenamine, was later given the name "salvarsan." Patients with advanced neurosyphilis, characterized by progressive paralysis and dementia, previously an invariably fatal condition, showed significant improvement after salvarsan injections, but the drug was most effective when given early in the disease process. Evaluating remedies for syphilis was, however, difficult because patients often experienced periods of remission, followed by new symptoms and complications. Salvarsan was associated with adverse reactions in some patients, but it remained the standard remedy for syphilis until it was replaced by penicillin after World War II.

In the 1920s, textbooks of therapeutics and pharmacology were still recommending ancient preparations for the treatment of infected wounds, along with relatively new disinfectants such as carbolic acid, hydrogen peroxide, iodoform, and the hypochlorites. Disinfectants and antiseptics like carbolic acid could be used to treat external wounds, but generally, such chemicals were too dangerous for internal use. Many chemicals killed pathogens in the test tube, but magic bullets like salvarsan were very rare.

Attempts to find safe and effective antibacterial drugs were largely unsuccessful until the 1930s, when Gerhard Domagk found that a sulfur-containing red dye called *prontosil* protected mice from streptococcal and staphylococcal infections. Domagk was the director of research in experimental pathology and bacteriology at a German chemical firm. Like Ehrlich, Domagk turned to the study of dyes as a means of understanding pathogenic microorganisms and their interaction with various chemicals. Preliminary studies of bacterial staining led to a systematic survey of the aniline dyes in the hope of finding chemicals that would kill bacteria. In a typical experiment, Domagk determined the quantity of bacteria needed to kill inoculated mice—the lethal dose. Then he inoculated mice with ten times the lethal dose and gave half of the animals a test substance, such as prontosil, a dye that had been synthesized and patented in 1932. When it was clear that prontosil protected mice against lethal doses of staphylococci and streptococci, Domagk conducted secret tests in human beings with life-threatening staphylococcal and streptococcal infections. Domagk's report, "A Contribution to the Chemotherapy of Bacterial Infections," was published in 1935.

While conducting tests of the antibacterial properties of prontosil, researchers at the Pasteur Institute proved that the intact molecule was inactive until it was broken down in the animal's body and the sulfonamide portion was released. Sulfanilamide, the antibacterial portion of prontosil, had been synthesized in 1908 and did not enjoy patent protection. Scientists synthesized and tested thousands of derivatives of sulfanilamide, which became known as the sulfa drugs. Optimism about the potential discovery of hundreds of miracle drugs faded when it became clear that very few of the new sulfonamide derivatives were both safe and effective. Nevertheless, the sulfa drugs were widely used in the treatment of gonorrhea and infections of unknown origin. As Ehrlich had anticipated, the effectiveness of the drugs was soon limited by the appearance of drug-resistant strains of bacteria. By the end of World War II, the sulfa drugs were considered essentially obsolete. In assessing the disappointment generated by the failure of the so-called miracle drugs of the 1930s, Domagk warned that the same problem would occur with the next generation of antibacterial drugs, unless physicians and scientists learned to appreciate the factors that led to the development and spread of resistant strains.

PENICILLIN AND THE GOLDEN AGE OF ANTIBIOTICS

The discovery of salvarsan and sulfonamide suggested that chemists might continue to synthesize valuable antibacterial agents, but some scientists thought that useful drugs might be found within the microbial world itself. By the 1870s, several scientists had called attention to the implications of what was called "antibiosis" (the struggle for existence between different microorganisms). The transformation of this vague idea into a new source of powerful therapeutic agents was the result of Alexander Fleming's study of the antibacterial effects of the mold *Penicillium notatum*. Fleming became interested in antibacterial agents while serving as a military physician during the first world war, but his experience in treating infected wounds convinced him that chemical antiseptics were generally more harmful to human tissues than to bacteria. After the war, Fleming devoted himself to bacteriological research.

In 1928, while conducting a study of staphylococci, Fleming discovered the remarkable effect of the mold *Penicillium notatum* on these bacteria. The mold was apparently killing staphylococci on one of Fleming's discarded petri dishes. Mold contamination of bacteriological preparations is a common laboratory accident, generally considered a sign of poor technique. Acknowledging this correlation, Fleming often said that he would have made no discoveries if his laboratory bench had always been uncluttered and overly tidy. When he went on vacation, Fleming left behind stacks of dirty petri dishes from old experiments. On his return to the laboratory, Fleming noticed that staphylococci growing on one of these petri diseases had been destroyed in the vicinity of a certain mold colony, which was identified as *Penicillium notatum*. Fleming assumed that the fungal colony was the product of a spore that had contaminated the bacterial culture and that something produced by the growing fungus had inhibited or killed the bacteria. Scientists who have attempted to recreate Fleming's discovery of the antibacterial properties of penicillin have called it the luckiest, greatest, and most improbable accidental discovery in the history of science. Very few species of mold actually produce useful therapeutic agents, and *Penicillium notatum* is fairly uncommon. Because penicillin cannot dissolve fully grown colonies of staphylococci, the mold must have been growing and releasing penicillin into the medium before the bacteria began growing.

Intrigued by the antibacterial properties of the mold that had killed his staphylococci, Fleming began a series of experiments, including some attempts to identify the active agent. Although his attempts to purify penicillin were unsuccessful, even in crude, dilute preparations, penicillin inhibited the growth of many different bacteria. Although penicillin was powerful enough to kill bacteria, Fleming noted that it was harmless to white blood cells in the test tube and to experimental animals. However, Fleming did not carry out the crucial kinds of experiments that would have demonstrated penicillin's effectiveness in fighting bacteria in infected animals and human beings. Fleming published an account of his studies of the antibacterial properties of penicillin and continued to use it in his research, but he later complained that bacteriologists and physicians ignored his work until the successful use of sulfanilamide transformed attitudes toward the treatment of bacterial infections.

The story of Fleming's accidental discovery of penicillin in 1928 is well known, but the fact that penicillin's therapeutic potential was not realized until World War II is often forgotten. Both aspects of the penicillin story were recognized in 1945 when the Nobel Prize for Physiology or Medicine was awarded to Alexander Fleming, Howard Walter Florey, and Ernst Boris Chain for the discovery of penicillin and for demonstrating its effectiveness in the treatment of infectious diseases. In 1938, Florey and Chain began a systematic study of naturally occurring antibacterial agents. They tested substances produced by various microbes before deciding that penicillin was particularly interesting. Within two years, Florey and his colleagues had partially purified penicillin and tested it in mice infected with virulent streptococci, staphylococci, and several other pathogens. Preliminary tests conducted on patients with deadly, untreatable infections caused by staphylococci and streptococci indicated that penicillin was safe and effective in humans. An account of their first successful clinical trial was published in the British medical journal *The Lancet*, but further studies of penicillin were classified until the end of World War II. Shortly before the United States entered the war, Florey and Norman Heatley flew to the United States, where they worked with American scientists to improve the production of penicillin. The mass production of penicillin became a major priority during the war because of its obvious importance to the armed forces as well as civilian populations.

Penicillin was effective against a host of Gram-positive bacteria, including pneumococci, staphylococci, and streptococci. By 1950, penicillin was widely available for use in the treatment of syphilis, gonorrhea, pneumonia, diphtheria, meningitis, strep throat, tonsillitis, rheumatic fever, boils, and abscesses. Although it was not effective against all pathogens, penicillin was generally seen as a revolutionary new therapeutic agent. Moreover, the successful use of penicillin provided proof of the concept that the microbial world itself might be the source of many valuable compounds that were too complex for chemists to synthesize in the laboratory. The term *antibiotic* was adopted to refer to this category of drugs, that is, compounds produced by microorganisms that inhibit the growth of other microorganisms. Most antibiotics are the products of filamentous fungi, like penicillin from *Penicillium notatum*, but some soil bacteria of the actinomycete group also produce important antibiotics. Antibiotics kill or inhibit pathogens by inhibiting nucleic acid or protein synthesis, damaging the plasma membrane, preventing cell wall synthesis, or interfering with cell metabolism. Streptomycin, which is produced by *Streptomyces griseus*, was discovered by Selman A. Waksman and his colleagues Elizabeth Bugie and Albert Schatz in 1944. Because it was effective against tuberculosis, streptomycin was especially valuable but neomycin, chloramphenicol, aureomycin, erythromycin, and nystatin also expanded the range of pathogens that could be treated with antibiotics.

In his systematic studies of soil microbes, Waksman, a pioneer in soil microbiology, discovered more than twenty antibiotics, but most were too weak or too toxic for human use. Streptomycin was toxic to many species of bacteria, including *M. tuberculosis* and the bacteria that cause typhoid, tularemia, and plague. Evaluating remedies for tuberculosis was very difficult because the disease is unpredictable, develops slowly, and is affected by nonspecific factors such as diet and rest. The failure of Koch's tuberculin led to considerable skepticism about other alleged miracle cures. William H. Feldman and Horton Corwin Hinshaw were conducting tests of various possible therapeutic agents, using guinea pigs as an experimental model for tuberculosis, when they learned about streptomycin's effect on *Mycobacterium tuberculosis*. After experiments with guinea pigs demonstrated that streptomycin was effective against tuberculous infections, tests were conducted on patients with pulmonary tuberculosis as well as deadly meningeal and miliary tuberculosis. Despite popular references to streptomycin as a miracle drug, early, impure preparations raised doubts about its safety and efficacy. Some patients suffered adverse effects, including nerve damage and deafness, but pharmaceutical companies were able to produce and market improved preparations of the drug by 1948. Waksman was awarded the Nobel Prize for the discovery of streptomycin in 1952, two years after the legal settlement of a complex royalty dispute initiated by his former associate, Albert Schatz. In 1994, Schatz, who insisted that he had not received sufficient credit for the discovery of streptomycin, received the Rutgers University Medal.

The success of penicillin and streptomycin stimulated the growth of the pharmaceutical industry and encouraged unprecedented support for biomedical research. Reflecting the optimism of the 1940s and 1950s, a period that has been called the golden age of antibiotics, Waksman predicted that future research would lead to the discovery of more powerful and less toxic antibacterial agents. By the 1960s, however, hopes that an ever-accelerating pace of discovery would continue seemed overly optimistic. Moreover, the overuse and misuse of antibiotics resulted in unanticipated adverse side effects and promoted the development of drug-resistant strains of bacteria. The prolonged course of treatment required to cure tuberculosis creates ideal conditions for the evolution of drug-resistant bacteria. Combination therapy using streptomycin, para-aminosalicylic acid, isoniazid, and rifampin transformed the management and treatment of tuberculosis. Clinical trials proved that combination therapies were more effective in the treatment of tuberculosis than individual drugs. Multidrug therapy helped avoid the proliferation and survival of drug-resistant bacteria. Although even with a combination of antibiotics, a complete cure took many months, a partial course of treatment generally arrested active tuberculosis infections, thus preventing the transmission of the disease.

Streptomycin and other antibiotics so revolutionized the treatment of tuberculosis that by the 1960s, infectious disease experts were optimistic about the prospects for controlling, or even eradicating, the disease. The major obstacles, as observed by nineteenth-century reformers, were associated with poverty and the consequent lack of medical and public health resources in areas where the burden of disease was greatest. As with any infectious disease, the persistence of the pathogen, even in isolated, impoverished populations, meant that the disease could still be a threat to wealthy countries where the incidence of tuberculosis had been drastically reduced. During the 1980s, public health authorities detected increases in the incidence of tuberculosis, especially in areas where poverty and the spread of HIV/AIDS facilitated the transmission of opportunistic infections. Despite improvements in the control of tuberculosis in some regions, significant increases in the incidence of the disease occurred in Africa and especially Eastern Europe during the 1990s, when WHO declared tuberculosis a global health emergency. Tuberculosis remains a serious problem in India, China, Indonesia, and Africa, especially South Africa and Nigeria. The emergence of drug-resistant bacteria is particularly likely to occur where treatment is inadequate, public health programs have been neglected, and antibiotics are widely available without prescriptions or medical supervision. Antibiotics generally affect a limited spectrum of bacteria, and they are all ineffective against viruses. Some antibiotics are quite toxic and are only prescribed when no other alternatives are available.

At the 2002 World Congress on Tuberculosis, experts estimated that about two billion people—about one-third of the global population—were infected with tuberculosis. Most tuberculosis infections are asymptomatic or latent, but about ten million people become clinically ill each year, and about two million people die of the disease. Globally, in 2006, about seven hundred thousand tuberculosis cases and two hundred thousand deaths caused by tuberculosis occurred among people with HIV/AIDS. Tuberculosis experts predict that unless all parts of the world cooperate in a coordinated global control plan, or establish a safe and effective vaccine, tuberculosis will infect an additional one billion people by 2020, raising the death toll to seventy million per year.

Drug-resistant strains of *Mycobacterium tuberculosis*—multidrug-resistant tuberculosis (MDR-TB) strains and extremely drug-resistant strains (XDR-TB)—are considered a growing threat to tuberculosis control programs throughout the world. Many of the drug-resistant microbes are resistant to at least three of the four first-line drugs recommended by WHO: streptomycin, isoniazid, rifampicin, and ethambutol. XDR-TB cases were most commonly found in Russia, India, Asia, and Africa. In 2008, when WHO released its fourth global report on tuberculosis and drug resistance, XDR-TB had been reported in forty-five countries.

Ordinary tuberculosis can be cured in about 95 percent of patients, but the cure rate is less than 70 percent for MDR-TB and falls below 30 percent for XDR-TB. Treating patients who are coinfected with tuberculosis and HIV/AIDS is particularly difficult. In an outbreak of XDR-TB in South Africa in 2005, fifty-two out of fifty-three HIV/AIDS patients with XDR-TB died. Like medieval lepers, patients with XDR-TB are often confined to institutions that are more like prisons than hospitals in an attempt to prevent the spread of XDR-TB. Protecting the public and respecting the rights of those already infected is a difficult balancing act for public health officials. Most countries rely on voluntary cooperation and outpatient treatment, but many health officials argue that it is sometimes necessary to isolate the sick to protect society. Because detecting drug resistance can take many months, patients may be taking useless drugs and infecting others before the extent of drug resistance is finally identified. If antibiotics fail because of drug resistance, traditional public health measures might provide the only useful approach to controlling the disease. International travel makes drug resistance a global threat. Guidelines issued in 2006 by WHO say that patients with MDR-TB should not travel by public air transportation until they have proved that they are noninfectious, but compliance and enforcement options are negligible. Tuberculosis is not considered highly contagious, but the lack of a serious, global response to XDR-TB suggests that international boundaries would not stop a highly contagious disease like influenza or SARS.

MODERN MEDICINE AND NOSOCOMIAL INFECTIONS

Modern hospitals are no longer associated with the so-called hospital fevers that Joseph Lister and his disciples wrestled with, but *nosocomial infections*—hospital-acquired infections—are now considered a very significant and increasing threat. Although it is difficult to quantify the morbidity and mortality caused by nosocomial infections, according to the National Nosocomial Infections Surveillance System, the overall infection rate is highest in large teaching hospitals and lowest in nonteaching hospitals. In all hospitals, the incidence of hospital-acquired infections is highest in surgical departments. Researchers consistently report that the most common and most preventable cause of nosocomial infections is a general neglect of hand washing by hospital doctors and staff members. Studies of hand-washing rates in various hospitals, including intensive care units, found that only 10 to 50 percent of doctors washed their hands before and after contact with patients. Efforts to raise awareness through education, monitoring, and feedback had little effect on hand-washing levels. Many health care practitioners think that hand washing is a nineteenth-century technique that has been superseded by modern advances such as the use of disposable gloves. But bacteria can contaminate the outside of gloves, which medical practitioners fail to change as often as needed.

The Centers for Disease Control and Prevention (CDC) estimates that about two million patients contract hospital-transmitted infections every year. Studies of nosocomial infection control in American hospitals indicate that about 6 percent of hospitalized patients developed a nosocomial infection. Investigators suggested that the true incidence of nosocomial infections was actually much higher because many were not properly reported. Tens of thousands of patients die directly from such infections, and in many more cases, nosocomial infections are a contributing cause of death. Overall, nosocomial infections may be causing more deaths per year in the United States than AIDS or breast cancer. Nosocomial infections add billions of dollars to annual health care costs in the United States, but when hospitals attempt to reduce costs, infection-control departments are common targets because they do not generate revenue. Although there is no doubt that nosocomial infections significantly add to morbidity and mortality rates and increase the costs of hospital care, it is difficult to determine the actual risk assumed when a patient enters a hospital. The proportion of extremely sick and vulnerable patients found in today's hospitals—transplant patients, premature infants, elderly patients with multiple disorders, cancer patients, burn victims, AIDS patients—has dramatically increased. Such patients would not have lived long enough to contract hospital infections in the not so distant past.

The life-threatening infections that Ignaz Semmelweis and Joseph Lister confronted in nineteenth-century hospitals were brought under control with relatively simple methods of disinfection and antibiotics. Despite the advances in hospital care and the introduction of a wide variety of antimicrobial agents, by the end of the twentieth century, hospital-acquired infections were once again considered a major problem. In the United States, nosocomial infections account for an estimated one hundred thousand deaths every year. The problem has been compounded by the emergence of drug-resistant bacteria, but other important factors are actually associated with some of the most successful advances in modern medicine. These include the ever-increasing range of difficult operations performed in hospitals and the growing population of immune-compromised patients. Organ transplantation has become remarkably successful since the introduction of effective antirejection drugs and improved surgical techniques. However, in the absence of effective screening procedures, blood transfusions and organ transplants provide unprecedented opportunities for the transmission of persistent infectious diseases such as HIV/AIDS, hepatitis, syphilis, babesiosis, and Chagas' disease. Acute but undiagnosed infectious diseases—such as rabies and West Nile fever—have also been transmitted by donated organs. Even soft-tissue implants, such as tendons, ligaments, cartilage, and heart valves, have transmitted life-threatening infections.

Experts call rabies a "sentinel disease" that reveals weak links in the system but argue that it is impossible to test every donor for rabies and other rare diseases. Unless a cluster of cases is detected, the true cause of death after organ transplantation may go undetected. In 1990, about twenty thousand people in the United States were on waiting lists for organs. Fifteen years later, that number was about eighty-eight thousand. Because of the shortage of donated organs, transplant specialists have relaxed the standards originally used to screen potential organ donors. As a result, the transplanting of so-called marginal organs—organs that once would have been considered unusable—has increased. Age, drug abuse, and even infectious diseases are no longer automatic disqualifiers. Hepatitis, for example, is so common in urban areas that few transplant surgeons will immediately turn down an organ from a donor with the virus.

The Sentry Antimicrobial Surveillance Program, established in 1997, rated the drug-resistance control record of the United States as among the worst among the industrialized nations participating in its surveys. The Sentry Program monitors the array of drug-resistant germs in hospitals and community settings. In general, staphylococcus bacteria are the most common cause of infections acquired in hospitals. About 2 percent of staph infections were drug-resistant in the 1970s, but by 2006, about 60 percent were caused by drug-resistant strains. One of the most dangerous, methicillin-resistant *Staphylococcus aureus* (MRSA), was cited as the cause of 22 percent of nosocomial staphylococcus infections in 1995. Within ten years, MRSA was responsible for at least 60 percent of hospital-associated staphylococcus infections. Although the vast majority of MRSA cases were originally acquired in hospitals, nursing homes, and other health care facilities, since 2000, significant numbers of MRSA infections have been traced to community settings, including prisons, athletic facilities, schools, and day care centers.

Staphylococcus aureus is widely distributed and generally harmless, but it can cause serious abscesses, joint infections, pneumonia, meningitis, septicemia, and death. In hospitals, the germ can enter the body via a catheter, a ventilator, an incision, or an open wound. Many people carry staphylococcus bacteria in their nose and on their skin without developing infections, but they can transmit the germ to vulnerable people with weak immune systems. Hospital patients who carry MRSA shed the germs on bedrails, wheelchairs, stethoscopes, blood pressure cuffs, and other surfaces, where MRSA can live for many hours. Doctors and other caregivers can pick up the germs on their hands, gloves, or clothing and carry them to another patient. There have been calls for MRSA screening of hospital patients and staff, but the 2006 CDC guidelines for nosocomial infection control did not include universal testing of patients for MRSA. In the 1980s, Denmark, Finland, and the Netherlands were confronted by very high rates of MRSA, but the problem was brought under control by screening patients and instituting strict infection control programs for all health care workers.

Attempts to improve the treatment of patients with uncertain diagnoses, such as pneumonia, through routine, rapid antimicrobial therapy results in millions of patients with nonbacterial diseases being unnecessarily treated with antibiotics. Infectious disease experts are attempting to minimize unnecessary antimicrobial treatment, while providing the best treatment for patients with uncertain diagnoses. The failure of antibiotics to cure an infection does not always mean the pathogen was antibiotic-resistant. Failure to determine the cause of disease or infection could mean that the infection was caused by a fungus or virus or a species of bacteria that was totally and predictably unaffected by the antibiotic.

The use of very large quantities of antibiotics for agricultural purposes is considered a significant source of antibiotic-resistant microbes. The Union of Concerned Scientists estimates that at least 70 percent of the antibiotics used in America are fed to animals living on factory farms. Without antibiotics, the spread of infectious diseases would make it virtually impossible to raise huge numbers of chickens, pigs, and cattle in close confinement. Moreover, the use of antibiotics increases the growth rate of animals, improving the production of meat and eggs. Many years ago, scientists predicted that the misuse of antibiotics for agricultural production would lead to the evolution of drug-resistant bacteria. Recent studies have found MRSA in the majority of large pig farms in Europe and North America. The strains of MRSA bacteria found in Ontario pigs and pig farmers included a strain common to human MRSA infections in Canada. Infected farmers have transmitted the bacteria to family members, veterinarians, and hospital staff. Based on evidence that the heavy use of antibiotics in industrialized livestock operations can select for resistant bacteria, scientists are calling for studies of the possible relationship between the use of antibiotics in agriculture and the surge in MRSA infections and deaths in the United States.

Although the antibiotics synthesized by microbes are clearly very useful to humans in the battle against infectious disease, the role of these chemicals in the microbial world itself is not so obvious. In terms of microbial ecology, these substances might be used to kill or inhibit the growth of the competing microbes, for communication and housekeeping functions, or to establish a balance between microbes and resources. Similarly, although the human use and abuse of antibiotics promotes the survival and selection of microbes with resistance genes, the evolution and exchange of such genes presumably played a role in the microbial world prior to and independent of the intervention of human beings. Thus, the appearance of significant levels of antibiotics and other drugs in soil and water supplies as an accidental by-product of medical and agricultural usage could be creating a dangerous environmental experiment. An increasing level of resistance to antimicrobial drugs throughout the microbial world could become the most pernicious infectious disease problem facing rich and poor countries in the future. Diseases that were considered easily curable would become as intractable and potentially lethal as they were before the introduction of penicillin. Nevertheless, a return to the era of rampant hospitalism of the nineteenth century is not inevitable because health care workers would presumably institute rigorous infection control techniques. People in wealthy countries—except for the immune-compromised—are likely to be better nourished, better educated, and healthier than their nineteenth-century counterparts. However, the situation would be very different in impoverished areas, where hospitals and clinics lack the resources needed to ensure good infection control procedures.

Microorganisms are continuously producing, exchanging, and collecting genes for virulence, toxins, and resistance to antibiotics. New antimicrobial agents may eventually be discovered as a result of genomic studies that reveal specific targets for new magic bullets that can attack microbes without damaging human beings. Scientists are also investigating interesting microbial agents that act as predators or parasites of other microbes in the hope of using them against disease-causing agents. Bacteriophages, the viruses that attack bacteria, have been of interest since they were discovered in the early twentieth century as possible therapeutic agents. Although this approach was overshadowed by the discovery of sulfonilamide, penicillin, and other antibiotics, phage therapy is still in use in some parts of the world. Since the discovery of *Bdellovibrio* in the 1960s, researchers have speculated about the possibility that this bacterial predator might eventually serve as a living antibiotic. *Bdellovibrio* attacks, kills, and digests other bacterial cells, including *Pseudomonas, Salmonella, Legionella,* and *Coliform* bacteria, but it does not seem to cause disease in humans and other animals. Nevertheless, the goal of turning living agents, such as bacteriophage and *Bdellovibrio,* into germ fighters remains elusive, and critics warn of the possibility of unforeseen adverse consequences.

PROBIOTICS: GOOD BACTERIA AND GOOD HEALTH

Popularized accounts of the germ theory of disease generally portray the relationship between microbes and human beings as a form of ceaseless warfare. But as scientists learn more about the natural history of microbial life and the relationship between humans and microbes, a more balanced picture is emerging. The concept of "good bacteria" is increasingly supported by studies of the microorganisms that inhabit the intestinal tract. Many of the microbes that normally reside within the human body are harmless, or even beneficial. Among the three hundred or so species of bacteria in the human gastrointestinal tract are species that help synthesize certain vitamins and amino acids, and others that are needed to digest some foods. Harmless bacteria also play a role in crowding out more dangerous germs such as salmonella.

Fear of bacteria has been tempered by interest in probiotic therapy, the idea that certain bacteria are beneficial to human health. Probiotics include bacteria that are used to ferment food such as yogurt and cheese. Supporters of probiotics claim that beneficial bacteria aid digestion, ameliorate inflammatory bowel diseases, boost the body's natural defenses, help control harmful bacteria, alleviate yeast infections, and moderate the adverse effects of antibiotics. Probiotic foods have been popular in Europe and Asia for many decades, but pills, capsules, and various forms of nutritional supplements claim to contain beneficial bacteria that can improve health and reduce gastrointestinal problems. These attempts to understand the relationship between the microbial world and the workings of the gastrointestinal tract are quite different from ancient doctrines about the need to completely evacuate or eliminate intestinal microbes. Nobel laureate Elie Metchnikoff, who is best known for discovering phagocytes, the white blood cells that attack and devour bacteria and other foreign bodies, thought of intestinal microbes as the worst sort of parasites. Metchnikoff blamed the putrefaction caused by bacteria inside the gastrointestinal tract for atherosclerosis, gray hair, senility, and death. In the future, Metchnikoff predicted, surgeons would routinely improve health and extend the human life span by removing the whole of the large intestine to eliminate the chronic poisoning caused by our intestinal flora.

Four

✥

VIRUSES AND VIRAL DISEASES

INVISIBLE MICROBES

By the end of the nineteenth century, microbiologists had determined the specific causative agents of many infectious diseases, but the pathogens that caused other diseases could not be identified, isolated, or cultured by conventional laboratory techniques. Some microbes that could be seen with the light microscope, but could not be grown in cell-free laboratory cultures, were eventually identified as bacteria and protozoans with unusual growth requirements or complicated life cycles. For example, the pathogens that cause typhus fever and Rocky Mountain spotted fever were identified as members of the unusual group of bacteria known as the rickettsia, in honor of the American pathologist Howard Taylor Ricketts. These bacteria act as intracellular parasites; that is, they multiply inside living cells and depend on arthropods, such as lice, ticks, mites, and fleas, to carry them to new victims.

Nineteenth-century scientists usually referred to pathogens that could not be identified as viruses, much as Fracastoro had used the term *contagion*. The ancient Latin word *virus* has undergone many changes in meaning over time. Originally, the word *virus* referred to slime: something that was unpleasant but not necessarily dangerous. In medical texts, the term was applied to substances that were hazardous to human health such as toxins, poisons, or unknown agents of disease. Medieval scholars generally used *virus* as a synonym for *poison*, whereas seventeenth-century physicians referred to a *virus pestiferum* or *virus pestilens* in discussing infectious diseases. Eighteenth-century medical writers applied the term *virus* to the contagion that transmitted an infectious disease, and nineteenth-century scientists often used the term for any and all microorganisms. Considerable confusion, therefore, arises when modern readers see the term *virus* in medical texts composed between the first century and the early decades of the twentieth century.

After the establishment of germ theory in the late nineteenth century, the term *virus* was used in discussions of unidentifiable entities with infectious properties. As with the term *contagion*, the lack of specificity made the term very useful. Louis Pasteur insisted that when searching for the causative agents of infectious diseases, it was clear that every virus—unknown infectious agent—was a microbe. Speculating about unidentified infectious agents, Robert Koch suggested that scientists might discover pathogens that were quite different from ordinary bacteria. In theory, these yet undiscovered pathogens might include entities smaller and simpler than bacteria or more complex organisms that were difficult to grow in laboratory cultures; that is, there might be some pathogens that could not be isolated, visualized, and cultured by existing laboratory methods. Therefore, it would be impossible to carry out the proofs known as Koch's postulates when working with unusual pathogens. Even Koch acknowledged that in some cases, it was appropriate to infer the causative relationship between specific microbes and specific diseases even if the microbe could not be cultured in the laboratory. Microbes that failed to grow in laboratory cultures might require very special media, unusual supplements, or peculiar growth conditions.

By the early twentieth century, the term *virus* was generally restricted to the class of filterable-invisible microbes—infectious agents that could not be seen under the microscope, or trapped by filters, or grown in laboratory cultures; that is, viruses were defined operationally in terms of their ability to pass through filters that trapped ordinary bacteria and their ability to remain invisible under the light microscope. The criterion of filterability was the outcome of work conducted by Pasteur's associate Charles Chamberland, who discovered that a porous porcelain column could be used to separate visible microorganisms from their culture medium. This technique could be used in the laboratory to prepare bacteria-free liquids and in the home to prepare pure drinking water. Defining classes of microorganisms in terms of laboratory techniques did not provide useful insights into the fundamental differences between viruses and other microbes. Furthermore, as scientists adopted new techniques, they sometimes found that operational criteria, such as invisibility, filterability, and the ability to grow under typical laboratory conditions, were not necessarily linked. Despite these uncertainties, invisible-filterable viruses were associated with many important diseases in humans and animals, including rabies, smallpox, and foot-and-mouth disease (FMD). However, it was primarily the study of a disease of plants known as tobacco mosaic disease that established the foundations of modern virology and led to an understanding of the fundamental characteristics of the invisible-filterable viruses. Adolf Eduard Mayer, Martinus Willem Beijerinck, and Dimitri Ivanovski are generally honored as the founders of virology because of their work with tobacco mosaic disease.

In 1886, Adolf Eduard Mayer discovered that he could transmit tobacco mosaic disease to healthy plants by inoculating them with extracts of sap from the leaves of diseased plants. Although the disease seemed to be caused by an infectious agent, Mayer could not identify or culture it in laboratory media. Preparations that were put through a filter were still infectious, but the invisible agent was inactivated when Mayer heated infectious sap. Mayer concluded that the infectious agent—the invisible-filterable virus of tobacco mosaic disease—must be a very unusual bacterium. In 1892, Dimitri Ivanovski described similar studies of tobacco mosaic disease. Like Mayer, Ivanovski demonstrated that the infectious agent for tobacco mosaic disease could pass through Chamberland filters that trapped bacteria. Filtered extracts of infectious tobacco leaves produced the same disease in healthy plants as an unfiltered extract. Ivanovski thought that a toxin or a very usual microbial agent in the filtered sap might explain these observations, but he was unable to isolate or culture the invisible microbe. Martinus Beijerinck, who began his study of tobacco mosaic disease as an associate of Adolf Mayer, was convinced that tobacco mosaic disease was caused by a living infectious agent because a very small quantity of filtered sap from an infected plant could transmit the disease to a very large number of plants. Unable to identify the infectious agent, he turned to other projects. When he resumed his studies of tobacco mosaic disease, Beijerinck discovered that the unknown infectious agent could only reproduce in the actively growing buds and shoots of living plants. Therefore, he concluded that the invisible-filterable agent, which he described as a *contagium vivum fluidum* (contagious living fluid), must be fundamentally different from bacteria; that is, the difference between bacteria and invisible-filterable viruses, or soluble germs, was not simply a matter of size or filterability. Viruses seemed to be infectious agents that could only reproduce within living cells; that is, they were obligate intracellular parasites of living organisms that could not grow in a cell-free medium. Based on reports in the botanical literature, Beijerinck thought soluble germs could cause many other plant diseases.

Tobacco mosaic virus (TMV) was the first virus to be purified and crystallized, a landmark achievement for which Wendell Meredith Stanley won the 1946 Nobel Prize in Chemistry. As a departure from the usual realm of microbiology, Stanley's achievement demonstrated that insights into the nature of viruses could be found by utilizing the methods of chemists and physicists. In the 1930s, Stanley laboriously purified crystalline material from a ton of infected tobacco plants. His purified crystals retained the infectious properties of the sap from infected plants. Initially, Stanley thought that TMV might be an unusual protein that could multiply in the presence of living cells, but the major implication of his work was that viruses could be thought of as living molecules, rather than conventional microorganisms. In 1939, the electron microscope provided the first portrait of TMV. Further work showed that TMV was actually a combination of protein and nucleic acid. Using the techniques that became available in the 1940s, including the ultracentrifuge and the electron microscope, scientists found that TMV consisted of a central core of RNA surrounded by a protein coat. High-speed centrifuges made it possible to concentrate and purify viruses. The electron microscope made it possible to see and characterize viruses in terms of their sizes and shapes.

By the end of the nineteenth century, microbiologists had identified diseases of animals that, like tobacco mosaic disease, were apparently caused by invisible-filterable viruses. Studies of FMD conducted by Friedrich Loeffler and Paul Frosch, disciples of Robert Koch, indicated that the causative agent could pass through a filter and could not be grown in laboratory cultures. Animals suffering from FMD develop characteristic blisters in their mouths and on their hooves. Although the disease seemed to be contagious, all attempts to isolate and culture the causative agent from the lesions of sick cattle were unsuccessful. In 1897, Loeffler and Frosch reported that they could transmit FMD to healthy cattle and pigs with bacteria-free filtrates of fluid taken from the blisters of infected animals. As a test of the effectiveness of their filtration system, Loeffler and Frosch added *Bacillus flourescens* to their preparations and demonstrated that filtration removed the added bacteria. Nevertheless, the agent that caused FMD passed through the filter. To prove that the causative agent was not a toxin, but a living agent that multiplied in sick animals, Loeffler and Frosch transmitted the disease through a series of six animals; that is, each healthy animal was injected with filtered material from the lesions of the previously infected animal. After proving that cattle could be immunized against FMD with mixtures of blood and lymph from the vesicles of sick animals, Loeffler and Frosch concluded that the disease might be caused by a very small and unusual microbe, and they suggested that other infectious diseases might be caused by similar filterable microbes.

Further studies of FMD proved that it is a highly infectious, airborne viral disease that attacks cloven-hoofed animals such as cattle, sheep, goats, and pigs. The FMD virus is a member of the picornavirus family, which includes many important human pathogens such as the poliovirus and the hepatitis A virus. The disease is generally not regarded as a threat to humans who consume meat or pasteurized milk from affected animals, but in rare instances, people in close contact with infected animals have contracted the disease. In the 1830s, scientists apparently infected themselves with FMD by inoculation and by drinking milk from infected cows. Proven cases of FMD in humans have occurred in Europe, Africa, and South America. Therefore, FMD is now defined as a *zoonosis*—a disease shared by humans and other animals.

After FMD was introduced into the Americas in the 1870s, outbreaks occurred in both North and South America. The Pan-American Foot-and-Mouth Disease Center, established in 1951, coordinated programs that led to the control and eradication of FMD in many participating countries. In countries where FMD is still endemic, vaccination is used as a control measure. Despite the availability of effective vaccines, FMD remains a threat to domesticated animals in many parts of the world. Vaccinated animals test positive for FMD antibodies and cannot be exported to countries that only accept animals certified as "disease-free."

Although many experts in animal diseases assumed that FMD had been essentially eliminated by the end of the twentieth century, in 2001, major outbreaks of the disease occurred throughout Europe. In Great Britain, where the disease was most prevalent, attempts to control the epidemic included the mandatory destruction of all sheep, pigs, and cows on infected farms. Ultimately, millions of animals were destroyed. Other European Union countries banned the importation of meats, milk, and livestock products from England, but outbreaks occurred in Ireland, France, and the Netherlands. When another outbreak was detected in 2007, British authorities acted quickly to destroy infected animals, quarantine farms, and ban the movement of cattle, pigs, and sheep. Ironically, the strain of virus that caused the outbreak seemed to be identical to virus used in the production of vaccine in veterinary laboratories near the affected farms. An investigation of the suspect facilities found deficiencies in the safety and containment procedures. FMD is only one of many viral diseases of domesticated animals that threaten international markets. Disease outbreaks among domesticated animals provide a clear warning about the way in which infectious diseases can spread. Tracing the movement of these diseases reveals many aspects of international cooperation, or the lack thereof, in tracking, reporting, and controlling infectious diseases.

BACTERIAL VIRUSES

Studies of disease-causing bacteria led to the remarkable discovery that even microorganisms could be attacked by invisible-filterable viruses. British bacteriologist Frederick Twort discovered this phenomenon in 1915, when he noticed that colonies of bacteria growing on agar in his petri dishes sometimes became glassy and transparent. When he deposited a tiny drop of material from the glassy colonies on normal bacterial colonies, they, too, became transparent. Twort speculated that he might be observing an ultramicroscopic virus that destroyed bacteria, but he could not rule out the possibility that his filterable bacteriolytic agent might be an enzyme produced by bacteria or a very unusual bacterial species. Two years later, Felix d'Hérelle independently discovered the same phenomenon while conducting research on dysentery. Both the dysentery bacillus and the invisible-filterable agent that attacked it were found in stool samples from patients recovering from bacillary dysentery. By taking a tiny sample of material from the clear spots, he could transmit the invisible agent to a series of petri dishes containing healthy bacteria, with the same results following each transfer. When bacteria-free filtrates were added to actively growing cultures of bacteria, growth stopped and the bacteria seemed to disappear. A trace of bacteria-free medium from this culture produced the same effect on fresh bacterial cultures. More than fifty such transfers gave the same results, indicating that a living agent—an antidysentery microbe—was responsible for bacterial death and dissolution (*lysis*). Because the invisible microbe could not grow on laboratory media or on heat-killed bacilli, but grew well in a suspension of washed bacteria in a simple salt solution, d'Hérelle concluded that the antidysentery microbe was an *obligate bacteriophage*, that is, an invisible microbe that could only grow and multiply by eating living bacteria. The term *bacteriophage*, or *phage*, was eventually universally adopted, but at first, some microbiologists preferred the term *Twort-d'Hérelle particles*.

Critics argued that d'Hérelle's bacteriophages were actually enzymes released by bacteria to kill other bacteria, rather than true microbial entities. The nature of phages and the question of whether there were separate and distinct species of phages remained controversial for many years. The lack of clear standards and definitions of phage types created considerable confusion when different scientists tried to compare their experimental results. Although d'Hérelle was fascinated by the possibility that phages might play a vital role in the natural control of bacterial infections, he had to address many basic questions about bacteriophages and their relationship to bacteria. Unlike chemical antiseptics and disinfectants, bacteriophages were remarkably specific in their attacks on bacteria. Indeed, phages have such strong specificity for their target bacteria that one of the early practical uses of phages was for identifying bacterial strains and species. Answering his critics took up much of his time and energy, but d'Hérelle's most cherished goal was the development of phage preparations that could be used as therapeutic agents for infectious diseases.

In 1921, d'Hérelle summarized the early work on phages in *The Bacteriophage: Its Role in Immunity*, which stimulated interest in phage therapy among European doctors and scientists. A series of lectures he delivered while visiting Stanford and other American universities was published in 1930 as *The Bacteriophage and Its Clinical Applications*. Speculating on the general implications of the phenomenon he had discovered, d'Hérelle predicted that bacteriophages would be found for many, if not all, pathogenic bacteria. Although bacteriophages collected from different sources seemed to attack only specific species of bacteria, d'Hérelle suggested that scientists would eventually learn how to transform naturally occurring phages into specially modified therapeutic agents that would destroy disease-causing bacteria.

Some proponents of phage therapy claimed that bacteriophage activity could explain some traditional Indian therapies and religious rituals. Europeans considered the widespread belief in the healing properties of the Ganges and Junna rivers super-stitious and illogical, given their obvious pollution and the large numbers of pilgrims who bathed and performed rituals in them. However, some scientists had already attempted to investigate the alleged healing powers of these much-revered rivers. In 1896, British bacteriologist Ernest Hanbury Hankin published an account of his experiments on the antibacterial action of water taken from the Ganges River. Ac-cording to Hankin, this antibacterial action was retained when river water was passed through a fine porcelain filter, but it was destroyed when the water was boiled. In particular, Hankin thought that this filterable antibacterial agent might have some influence on the severity of the cholera epidemics that were so prevalent in India. Similar observations were made in the 1910s by George Eliava, who was investigating the anticholera properties of water from the Mtkvari River, which flows through Tbilisi in the Georgian Republic. The implications of these observations were not appreciated until Frederick Twort and Felix d'Hérelle demonstrated the existence of bacterial viruses.

Like Hankin, Eliava could not explain the antibacterial properties found in river water, but after learning about the properties of bacteriophages, Eliava went to the Pasteur Institute to work with d'Hérelle. Their collaboration led to the establishment of the Tbilisi Institute of Bacteriophage Research in 1923. Joseph Stalin, leader of the Union of Soviet Socialist Republics (USSR) from 1922 to 1953, who was born in Georgia, was very interested in the work of the institute. *Bacteriophage and the Phenomenon of Recovery* (1935), which d'Hérelle wrote while working in Tbilisi, was dedicated to Stalin. D'Hérelle's plans for a permanent move to Georgia ended in 1937 when Eliava was arrested by the Soviet Union's secret police as an "enemy of the people" and executed. By the time d'Hérelle died in Paris in 1949, phage therapy was essentially forgotten in the West. The Tbilisi Institute, however, continued to provide bacteriophages for therapy and bacterial typing. Several other centers for phage studies were established in other parts of the USSR. Soviet scientists collected bacteria and phages, often from sewage, analyzed the phage sensitivity of different strains of pathogenic bacteria, and established collections of phages that could be used to identify bacteria.

When antibiotics became widely available, phage researchers reported that in some cases, a combination of phage therapy and antibiotics was more effective than either alone. Phage treatment was considered the answer to the problem of antibiotic-resistant bacteria. Researchers tested hundreds of different phages against infections caused by *Staphylococcus, Klebsiella, Proteus, Escherichia, Shigella, Pseudomonas*, and *Salmonella*. Therapeutic phages were used to treat dysentery, typhoid fever, parathy-roid fever, and cholera as well as wound infections and diseases of the urinary tract. Soviet researchers claimed that patients were successfully treated with phage prepara-tions after antibiotics failed to cure abscesses, furunculosis, septicemia, lung infections, bronchopneumonia, peritonitis, and surgical wound infections. Phages were administered in tablets, liquids, sprays, enemas, and injections and were also applied directly to wounds. Phage preparation was carried out on an industrial scale, and before the breakup of the USSR, large quantities of liquid and solidified phage preparations were shipped to hospitals and pharmacies throughout the former Soviet Union. Military doctors were especially interested in phage therapy for infections associated with wounds and burns and as a means of preventing outbreaks of gastrointestinal diseases in military camps.

American novelist Sinclair Lewis, in collaboration with science writer Paul de Kruif, introduced the American public to the concept of phage therapy in *Arrowsmith* (1925), a popular and successful novel about Dr. Martin Arrowsmith, an idealistic young physician conducting biomedical research. In this Pulitzer Prize–winning novel, Arrowsmith attempted to end an outbreak of bubonic plague on a Caribbean island with a phage he had discovered. In 1931, the novel was made into a film that was nominated for the Academy Award for Best Picture. The novel and the film played a significant role in raising popular interest in phage therapy and biomedical research. During the 1930s, Eli Lilly and other American pharmaceutical companies conducted phage research and considered marketing therapeutic phage products. Enthusiasm for phage therapy was high before the discovery of penicillin, but despite the publication before the 1960s of some eight hundred papers on phage therapy, overall results were inconsistent. Although many claims had been made for phage therapy, consistent success seemed to be limited to the treatment of staphylococci infections of the skin. Many success stories were anecdotal accounts published by entrepreneurs trying to market phage products or by doctors with little or no research experience. Most of the publications concerning phage therapy were from the USSR. Many of these reports claimed high rates of success in the treatment of infected wounds and infectious diseases, but this work was generally ignored outside the Soviet Union. During the Cold War, Russian publications were rarely accessible to Western scientists and physicians, who tended to distrust Russian biology and clinical medicine. Skeptics argued that because phage therapy had not been submitted to rigorous clinical trials, its safety and efficacy remained uncertain.

In 1931, the American Medical Association commissioned a review of bacteriophage therapy to be carried out by its Council on Pharmacy and Chemistry. For the most part, the report by the council indicates that very little was known about viruses at the time, and doubts remained concerning d'Hérelle's theory that phages were parasitic entities that reproduced within living bacteria. Indeed, critics of d'Hérelle favored the hypothesis that phages were probably enzymes, rather than a new kind of microbe. Therefore, any beneficial activities associated with d'Hérelle's bacteria-free filtrates might be caused by enzymes or factors that stimulated the immune system, rather than his so-called bacteriophages. Skepticism about phage therapy was often based on the belief that researchers at the Eliava Institute and other Soviet centers did not conduct controlled clinical trials.

With the successful introduction of penicillin and other antibiotics in the 1940s, studies of phage therapy were essentially abandoned in Europe and the United States. Many biomedical scientists later incorrectly assumed that phage therapy had been thoroughly tested and found ineffective before World War II. For most scientists, bacterial viruses were little more than laboratory curiosities until they became the favorite experimental animal of molecular biologists. In contrast, researchers at the Eliava Institute and similar institutions continued to study the growth, biochemical characteristics, and phage sensitivity of hundreds of strains of bacteria, including drug-resistant strains. During World War II, phage therapy was used to treat Russian soldiers suffering from dysentery, gangrene, and other kinds of wound infection. Soviet scientists also attempted to use phages to fight pathogens in farm animals, fish farms, plants, and raw foods. After the war, phage therapy remained a widely accepted part of preventive and therapeutic medicine throughout the Soviet Union. During the 1970s and 1980s, hundreds of people worked at the Eliava Institute, making tons of phage products for military and civilian uses throughout the Soviet Union, analyzing hundreds of thousands of bacterial samples, isolating and characterizing new phages, and testing therapeutic phage preparations. Phages were also used to destroy bacteria in food and water and on surfaces and equipment in homes, nursery schools, and hospitals. With the collapse of the USSR in the 1990s, many phage research centers disappeared, along with other components of the health care and public health services. The George Eliava Institute of Bacteriophages, Microbiology, and Virology, however, survived the fall of the Soviet Union.

In the Western world, by the 1990s, the growing threat of antibiotic-resistant bacteria revived interest in phage therapy. Since the introduction of sulfanilamide, scientists have issued warnings about the evolution of drug-resistant pathogens. Yet, even as resistance to penicillin, streptomycin, and other drugs appeared, the public and the medical community generally assumed that the discovery of more powerful antibiotics would continue. As multidrug-resistant pathogens became increasingly prevalent, the possibility of returning to a preantibiotic era of untreatable infections and epidemic diseases led some Western scientists to begin a reevaluation of phage therapy and the role of phages in nature. By the beginning of the twenty-first century, Western companies were involved in collaborative projects at the Eliava Institute and other phage production companies in the newly independent republics of the former Soviet Union in the hope of bringing phage products to Western markets. Cooperation between phage advocates in Russia and the West resulted in the publication of English translations of previously unknown Russian research and review articles on phage therapy.

Although scientific issues and obstacles may inhibit work on phage therapy, advocates of this approach argue that in the United States, economic factors and regulatory considerations are more significant barriers. The research and testing required to market new drugs is extremely costly, time consuming, and difficult. The standards and documentation required in the United States for drug approval will presumably inhibit the development and marketing and increase the costs of phage therapy. Leaders of fermentation industries that depend on microbes warn that phages could cause serious problems if production facilities become contaminated by destructive phages, either by accident or deliberate sabotage. Critics of phage therapy warn that unless phage preparations are carefully purified, they might contain dangerous debris and toxins released by dead bacteria.

Advocates of phage therapy point out that there were many problems in the development and testing of the first antimicrobial agents, but the success of penicillin encouraged continued efforts to find other broad-spectrum antibiotics. Antibiotics were accepted as miracle drugs that could be prescribed for a wide range of infectious diseases, without overly specific identification of the causative organism. In contrast, therapeutic phages must be continuously evaluated and selected to target rapidly evolving strains of bacteria. The specificity of phages for particular bacteria might be a problem for doctors, who have come to rely on broad-spectrum antibiotics. By sequencing phage genomes to determine how they seek out, enter, and take over the machinery of their target hosts, scientists might be able to engineer safe and effective therapeutic phages. Presumably, such phages would be far more specific for the pathogenic bacteria attacking the patient than any known antibiotic.

Critics of phage therapy warn that most of our information about phages and bacteria is the result of laboratory studies; much less is known about their interaction in a more natural environment and their potential effect on the immune system of the patient. Theoretically, phages will disappear from the patient after all the vulnerable bacteria have been killed, but phages might acquire genes from other viruses, their bacterial targets, or other cells. Phages might spread from treated patients to other people or into the environment, with unpredictable results. As they replicate, phages might exchange genes, including genes for toxins and antibiotic resistance, with other microbes. Novel pathogenic viruses might arise through recombination or mutation and might attack the patient or the normal microflora in the gastrointestinal tract. Researchers hope to engineer viruses that kill their intended bacterial targets but are incapable of lysing the dead bacterial cell after they have destroyed it, which would make it impossible for them to undergo further cycles of replication. Nevertheless, it is probably impossible to be absolutely sure that therapeutic phages will not acquire mutations that would overcome attempts to establish protective mechanisms.

Many scientists believe that it is time to look more carefully at the potential of phage therapy, reexamining the existing literature and planning research based on modern methods and knowledge. The use of specific phages to treat the environment—in agriculture, animal husbandry, food processing, food products, water treatment facilities, and so forth—might be more acceptable to those who worry about phage therapy for people. If successful, the use of phages to prevent infections in domesticated animals could reduce the inappropriate use of antibiotics and the development of antibiotic-resistant strains of bacteria. Applying phage preparations to hospital equipment, instruments, and surfaces might help reduce the problem of nosocomial infections. Phages could be used in feedlots and meatpacking plants and sprayed on meat to kill bacteria, and they could be inactivated after use to reduce their transfer to people. Some experts argue that phages against certain common bacteria belong to the category of agents that scientists have already generally recognized as safe (GRAS status). However, people might be as suspicious of phage-treated meat and poultry as they are of genetically modified foods. Since the early 1980s, scientists in Britain and the United States have been studying the effect of therapeutic phages in systemic infections, diarrheal disease, and burns in various experimental animals. Promising results in experimental animals, reviews of the clinical literature from Eastern Europe, and reports in the popular media contributed to increased interest in phage therapy in the scientific community and greater awareness of the field in the general community.

Researchers expect to isolate and characterize many more phages in the future. Scientists have traditionally collected phages from sewage treatment plants, zoo animals, and convalescing patients, but they may be able to find phages that can attack bacteria in almost any environment—soil and sewage, oceans and rivers, swamps and hot springs. Although thousands of phages have been isolated, relatively few have been fully characterized or classified. Preliminary studies of the microbial life in seawater samples suggest that phages play a critical role in determining the life of the oceans. Even in an area like the Sargasso Sea, which was thought of as an ocean desert devoid of nutrients and microbial life, J. Craig Venter, best known for his pioneering work in genomics, has discovered traces of millions of unique species, single-celled organisms, and viruses. According to Venter, the activity of phages might affect the distribution and population density of microbial life—including potential pathogens—in oceans, rivers, lakes, and so forth. D'Hérelle's goal of turning phages into disease fighters might seem modest in comparison to Venter's predictions about the potential applications of an approach he calls *synthetic genomics*, that is, designing microbes that could perform a wide range of specific tasks, from making medicines to creating new energy sources.

MOLECULAR BIOLOGY AND BACTERIOPHAGES

During the 1930s, virology gradually separated itself from bacteriology and became a scientific discipline in its own right. Philosophical debates about viruses and the nature of life remained unresolved, but viruses were analyzed by means of chemical and physical techniques that were used to study proteins and other large, complex molecules. It was not until 1953, however, that Salvador Luria published *General Virology*, the first major textbook devoted to this branch of microbiology. Textbook descriptions of viruses made it clear that the fundamental difference between viruses and other microbes was that a virus could only reproduce by entering a living host cell and taking over its metabolic apparatus. Viruses were, therefore, defined as "infectious obligate intracellular parasites." Like other microorganisms, viruses contain genetic information, but they need to use the biosynthetic machinery of living cells to produce new virus particles; that is, viruses are infectious agents that can only reproduce by entering a living host cell and taking over its metabolic apparatus. Viruses have therefore been described as "living molecules" on the borderline between macromolecules, genes, and cells.

All viruses consist of a nucleic acid core that serves as the viral genome, either deoxyribonucleic acid (DNA) or ribonucleic acid (RNA), and a protective protein coat. Despite their small size and relative simplicity, viruses are diverse in shape, structure, and their ability to infect host species ranging from bacteria, fungi, and algae to plants, animals, and humans. Viruses differ considerably in the size of their genome and the time it takes to undergo replication. For example, some bacteriophages produce new viral particles in less than an hour, whereas some animal viruses take several days to complete the process.

The origin of viruses is obscure, but they may have evolved from microorganisms that lost many of their cellular components or from genes that escaped from an ancestral cell and gained the ability to infect other cells. The behavior of viruses, even those that only attacked bacteria, proved to be more complicated than originally anticipated. During the 1940s, scientists were able to demonstrate the existence of two quite different groups of bacteriophages: lytic phages and lysogenic phages. *Lytic phages* take over a bacterial cell, replicate, and lyse the host cell to release a burst of new phages. Instead of immediately replicating and killing their target cells, *lysogenic phages* can either replicate in their target cell or integrate their DNA into the host's DNA. In this case, the phage remains hidden in the genome of the host and its daughter cells until some stimulus triggers its reactivation. The existence of lysogenic phages was unknown to early phage workers, who assumed that all phages simply attacked and killed their bacterial targets. Eventually, researchers discovered that some of the viruses that cause disease in humans, such as the herpes virus, are also capable of establishing latent infections in human cells. After remaining dormant for long periods, a latent virus may become active and begin to replicate, producing new viruses that attack other cells.

The French microbiologist André Lwoff, who won the 1965 Nobel Prize for his work on lysogeny, was primarily interested in the physiology, biochemistry, and life cycle of microorganisms. Ultimately, Lwoff's interest in lysogeny as the prototype for persistent, but hidden infections led to work on *oncogenes*, cancer-causing genes that might have originated as viruses. Through his painstaking studies of lysogenic strains of bacteria, Lwoff proved that the genetic material of these bacteria contained a virus in a form he called the *prophage*. Although the prophage and its host could coexist peacefully for many generations, if the latent virus was activated, it began to replicate. Eventually, the infected bacterial cell lysed, releasing large numbers of new viruses, some of which carried bits of genetic material from their former bacterial host. In 1953, Joshua Lederberg and Norton Zinder demonstrated that bacteriophages could therefore transfer bacterial genes from one bacterium to another, a phenomenon now known as transduction. A therapeutic phage cocktail that contained lysogenic phages could lead to the transduction of genes for toxins or drug resistance into previously harmless bacteria.

In the early 1940s, Max Delbrück, Alfred Hershey, Salvador Luria, and other pioneers of molecular biology adopted bacterial viruses as their model system for exploring the basic nature of the gene, its chemistry, and its role in heredity. Bacterial viruses provided the perfect "experimental animal" for a new approach to genetics that was especially appealing to scientists who had originally been trained as physicists. Using a narrow range of lytic phages, scientists were able to explore questions about gene structure, mutation, gene regulation, and the transmission of information at the molecular level. The Phage Group associated with Delbrück was instrumental in shifting the focus of phage research in the United States and Europe toward basic research that used *Escherichia coli* and a limited number of lytic phages as tools in the study of the physical basis of genetics. Studies of this model system led to the demonstration that DNA is the genetic material, recognition of the role of messenger RNA in gene expression, the elucidation of the genetic code, and many other core concepts of molecular biology. In 1969, Delbrück, Luria, and Hershey shared the Nobel Prize for their fundamental insights into viral genetics.

During the 1940s, most chemists, physicists, and geneticists thought that the genetic material must be a protein, but studies of what Oswald T. Avery called the *transforming principle* in bacteria suggested that nucleic acids might serve as the genetic material. Most scientists were skeptical about this possibility until the 1950s, when experiments using bacterial viruses appeared to confirm Avery's suggestion. Phage workers suspected that bacteriophages might act like tiny hypodermic needles that injected their genetic material into their bacterial victims and left their empty viral coats outside. To test this possibility, Hershey and his associate Martha Chase used radioactive isotopes to label phage proteins and DNA. Their experiments indicated that it was the phage's DNA, not its protein, that entered the bacterial cell. In 1953, James D. Watson and Frances Crick proposed a model for the structure of DNA that helped explain its biological role in heredity. Phage studies led James Watson to what he called the *central dogma* of the molecular biology of the gene: "DNA makes RNA makes protein." However, within ten years—largely through studies of animal and tumor viruses—it became clear that the central dogma, at least in its original form, had failed to predict the possibility that information could be transferred from RNA to DNA.

CANCER AND VIRUSES

Francis Peyton Rous's report of an association between a virus and cancer in chickens led to the identification of the first tumor virus. In 1909, Rous began a series of experiments on a large tumor that had appeared on a Plymouth Rock hen. After successfully transplanting the tumor to other chickens, Rous demonstrated that it could also be transferred by cell-free filtrates of tumor tissue. Virologists later identified the causative agent as a retrovirus, which is now known as the Rous sarcoma virus (RSV). Until the 1950s, Rous's suggestion that a filterable virus caused at least one form of cancer was generally ignored, but since that time, many other viruses have been associated with cancers in humans and other animals. These viruses have been called oncogenic, carcinogenic, tumorigenic, or transforming viruses. In 1966, Rous was awarded a Nobel Prize for his pioneering studies of RSV and the possible relationship between malignant tumors and viruses.

Studies of tumor viruses led to the discovery of the enzyme known as reverse transcriptase and proof that, contrary to the original version of the central dogma of molecular biology, genetic information could flow from RNA to DNA. Howard Temin and David Baltimore independently discovered reverse transcriptase, an enzyme encoded in the genes of viruses that can transcribe RNA sequences into DNA sequences. This discovery has been critical to understanding a group of viruses called retroviruses, one of which is the human immunodeficiency virus (HIV), the virus that causes acquired immune deficiency syndrome (AIDS). In 1975, the Nobel Prize in Physiology or Medicine was awarded to Howard Temin, Renato Dulbecco, and David Baltimore for their discoveries concerning the interaction between genes and tumor viruses and the relationship between viruses and cancer. While working on RSV, Temin noted that the inhibition of DNA synthesis and DNA-dependent RNA synthesis blocked RSV infection. This observation was surprising because the RSV genome is single-stranded RNA, and it was assumed that the RNA served as the genetic material. To explain his observations, Temin suggested that a DNA intermediate must be involved in RSV infection. As an explanation for his findings, Temin proposed the *provirus hypothesis*.

According to the provirus hypothesis, after an RNA virus enters a host cell, a DNA provirus is synthesized. The DNA provirus contains the genetic information of the RNA viral genome, and progeny viral RNA is synthesized from the DNA provirus. This hypothesis could also account for the integration of RSV genetic material into the genome of the host. In 1970, Temin and Satoshi Mizutani proved that RSV infection involves an enzyme that transcribes single-stranded viral RNA into DNA. An anonymous reviewer for the journal *Nature* gave the enzyme the name "reverse transcriptase." At about the same time, David Baltimore demonstrated the existence of reverse transcriptase in Rauscher murine leukemia virus. RNA tumor viruses and reverse transcriptase quickly became basic tools for studying the molecular biology of mammalian cells. Virologists suggested that the modern human genome might still contain retroviruses that were integrated into the genome of the primate ancestors of humans.

Despite the discovery of tumor viruses in chickens and other animals, there was considerable skepticism in the biomedical community about the relevance of these findings for cancers in humans. However, some epidemiological studies suggested that infective agents, including viruses, bacteria, protozoa, and parasites, might play a role in the initiation and development of human cancers. In particular, the discovery of the Epstein-Barr virus (EBV) in pathological samples from Burkitt's lymphoma patients supported the hypothesis that viruses had a significant role in the development of human cancers. Burkitt's lymphoma was first identified by Denis Parsons Burkitt, who served as a British army doctor in Africa during World War II. In addition to his missionary calling, Burkitt was interested in medical geography and epidemiology. He remained in Africa as a general practitioner in Kampala, Uganda, until 1966, when he accepted a position at the Medical Research Council in London.

In 1957, Burkitt examined several children with unusual, fast-growing tumors of the head and neck. Suspecting that he had discovered a childhood cancer that had not been previously described, Burkitt sent queries to doctors in other African hospitals and traveled widely in search of additional cases. After analyzing the incidence and geographical distribution of this new form of lymphoma, Burkitt concluded that it was the most common cancer of children in tropical Africa. Finding a close correlation between the geographic distribution of this cancer and that of malaria, Burkitt speculated that, like malaria and other tropical diseases, the cancer might be associated with an insect vector. (Other comparative studies of patterns of disease in Africa and Europe led Burkitt to the conviction that the lack of fiber in the typical Western diet contributed to the development of diseases such as diabetes, diverticulosis, gallstones, obesity, high cholesterol levels, and colon cancer. He published several books devoted to this hypothesis.)

Through his journal articles and lectures, Burkitt succeeded in drawing attention to his studies of lymphoma in African children. After attending one of Burkitt's lectures in 1961, English virologist Michael Anthony Epstein asked Burkitt for samples of tissue from some of his African patients. In 1964, Epstein and his colleague Yvonne Barr identified a herpes virus—now known as the Epstein-Barr virus—in cultured lymphoma cells. Although EBV was discovered as a result of Burkitt's work on childhood cancer in Africa, the virus is very common throughout the world. Moreover, children and adolescents rarely experience any symptoms when first infected.

If the virus is acquired by young adults, about half suffer from a generally mild illness referred to as infectious mononucleosis. Healthy people seem to carry the virus throughout their lives, but the virus is clearly associated with the development of certain cancers, most notably Burkitt's lymphoma, Hodgkin's lymphoma, and nasopharyngeal carcinoma.

About twenty years after Epstein and Barr identified the virus, its entire genome was successfully sequenced. Thus, scientists have been able to analyze the organization of the viral genes, their functions, their pattern of expression, and the interactions between the virus and the human cells that it infects. Although the immune system attempts to attack the virus, EBV has evolved many strategies to evade the immune response. Nevertheless, many questions about the way in which the virus induces cancer and the striking geographic differences in the incidence of various forms of cancer associated with EBV remain. Epidemiological studies of other cancers suggest that viruses may be associated with about 15 to 20 percent of the global burden of cancer. As in the case of cancers linked to EBV, the incidence of other cancers associated with infectious agents seems to vary in their geographic distribution. Many different direct and indirect pathways—from chronic inflammation and inhibition of cellular repair mechanisms to immunosuppression and oxidative stress—seem to link infectious agents and the development of cancer. Researchers are increasingly interested in studying the complex problem of how viruses establish latent infections that may eventually cause serious diseases, including cancer. Such studies have been extremely difficult and the results ambiguous.

Despite intensive efforts to deal with major and minor viral diseases, from influenza to AIDS, viral diseases have no specific cure, although antiviral agents are improving the treatment and prognosis for some viral diseases. Preventive vaccines remain the most important means of controlling viral diseases, but safe and effective vaccines are not available for all viral diseases. Many public health experts have become very pessimistic about the possibility of developing a vaccine for certain intractable viral diseases such as AIDS. (For a more detailed discussion of AIDS, see Chapter 7, "Emerging Infectious Diseases.") Certain viruses, such as HIV, the virus that causes AIDS, and the influenza virus, are constantly changing because of their high mutation rate. Understanding viruses and finding ways to prevent and cure viral infections are vital to dealing with viral diseases, especially as viruses increasingly becoming suspects in complex chronic diseases—as causes or contributing factors—such as multiple sclerosis, Epstein-Barr syndrome, chronic fatigue syndrome, autoimmune diseases, diabetes, cancers, heart disease, degenerative brain disorders in the elderly, and so forth. Evidence of the global distribution and movement of viruses among wild and domesticated animals and humans is also increasing.

The relationship between three common human cancers and specific pathogens seems to be well established: liver cancer and hepatitis B or C; cancer of the cervix and papillomaviruses; and stomach cancer and *Helicobacter pylori*. Studies of the relationship between viruses and cancers have already led to the development of preventive vaccines. The hepatitis B vaccine was initially developed to prevent acute hepatitis B, but the vaccine may also prevent the induction of liver cancer. In Taiwan, for example, statistical studies conducted ten and twenty years after the introduction of hepatitis B vaccination programs in the 1980s demonstrated a significant decrease in the incidence of hepatitis B infections and liver cancers among those who had been vaccinated. Virologists suspect that viruses are involved in various forms of leukemia, lymphatic cancers, and some brain tumors. Human herpes virus 8 has been implicated as the cause of Kaposi's sarcoma, a cancer often found in AIDS patients. A polyoma virus seems to be linked to a rare form of skin cancer known as Merkel cell carcinoma. Both Kaposi's sarcoma and Merkel cell carcinoma were originally described as rare cancers that typically affected people over sixty-five, but these cancers are increasingly found in people whose immune systems have been compromised, either by HIV/AIDS or the drugs used by organ transplant recipients.

SUBVIRAL INFECTIOUS AGENTS: VIROIDS AND PRIONS

Viruses were once considered the simplest of all possible pathogens, that is, so-called living molecules inhabiting a unique place in the world of infectious agents—the borderline between macromolecules, genes, and cells—but research on diseases once attributed to atypical viruses led to the discovery of even smaller infectious entities that, despite their apparent structural simplicity, cause devastating diseases. Indeed, the discovery of radically new infectious agents known as viroids and prions provided an unanticipated challenge to classical microbiology and the central dogma of molecular biology. These discoveries extended the scope of the germ theory of disease, stimulated the search for still-unknown subviral particles that might interact with living cells, and raised new questions about the role of such agents in the natural world.

VIROIDS

Studies of potato spindle tuber disease, an infectious disease that plant pathologists assumed must be caused by a virus, led to the discovery of viroids. Thus, this little-known plant disease was as important to the discovery of viroids as tobacco mosaic virus was to the discovery of viruses. Spindle tuber disease develops very slowly in potatoes, but by transmitting the disease to tomato plants, William B. Raymer and Muriel O'Brien developed a relatively rapid bioassay for the infectious agent. Attempts to isolate a virus from diseased tomato plants were, however, totally unsuccessful. In

1965, Theodor O. Diener began working on this problem with Raymer. Their findings led to the surprising conclusion that the infectious agent that caused potato spindle tuber disease was not a virus. Diener called the new agent a *viroid* because it was like a virus, but it seemed to be much smaller than any known virus. Enzymes that attack RNA destroyed the viroid's infective properties, but enzymes that break up DNA or proteins had no effect. Therefore, the physical and chemical properties of the infectious agent indicated that, unlike typical RNA viruses, the viroid did not have a protein overcoat. Because the properties of the viroid contradicted prevailing ideas about infectious agents, Diener spent six years confirming the existence of an entirely new kind of plant pathogen.

In 1971, Diener reported that potato spindle tuber disease was caused by a novel infectious agent consisting of naked, single-stranded RNA molecules that could only replicate within the cells of its specific host. Although Diener's concept was originally quite controversial, within thirty years, scientists discovered dozens of additional viroid species and hundreds of variants, including avocado sunblotch viroid, peach latent mosaic viroid, tomato plant macho viroid, citrus bent leaf viroid, and pear blister canker viroid. Like a virus, the viroid invades a cell and uses the host cell's metabolic and reproductive apparatus to replicate viroid RNA. All viroids are comprised of single-stranded RNA, but unlike RNA viruses, viroids do not have a protective protein coat. Unlike the RNA of retroviruses, such as HIV, the virus that causes AIDS, viroid RNAs do not code for genes. Despite the absence of a protective protein coat, viroid RNA seems to be remarkably stable.

Most viroids seem to replicate within the cell nucleus and trigger a biochemical chain of events that leads to disease symptoms such as stunted growth. Although plant diseases led to the discovery of viroids, researchers subsequently realized that these novel infectious agents could be used to investigate the roles played by various kinds of RNA molecules within plant cells and cell organelles. Plant scientists hope to find ways of preventing diseases caused by viroids, but they also think that viroids, like bacteriophages and retroviruses, might become useful tools for molecular biology. Viroids could serve as probes to study the ways in which plant proteins and nucleic acids move in and out of cell nuclei. If viroid infections could be strictly controlled, viroids that cause stunting might be used to create very desirable varieties of dwarf trees.

Although there is still much confusion about the mechanisms by which viroids multiply, move from cell to cell, and cause disease in plants, the discovery of these naked RNA pathogens has stimulated research into the interaction between foreign nucleic acid molecules and human diseases. Such studies led to the discovery of subviral entities similar to viroids in animals and humans. An especially dangerous form of hepatitis known as hepatitis D is apparently caused by a viroidlike entity, which was previously known as the hepatitis Delta virus. Hepatitis D, which only occurs in people who contract the hepatitis B virus as well as the hepatitis D agent, can lead to liver failure. Researchers are attempting to clarify suggestive evidence that the subviral world contains other esoteric disease-causing entities, some of which operate on their own and others that seem to require helper viruses to multiply and cause disease.

PRIONS

Viroids may differ from viruses in many ways, but because they contain nucleic acid, they still seem to fit into the fundamental framework of molecular biology. Prions, a radically new kind of infectious agent discovered in the 1980s, raise fundamental questions for virology, microbiology, and molecular biology because they do not contain nucleic acids. All known infectious agents, prior to the discovery of prions, contained genetic material in the form of nucleic acids, either DNA or RNA. Diseases now known to be caused by prions were originally attributed to an elusive infectious entity that Carleton Gajdusek, physician, virologist, and anthropologist, described as a "slow virus." During the 1950s, Gajdusek became involved in studies of kuru, a neurological degenerative disease that seemed to occur only among the Fore people of New Guinea. This devastating disease, which began with uncontrollable trembling and progressed to dementia, killed hundreds of Fore people each year. Most of the victims were women and children.

Given the pattern of disease among the Fore, Gajdusek suggested that kuru might be caused by an infectious agent that was acquired during mourning rituals in which women and children consumed the brains of deceased relatives as a sign of respect and grief. Using brain tissue from victims of kuru, Gajdusek and his associates were able to transmit the disease to a series of chimpanzees. Because symptoms did not appear for about two years, Gajdusek suggested that kuru was caused by an unconventional infectious agent that he called a slow virus. While conducting his research on kuru, Gajdusek learned that similar lesions occurred in the brains of sheep that succumbed to a progressive neurological disease known as scrapie. Although the disease had been seen in sheep since the eighteenth century, people who worked with sick animals did not seem to contract the disease. Searching the medical literature for diseases that resembled kuru and scrapie, Gajdusek began a study of a rare, progressive, fatal dementia known as Creutzfeldt-Jakob dementia (CJD). As in the case of kuru, Creutzfeldt-Jakob disease could be transmitted to chimpanzees, and the onset of symptoms occurred after a long incubation period.

When he accepted the 1976 Nobel Prize in Medicine or Physiology for discovering new ways of understandings the origin and dissemination of persistent, chronic infectious diseases, Gajdusek summarized his work in a lecture titled "Unconventional Viruses and the Origin and Disappearance of Kuru." Prions, the agents that cause kuru, scrapie, and CJD, proved to be much more unconventional than Gajdusek and other scientists had ever anticipated. Stanley Prusiner, who discovered prions and introduced a controversial hypothesis to account for the origin and dissemination of prion diseases, was awarded the Nobel Prize in 1997.

In 1972, after one of his patients died of CJD, Prusiner began studying the literature that linked CJD to kuru and scrapie. CJD is a rare disease that generally affects elderly people. However, Gadjusek's work suggested that it might be caused by a slow virus like the obscure agents associated with kuru and scrapie. Using scrapie as his experimental model, Prusiner found that he could transmit the infectious agent to hamsters. When Prusiner tried to isolate and characterize the infectious agent from the brains of diseased hamsters, he found that it was sensitive to enzymes that digest proteins but was unaffected by procedures that destroy nucleic acids. Prusiner began to suspect that the scrapie agent might not contain nucleic acid, although the genetic material of all known infectious agents, even the smallest virus, was either RNA or DNA. To characterize the unique nature of the scrapie agent, in 1982, Prusiner introduced the term *prion*, which stood for "proteinaceous infectious particle." Studies of prion proteins indicated that they were remarkably stable; they resist boiling, hospital detergents, heat, and ultraviolet radiation, which would kill other kinds of pathogens. Prusiner's protein-only prion hypothesis was extremely controversial, but intensive attempts by advocates and critics to find nucleic acids associated with the scrapie agent were unsuccessful.

Despite continuing skepticism and controversy, by the early 1990s, many scientists had accepted Prusiner's protein-only prion hypothesis. Prusiner's hypothesis led to the discovery of genes that encoded prion proteins in all animals tested, including humans. According to Prusiner's theory, prion proteins can exist in two distinct conformations, one of which is a harmless cellular protein. In their alternative conformation, prion proteins force their benign counterparts to undergo transformation and aggregate. After an incubation period that may vary from months to years, the aggregates of altered proteins form threadlike tangles that ultimately destroy brain cells and cause fatal brain diseases. Unlike bacteria and viruses, prions provoke little or no immune response because they are not recognized as foreign invaders. The characterization of prions as "proteinaceous infectious particles" without nucleic acids established a new category of disease-causing agents and raised the possibility that other bizarre infectious entities may exist in obscure corners of the environment or hidden in a latent state within the cells and genes of plants and animals.

All of the diseases attributed to prions are known as *transmissible spongiform encephalopathies*, that is, progressive, degenerative diseases of the central nervous system. Extracts of diseased brains can transmit these diseases to previously healthy animals. Prion diseases of animals include scrapie in sheep and goats, transmissible mink encephalopathy, chronic wasting disease of mule deer and elk, feline spongiform encephalopathy, and bovine spongiform encephalopathy (BSE, commonly known as mad cow disease). Human diseases attributed to prions include CJD, fatal familial insomnia, Gerstmann-Sräussler-Scheinker syndrome, and kuru. Unlike kuru, which was only found among the Fore people of New Guinea, CJD appears to strike sporadically, affecting about one in a million people over the age of sixty throughout the world. CJD seems to have a genetic basis in about 10 to 15 percent of known cases, but the vast majority of all cases seem to arise spontaneously. Some cases have been associated with medical interventions such as organ transplantation, the implantation of electrodes in the brain, and the use of contaminated surgical instruments. In the 1970s, an unusual cluster of CJD cases was diagnosed in people treated with human growth hormone harvested from the pituitary glands of human cadavers. The outbreak ended after genetically engineered growth hormone became available.

Until the 1980s, when mad cow disease (BSE) first appeared in England, there was no historical evidence of the transmission of scrapie to cows, humans, or other animals. The first recorded case of mad cow disease occurred in 1984, when several English dairy cows died of a previously unknown illness. By 2001, cattle in Italy, Spain, Germany, France, Portugal, Belgium, and Denmark as well as England were dying of mad cow disease. Almost two hundred thousand cattle were affected by the disease, and millions were destroyed in an effort to end the outbreak. The BSE epidemic apparently began when a nutritional supplement containing rendered meat and bone meal from sheep and cows was added to cattle feed as a nutritional supplement. By essentially transforming domesticated herbivores into carnivores—or cannibals, like the kuru victims in New Guinea—the new dietary regimen presumably created an unprecedented opportunity for scrapie agents to infect cattle. As the mad cow epidemic reached its peak in 1992, millions of cattle were destroyed, but by then, contaminated meat products had probably entered the food chain. The British government banned the use of animal-derived feed supplements in 1988, but by 1994, a condition that appeared to be related to BSE and CJD was diagnosed in people. The disease was labeled vCJD, to indicate that it appeared to be a new variant of CJD. The total number of cases of vCJD, about 120, was relatively small, considering the millions of people who may have eaten contaminated meat, but the disease was invariably fatal. BSE also spread to house cats and some zoo animals.

Since the mad cow outbreak, other examples of prion transmission across species barriers have been discovered. A transmissible spongiform encephalopathy called chronic wasting disease is endemic in deer and elk in parts of the United States and Canada. Thus, the occurrence of a CJD-like condition among deer hunters suggested that people could contract a prion disease by eating meat from infected deer. In the 1980s, thousands of mink contracted a fatal spongiform encephalopathy after they were fed meat from so-called downer cows, that is, cows that lie down because they are close to death. Although it was the panic caused by mad cow disease that raised public awareness of prion diseases, the discovery of prion diseases in wild animals suggests that these diseases may be more widely distributed than originally suspected. Moreover, the emergence of new diseases, such as BSE and vCJD, seem to be particularly striking examples of the unanticipated consequences of changes in agriculture, food production, and the global redistribution of previously isolated plants, animals, and infectious agents.

MICROBIAL ECOLOGY

Since the 1990s, pioneers of a field known as microbial ecology have been exploring the complex microbial populations found in natural ecosystems. These studies prove that only a tiny fraction of the microbial species present in most environments has ever been identified. Many of the unknown organisms cannot be cultured by traditional laboratory techniques, but the techniques of molecular biology are beginning to reveal the genetic diversity of microbial communities in different habitats. Through DNA and RNA sequencing, scientists are assessing the relative abundance of microbial species found in various habitats. The discovery of prions suggests, however, that researchers will have to look beyond entities characterized by their nucleic acids as they explore submicroscopic ecosystems.

FIVE

༄࿐

SANITARY REFORM, PUBLIC HEALTH, AND THE BATTLE AGAINST FILTH AND EPIDEMIC DISEASES

SANITARY REFORM AND THE BATTLE AGAINST FILTH

By the end of the nineteenth century, microbiology made it possible to identify the specific cause and means of transmission of many infectious diseases. For a very few diseases, scientists and physicians had developed preventive vaccines and serum therapy, but microbiology had little impact on therapeutics. Because of anesthetics and aseptic techniques, surgeons could perform more complicated operations than their predecessors. Nevertheless, when confronted with infected wounds, they were as helpless as their medieval counterparts. Thus, the major public health benefit of nineteenth-century germ theory was the guidance it provided in dealing with epidemic diseases. Once the causative agent had been identified, investigators could search for it in food and water, droplets or dust particles in the air, mosquitoes and ticks, and the people who came in contact with the sick. Public health measures that directly affected individuals, such as mandatory vaccination and the isolation of the sick, were controversial and not always effective, but improved sanitation, food inspection, and pasteurization helped reduce the universal threat of diseases spread by contaminated food and water. Public health advocates needed reliable data to assess the incidence of various diseases and the effectiveness of preventive measures.

Throughout history, the social, economic, and environmental origins of threats to human health have been among the central issues of public health policy. Important trends in morbidity and mortality were already obvious in John Graunt's *Observations upon the Bills of Mortality* (1662), which is considered a landmark in the use of vital statistics to analyze the factors that determine the health of societies. Graunt attempted to derive general trends from the local "Bills of Mortality" (weekly lists of burials) and the records of marriages and baptisms kept by parish clerks. According to Graunt's calculations, the urban death rate was greater than that of rural areas. The death rate for infants and children was particularly striking: about 40 percent of all infants died before reaching their second birthday, and only half of all babies would reach their seventeenth birthday. Evidence of the heavy burden of disease stimulated the search for practical means of preventing disease and improving the human condition.

The goals and ideals as well as the sometimes authoritarian methods that characterized the developing field of public health medicine are reflected in the work of Johann Peter Frank, a pioneer of public health and social medicine. His philosophy was summarized in his essay "The People's Misery—Mother of Diseases" and in his *System of Complete Medical Police* (six volumes, 1777–1817). This monumental work was a widely known and influential exploration of the social, economic, and political problems that affected health and disease. Weaving together the noblest ideals of Enlightenment philosophy and pragmatic public health goals, Frank attempted to convince Europe's rulers that their people constituted the state's greatest wealth. The power and prosperity of the state, therefore, depended on improving the health and productivity of its subjects through regulations and programs to protect the population against disease and promote health. Frank called for a national system of medical police, training schools for midwives and surgeons, and hospitals for the poor. According to Frank, diseases were generated by a social system that kept peasants and workers in conditions of permanent misery.

Until the acceptance of modern germ theory, the miasmatic theory of disease was generally more influential than any competing theory, including the belief that disease was transmitted by contagion. Even in the late nineteenth century, the miasmatic theory of disease was vigorously defended by eminent public health reformers, who insisted that poor sanitary conditions, filth, and noxious air caused the epidemic diseases that flourished in the rapidly growing cities of Europe. Many critics of germ theory were actively involved in sanitary or hygienic reform movements and could claim significant successes in improving the health of cities. By the end of the nineteenth century, many physicians and surgeons accepted the germ theory of disease, and the battle for sanitary reform incorporated scientific discoveries that made it possible to understand, explain, and prevent epidemic disease. Whatever theory motivated sanitary reform movements, comprehensive attacks on filth and pollution were critical to reducing the burden of epidemic and endemic diseases, as demonstrated by the work of Max von Pettenkofer, the founder of Munich's Institute of Hygiene. Highly respected for his pioneering work on hygiene and epidemiology, Pettenkofer believed that the modern science of hygiene would provide more useful information about the origins of infectious diseases than the germ theory of disease. Rejecting the major conclusions drawn by Pasteur and Koch, Pettenkofer argued that poisonous miasmata, soil conditions, and climatological disturbances were primarily responsible for the generation of disease. Therefore, he concluded, sanitary reforms were the most effective means of preventing epidemic diseases. Despite the conflict between Pettenkofer's miasmatic theory and Robert Koch's germ theory, both were dedicated to the idea that the scientific study of hygiene would have a great and beneficial impact on the battle against infectious diseases.

Leaders of the public health movement were generally confidant that the causes of epidemic disease were well enough understood to make the conquest of disease possible. All that was necessary was to devote sufficient resources to improving individual and public hygiene and relief of the miserable social conditions that allowed disease to flourish. Implementing sanitary reform measures required the work of sanitary engineers, politicians, and bureaucrats as well as scientists and physicians. Edwin Chadwick, one of the leaders of Britain's sanitary reform movement, was a disciple of moral philosopher Jeremy Bentham, the champion of the doctrine known as utilitarianism. What Chadwick called his "sanitary idea" was, however, already implicit in articles he had written before meeting Bentham. Public health policy, or the sanitary idea, can be seen as a perfect example of the utilitarian doctrine that society should be organized for the greatest benefit of the greatest number.

After his appointment to England's Poor Law Commission in 1832, Chadwick devoted the rest of his life to analyzing the sanitary condition of the working people of Great Britain, reducing the costs of poor relief, and managing public health policy. In his famous 1842 report for the Poor Law Commission, Chadwick recommended improving the urban environment by constructing drains and sewers. In crowded urban slums, epidemic and endemic diseases were caused and disseminated by atmospheric pollution that could invariably be traced to the putrefaction of animal and vegetable wastes, dampness, filth, and overcrowded dwellings. To demonstrate the contamination found in London's drinking water, Chadwick included illustrations of water samples laden with debris, filth, and microbes. Diseases caused by pollution and filth, Chadwick concluded, caused more death and disability than any wars fought by Great Britain, destroying families and sending impoverished men, women, and children to workhouses and orphanages. Government officials could therefore improve the health of working people by building drains and sewers; removing filth and refuse from houses, streets, and roads; and improving water supplies for domestic use and for washing away refuse. The expense of such projects, he argued, would be more than compensated for by significant decreases in the burden of epidemic and endemic diseases. Improving the health of the working classes would decrease the numbers of people seeking poor relief. Comparative studies of different towns, cities, and districts demonstrated that if filth and putrefaction were thoroughly removed by drainage, proper disinfection, and improved ventilation, epidemic and endemic diseases virtually disappeared.

According to Chadwick, noxious smells, so prominent in the city slums, were a direct threat to human health. Many public health reformers were sure that polluted air caused epidemic disease, but it was difficult to understand why some people, including the scavengers who worked in sewers and cesspits, were often quite healthy, despite their exposure to offensive smells. Nevertheless, when the Great Stink of London struck during the unusually hot summer of 1858, the stench made it impossible for government officials to avoid the fact that the River Thames and other rivers flowing through London had become open sewers. Although heavy rains and cooler weather eventually ended the crisis, the Great Stink demonstrated the need to construct new sewer systems to carry away the wastes of the city. Paris suffered through a Great Stink in 1880 that generated widespread fear of potentially deadly epidemics triggered by foul odors. By the time of the Great Stink of 1895, fear of foul odors as a source of epidemic diseases had diminished because of the growing influence of Louis Pasteur's germ theory of disease.

The germ theory of disease did not completely displace the sanitarian concept that linked epidemic disease to filth or the fear of noxious odors, but the work of Pasteur, Koch, and their disciples gradually led to the integration of biomedical research into public health and sanitary engineering. For example, bacteriological laboratories were established for the analysis of food and water and the diagnosis of specific infectious diseases. Public health bacteriological laboratories were dedicated to the identification of pathogenic microbes, rather than the search for environmental filth and pollution.

WATERBORNE DISEASES

Sanitary reformers throughout the Western world were inspired by Chadwick's *Report on the Sanitary Condition of the Labouring Population of Great Britain* (1842). In the United States, Lemuel Shattuck, the founder and first president of the American Statistical Association, conducted a similar survey of sanitary conditions. His *Report of a General Plan for the Promotion of Public and Personal Health* (1850) included a model state public health law. However, it could be argued that it was the fear generated by a disease that Europeans called *Asiatic cholera* that forced city governments to establish programs to fight filth and establish safer water supplies. Deaths that were due to cholera were actually a small part of nineteenth-century mortality, but the terror provoked by the disease was as great as that previously caused by rumors of bubonic plague.

Asiatic cholera was unknown to Europeans until the nineteenth century, when warfare, trade, and travel broke down regional barriers that had previously confined the disease to limited areas of India. In 1817, cholera apparently escaped from South Asia and began spreading from seaport to seaport, presumably carried by infected sailors and merchants, until it reached Russia, the Middle East, Europe, and North America. At first, European physicians thought that Asiatic cholera might be a more virulent form of previously known, nonspecific gastrointestinal conditions variously referred to as cholera morbus, cholera nostra, autumnal cholera, or dysentery. Further experience with cholera epidemics convinced doctors that the disease was quite different from other gastrointestinal disorders. An attack of cholera generally began with a sudden attack of diarrhea, vomiting, and cramps. Many victims rapidly progressed from mild discomfort to violent vomiting and a watery diarrhea called *rice water stools* that contained bits of the intestinal lining and huge numbers of bacteria. The catastrophic loss of fluids and electrolytes led to dehydration and shock as the kidneys failed and the circulatory system collapsed. In severe cases, shock, coma, and death occurred within twenty-four to forty-eight hours of the onset of symptoms.

Attempts to explain the origin and transmission of cholera reflected the general divisions in the medical community concerning epidemic diseases. Contagion seemed the least likely explanation because it was clear that doctors who examined the sick or performed autopsies on cholera victims rarely contracted the disease. Most doctors believed that cholera epidemics were the result of local, environmental conditions—such as filth, heat, and humidity—that generated noxious airs or miasmata. Sanitary reforms that established cleanliness of air, water, streets, houses, and people should, therefore, control and prevent outbreaks of cholera. Thus, cholera outbreaks led to widespread fear of filth, contamination, and polluted water long before the causative agent was finally established.

In urban areas, cholera became the focal point of pioneering studies of epidemiology and the friend of the public health movement. The study of cholera carried out by British physician John Snow has served as a model for epidemiological investigation and reasoning. Snow's study of the 1854 cholera outbreak in London, known as the Broad Street epidemic, has become a landmark in the history of epidemiology, although it was only part of Snow's analysis of the causes and dissemination of the disease. Six years before the Broad Street outbreak, London had experienced a cholera epidemic that, according to the *Report of the General Board of Health on the Epidemic Cholera of 1848–9*, killed more than fourteen thousand residents of London. As Snow analyzed the distribution of cases in this epidemic, he began to suspect that contaminated water might link all the people who had contracted cholera. Snow concluded that the specific cause of cholera was introduced into the digestive system via the mouth. It was subsequently transmitted to new victims by water that had been contaminated by the excretions of cholera patients.

When the Broad Street outbreak occurred, Snow immediately suspected the local water supply. A detailed study of the outbreak, especially the pattern of deaths, revealed that almost every known case was linked to the Broad Street pump. Snow concluded that the well had been contaminated by cholera excretions. After Snow presented his analysis of the outbreak, the local Board of Guardians agreed to remove the handle of the Broad Street pump, although the outbreak was already beginning to subside. Motivated primarily by skepticism, the Reverend Henry Whitehead conducted his own detailed study of the Broad Street outbreak. In addition to confirming Snow's hypothesis, Whitehead's painstaking interviews of essentially all the people affected by the outbreak led to the discovery of how the well had become contaminated. During his interview of Mrs. Lewis, who lived in the house at 40 Broad Street, Whitehead learned that her infant daughter had contracted a virulent case of diarrhea shortly before the beginning of the cholera outbreak. Undifferentiated fevers and fluxes (diarrheal diseases) were, of course, quite common and life-threatening aspects of childhood at the time. Mrs. Lewis had soaked the baby's soiled diapers and dumped the wash water into the cesspool (septic tank) in the yard in front of the house. Most residents of this house threw waste materials into the courtyard at the back of the house rather than into the cesspool. The cesspool, Whitehead noted, was only a few feet from the Broad Street well. About two days after baby Lewis died, the cholera outbreak began. When Mr. Lewis became ill with cholera, the soon-to-be-widowed Mrs. Lewis again tossed her buckets of contaminated wash water into the cesspool. Fortunately, by this time, the handle had been removed from the pump, and the well was no longer being used as a source of drinking water. Thus, although removing the handle did not end the infamous Broad Street cholera epidemic, it probably saved the neighborhood from a second outbreak. Subsequent inspections of the cesspool found a partially blocked drain and crumbling walls that allowed its contents to seep into the nearby well. Presumably, Mrs. Lewis and her wash water had added a deadly pulse of contamination to the cesspool and the well.

When another cholera outbreak struck London in 1866, William Farr, epidemiologist and medical statistician, concluded that there was a clear relationship between cholera deaths and water supply lines. His investigation demonstrated that the epidemic in the Whitechapel area of London was caused by water supplied by the East London Water Company, which sold water taken from the Lea River. When Farr testified before Parliament about the outbreak, he apparently could not resist expressing his cynicism about the continuing support for the miasma theory. He pointed out that blaming cholera outbreaks on polluted air perfectly suited commercial interests because, although no one could sell the air that people breathed, business people could make large profits by selling drinking water.

John Snow did not identify a specific causative agent for cholera, despite his indictment of contaminated water. Suggestive evidence that a microbe found in the intestines of cholera victims caused the disease was presented by the Italian histologist Filippo Pacini in 1854. Although the discovery of the comma-shaped bacterial form that causes cholera is usually attributed to Robert Koch, in 1965, the international committee on nomenclature proposed the name *Vibrio cholerae Pacini* in honor of Pacini. In 1884, Koch announced that he had discovered the agent that caused cholera; it was referred to as the comma bacillus, or cholera vibrio because of its active, vibrating movements. Subsequently, he proved that it could survive in water, food, soiled clothing and bed linens, and damp earth. Although Koch was unable to find an animal model that would allow him to establish unequivocal proof that he had isolated the specific causative agent for cholera, the circumstantial evidence linking the cholera vibrio to the disease was strong enough to convince many bacteriologists that cholera outbreaks were caused by contaminated water.

Dismissing the significance of Koch's study of the cholera vibrio, Max von Pettenkofer, an eminent German chemist and epidemiologist, argued that cholera outbreaks were the result of miasmata generated by peculiar conditions in damp soils or groundwater and disseminated in noxious air. Sanitary reforms prescribed by Pettenkofer and stimulated by the fear of disease-causing miasmas had improved Munich's sewage system, resulting in a significant reduction in the burden of intestinal diseases. Cholera excrements and cholera germs might be among the many factors that promoted the development of a cholera miasma, but, Pettenkofer argued, germs or contagion alone could not account for cholera epidemics. For practical and philo-sophical reasons, when thinking about epidemic diseases, physicians had to consider a more complex and interacting series of predisposing and exciting causes, including miasmata; corrupt habits; immoral behaviors; poor living conditions; overcrowding; polluted water; noxious odors, especially those arising from cesspits; and the lack of ventilation and sunlight. In 1892, Pettenkofer publicly challenged Koch and his germ theory of disease by swallowing a culture of cholera vibrios. Perhaps as a result of prior infection, Pettenkofer survived without experiencing any significant discomfort.

Despite many years of controversy concerning the specific cause of cholera and the factors that contributed to epidemics, fear of this disease was a critical factor in the establishment of public health boards and municipal laboratories for the routine bacteriological diagnosis of disease. By studying cholera outbreaks and searching for the vibrio in areas where the disease frequently appeared, bacteriologists discovered that the cholera vibrio does not need people, cesspits, and wells to survive. The vibrio can grow and multiply in fresh or brackish water in association with zooplankton, shellfish, and crustaceans, including edible species such as oysters and blue crabs. Cholera vibrios flourish in the Ganges River, the Gulf of Mexico, the Chesapeake Bay, and other waterways. When conditions are unfavorable, the vibrios enter a sporelike state. Using tiny crustaceans as their hosts, cholera vibrios are able to survive and travel until conditions allow them to cause new outbreaks. Many different strains of the cholera vibrio, which differ significantly in their virulence, have been discovered. Virulent cholera vibrios colonize the intestines and produce a toxin that disrupts the body's ability to regulate water intake and outflow. An important subtype of the cholera vibrio was first identified in 1960 at the El Tor quarantine station in Saudi Arabia. The El Tor biotype is less virulent than the classic biotype, but it produces more asymptomatic carriers, who continuously excrete the vibrio. Epidemiologists think that it is now more widely disseminated than the classic subtype, except on the Indian subcontinent. The genome of the cholera vibrio, including the genes that code for the synthesis of the toxin, was sequenced in 2000.

Cholera led to an understanding of the fact that urbanization amplified the danger of epidemic diseases, but when scientists discovered the causes and means of dissemination of these infectious diseases, they could design public health measures to bring them under control. Cholera outbreaks enhanced support for massive, costly public works projects to bring clean water to major cities. With the installation of sanitary water systems, cholera was essentially banished from most industrialized nations by the 1930s, although cholera was still a serious public health threat in Russia, the Middle East, Africa, and Asia. Chlorine helped to make water safe from pathogenic microbes, but with the threat of cholera forgotten, people in wealthy countries tend to worry more about chlorine in their water supply than microbial contamination. Public health experts are concerned about the possibility that the growth of the bottled water industry might result in neglect of the infrastructure that maintains public water supplies. This could lead to the kind of situation that allowed cholera to flourish in nineteenth-century slums: safe water for the rich and questionable supplies for the poor.

Cholera is still a public health problem in many parts of the world because more than one billion people do not have access to safe water. In many poor countries, drinking water in rural areas as well as city slums is heavily contaminated with parasites, bacteria, and viruses. Public health experts estimate that about half of the world's poor still suffer from waterborne diseases. Thousands died of cholera in India and Bangladesh in the 1960s and 1970s. Cholera outbreaks also occurred in Cambodia, Angola, Zimbabwe, Iraq, Sudan, Ethiopia, Somalia, Kenya, Uganda, and Peru. Sporadic cases of cholera in the United States were generally traced to consumption of seafood from the Gulf of Mexico. Travelers to areas where cholera is endemic have acquired the disease by drinking contaminated water or consuming contaminated food, particularly raw shellfish.

During serious cholera epidemics, mortality rates of about 50 to 60 percent are usually reported, but mortality rates as high as 80 percent have occurred during some outbreaks. Infectious disease experts believe that almost all cholera patients could be saved through the administration of intravenous liquids. Unfortunately, the medical resources needed for intravenous infusions are almost nonexistent in areas where cholera outbreaks and diarrheal diseases are common. Liquids given by mouth (oral hydration) are usually ineffective in cases of severe dehydration, but in the 1970s, researchers discovered that appropriate solutions of glucose and salts given by mouth were absorbed rapidly enough to save victims of cholera. Oral rehydration can also prevent most deaths from severe infantile diarrhea, even in the most primitive settings, if safe water is available. With proper oral or intravenous rehydration therapy, the case fatality rate is less than 1 percent.

The first twentieth-century cholera epidemic in South America was detected in Peru in 1991. About fourteen million people in Peru were infected, and 350,000 were hospitalized. Although the fatality rate was only about 1 percent, about thirty-five hundred people died. Some cases were traced to contaminated food served in airplanes leaving Peru, proving again that an infectious disease anywhere in the world is just a plane ride away from any other point on the globe. The Pan American Health Organization reported that within six years of the 1991 outbreak in Peru, cholera had become established in fourteen countries because of inadequate water quality, sanitation, and hygiene. Thousands of cases and hundreds of deaths were reported, but experts suspect that only a fraction of all cholera cases are ever reported. Epidemiologists suggested that the cholera outbreaks were associated with unusually warm ocean currents that promoted the growth and spread of cholera vibrios carried by plankton, the mixture of microscopic plants and animals that drift in the ocean. Warmer waters promote their growth, thus increasing the chance of cholera epidemics wherever people lack access to safe water supplies and proper sanitary facilities. Misinformation about the 1991 cholera epidemic in Peru included claims that the disease appeared after chlorination of the water supply was discontinued. This was untrue because the water supply in the areas where the disease was most prevalent was quite primitive and was seldom, if ever, chlorinated or otherwise treated. Except in the capital city of Lima, Peru's drinking water supplies at the time of the epidemic were generally not chlorinated.

At the beginning of the twenty-first century, cholera was still present in seventy-five countries and on all continents. Epidemiologists estimate that hundreds of thousands of people contract cholera every year, but the true extent of the threat is unknown because governments prefer to list deaths from cholera as gastroenteritis, intestinal flu, food poisoning, or other euphemisms for diarrheal diseases. A United Nations report published in 2006, *Beyond Scarcity: Power, Poverty and the Global Water Crisis*, estimated that more than one billion people get water for drinking, washing, and cooking from sources polluted by human and animal wastes. Diseases associated with the lack of safe water and adequate sanitation kill more than two million people in poor countries every year. Diarrhea and other diseases associated with dirty water and inadequate sanitation kill more than two million children every year. Many medical experts agree that Chadwick's sanitary idea has contributed more to the health and welfare of human populations as a whole than any other medical advance, including the discovery of antibiotics and the development of vaccines. Cholera outbreaks continue to vindicate the sanitarian doctrine that poverty, pollution, and the lack of hygienic conditions are the most significant factors in generating and disseminating epidemic disease. Even prosperous, modern cities are vulnerable to the epidemic diseases that can emerge after natural disasters, such as floods, and man-made catastrophes, such as war and military occupation. When basic services—drinking water, sanitation, and health care—are disrupted, cholera and typhoid fever become significant public health risks, especially among refugees and displaced people.

TYPHOID FEVER

Cholera and typhoid fever outbreaks are generated by similar conditions. Both are waterborne bacterial diseases that challenged conventional public health measures because quarantine measures and the isolation of the sick do not necessarily break the chain of transmission. As in the case of cholera, the bacteria that cause typhoid fever are typically transmitted by water and food contaminated by the excretions of infected people. Symptoms of typhoid fever include fever, headache, pinkish rash, nausea, vomiting, diarrhea or constipation, mental confusion, stupor, delirium, and coma. Perforation of the intestinal wall and damage to blood vessels can lead to painful, life-threatening peritonitis (infection in the abdominal cavity caused by the escape of materials from the intestinal tract) and internal hemorrhages. Physicians generally estimated the mortality rate for typhoid at between 8 and 15 percent.

Characteristic lesions, signs of inflammation, and ulcerations are usually found in the small intestines during an autopsy. Initially, typhoid bacteria multiply in the intestines, but bacteria that enter the bloodstream can attack the spleen, bone marrow, and other organs. Typhoid fever is typically associated with poverty and lack of sanitary facilities, but the disease was a threat to the rich and famous. Queen Victoria's beloved husband, Prince Albert, contracted typhoid and died in 1861 after weeks of increasingly severe gastrointestinal problems, fever, and delirium, leaving the queen in mourning until her death in 1901.

Like John Snow's work on cholera, William Budd's *Typhoid Fever; Its Nature, Mode of Spreading, and Prevention* (1873) is a remarkable example of the painstaking detective work that established the art and science of epidemiology. William Budd, an English country doctor, had studied medicine in Paris with Pierre Charles Alexandre Louis, the eminent pathologist who used statistical methods to establish the foundations of what is now called *evidence-based medicine*. Louis's studies of enteric fevers (intestinal diseases) had linked clinical observations of symptoms with characteristic signs of inflammation and ulceration found at autopsy. Typhoid had been associated with intestinal lesions known as Peyer's patches, which were first described by Johann

Conrad Peyer and other anatomists in the 1670s. At the time, typhoid was not clearly differentiated from other febrile diseases, but some doctors thought that the "slow nervous fever" (typhoid) could turn into the deadly disease known as putrid fever, war fever, ship fever, or typhus. (For more about typhus, see Chapter 6.) Because typhoid, typhus, dysentery, and other contagious diseases were likely to flourish among soldiers and sailors living in crowded, unsanitary conditions, military doctors probably diagnosed some cases of typhoid as malaria or dysentery.

While serving as a doctor in several small villages, Budd had the opportunity to investigate the course of several typhoid outbreaks. His observations convinced him that typhoid was communicated from person to person through some common factor, which he deduced was contaminated water. To prevent the transmission of typhoid, Budd recommended the disinfection of contaminated privies, drains, and sewers with chloride of lime (also known as bleaching powder), carbolic acid, or green vitriol (sulfate of iron). The first of Budd's classic papers, "On Intestinal Fever," was published in the British medical journal *The Lancet* in 1859, but his landmark treatise *Typhoid Fever* did not appear until 1873.

According to Budd, physicians who practiced in large towns and cities tended to be anticontagionists, but country doctors had better opportunities to follow the sequential appearance of individual cases of typhoid and other diseases. Indeed, other country doctors, who had observed similar patterns, supported his conclusion that the disease was transmitted by a contagion found in the excretions of typhoid patients. Anticontagionists, however, continued to argue that even if typhoid was sometimes transmitted by contaminated water, it could also be spontaneously generated by environmental conditions and miasmas generated by filth. No matter how thorough the detective work carried out by Budd and other advocates of the contagion theory might have been, it was not always possible to determine the initial source of the disease. Even in isolated communities, it was sometimes impossible to point to the first "imported" case. At the time, the concept of the healthy, asymptomatic disease carrier was unknown.

The causative agent for typhoid, *Salmonella typhi*, was discovered by Carl Joseph Eberth in 1880, the year in which Budd died. Robert Koch and George Gaffky confirmed the identification of Eberth's microbe, but it was not until 1886 that bacteriologists were able to grow pure cultures in the laboratory. By studying urban epidemics, public health physicians learned that contaminated water was not the only factor involved in amplifying the spread of *Salmonella typhi*. Early in her career, Alice Hamilton, who is best known as the founder of occupational medicine in America, carried out studies of a typhoid fever outbreak that occurred in Chicago, Illinois, in 1902 that demonstrated the relationship between inadequate sanitation and the disease. Her work proved that the flies that infested the outhouses and toilets shared by the impoverished inhabitants of filthy, overcrowded city slums could also transport typhoid. As a result of Hamilton's proof that flies could transport germs and contaminate food, public health workers came to think of flies as dangerous "germs with wings," rather than just a petty nuisance. In addition to efforts to clean city slums, public health workers in Chicago called for the pasteurization of milk because of evidence that contaminated milk could be a source of typhoid and other infectious diseases.

During the first decade of the twentieth century, several bacteriologists identified active, infectious typhoid bacteria in the feces of healthy individuals, long after they had recovered from the disease. In fact, perhaps as many as 3 to 5 percent of those who contract the disease become carriers. Robert Koch and his disciples became convinced that healthy carriers of infection were important factors in the epidemiology of typhoid. Testing for carrier status was complicated by the discovery that some carriers shed bacteria intermittently.

When physicians and public health workers realized that viable *Salmonella typhi* could be found in the feces of apparently healthy people, the disease came to symbolize the problem of the healthy carrier as the enemy of the public health. Carriers are defined as people who excrete typhoid bacilli more than twelve months after suffering from typhoid fever, but some chronic carriers are classified as intermittent carriers because they only shed typhoid bacilli at irregular intervals. This phenomenon makes it difficult to detect and effectively monitor typhoid carriers. After victims of typhoid fever had apparently recovered from the disease, about 10 percent continued to excrete bacteria for several months, and about 5 percent appeared to become chronic carriers. The factors that allowed the bacteria to establish chronic infections remain unclear, but the age and sex of the patient and prior gallbladder disease seem to play a role. Attempts to cure chronic carriers were generally unsuccessful, despite the usual unsubstantiated claims from assorted quacks. Tests conducted in the 1950s, when antibiotics were still seen as miracle drugs, found that sulfonamides, penicillin, chloramphenicol, and combinations of these drugs generally had little or no effect on preventing or permanently curing the carrier state. Only the surgical removal of the gallbladder (cholecystectomy) was somewhat effective because in carriers, the bacteria apparently remain hidden in the biliary system (the gallbladder and bile ducts).

The most notorious example of a healthy carrier, a cook named Mary Mallon, was associated with at least forty-seven cases of typhoid and three deaths. *Typhoid Mary* has become a generic term for an apparently healthy person who knowingly endangers others by refusing to take appropriate precautions against the transmission of an infectious disease. Mallon, who was born in 1869 in County Tyrone, Ireland, immigrated to the United States at the age of fifteen in search of a better life. After arriving in New York, she quickly found employment, first as a domestic servant and, eventually, better-paying positions as a cook. In 1906, she was cooking for a well-to-do family spending the summer on Long Island. Within a few weeks, six of the eleven members of the household contracted typhoid fever. George Soper, a civil engineer hired by the family to investigate the source of the illness, suspected that Mallon was to blame. By tracing her previous job history, Soper discovered that her service in seven different households in the New York area was associated with more than twenty cases of typhoid and at least one death.

After Mallon refused to provide blood and stool samples for analysis, officials at the New York City Health Department arranged for Dr. Sara Josephine Baker and several police officers to forcibly take Mallon to a hospital, where bacteriological tests were conducted. Baker, who dedicated her life's work to public health and child welfare, believed that the public health authorities had to use the power of the state to prevent the spread of epidemic diseases. Although the tests were positive for typhoid bacteria, Mallon insisted that she was completely healthy, had never suffered from typhoid, and demanded to be released. Instead, she was confined to a hospital on Brother Island in the East River. Despite significant public sympathy for her situation, Mallon was kept in isolation for about three years. New York City's new Health Commissioner, Ernst J. Lederle, agreed to release Mallon if she swore that she would never again work as a cook. Lederle expected Mallon to work in a laundry, instead of a kitchen, and to keep the authorities informed about her employment. Once free, Mallon took a new name and returned to her career as a cook, which she saw as the only practical option available to a poor, uneducated woman who had to support herself.

In 1915, while she was working in the kitchen of Sloane Maternity Hospital in Manhattan, twenty-five cases of typhoid, including two that ended in death, led the authorities back to Mallon. The public had little sympathy for Mallon after this outbreak. The American Public Health Association used the case of Typhoid Mary to campaign for granting public health authorities more power to examine and manage people who handled foods in restaurants, hotels, public institutions, dairy farms, and so forth. By 1916, the New York City health department had performed bacteriological examinations of thousands of food handlers, but unlike Mallon, other typhoid carriers were rarely, if ever, incarcerated. Mallon was confined to Brother Island until she died of pneumonia in 1938. The autopsy report confirmed the speculation that her gallbladder still harbored *Salmonella typhi*.

Although Mary Mallon was certainly not the only healthy carrier of typhoid to leave a trail of illness and death among those who crossed her path, she was the one who became notorious as Typhoid Mary. Typhoid outbreaks that occurred from 1899 to 1909 in Folkestone, England, for example, were eventually traced to a man who milked cows at various farms in the area. Until 1909, the authorities failed to associate the spread of disease with the healthy carrier, who was only identified as "Mr. N." Although Mr. N, who was sixty when he was finally identified as the source of at least two hundred cases of typhoid, claimed he had never suffered from the disease, bacteriological tests found *Salmonella typhi* in his feces. Unlike Mallon, Mr. N was not incarcerated, but he did agree to leave Folkestone and the dairy business.

Contrary to the mythic version of the life of Typhoid Mary, Mallon was not the only healthy carrier involuntarily imprisoned for life as a danger to the public health. Investigative reporters and historians have discovered evidence of other typhoid carriers who were forced into lifelong quarantine. When Dr. Thomas Bewley accepted a position at Claybury Hospital in Woodford Bridge (now a suburb of London) in the 1950s, he discovered that two wards still housed fourteen patients classified as typhoid carriers, despite the fact that each one had undergone a cholecystectomy (surgical removal of the gallbladder). Surprised that these patients were still being kept in isolation long after their initial diagnosis, Bewley had them retested and discovered that their stool samples were negative for typhoid bacteria. In 2008, an investigation conducted by the British Broadcasting Corporation provoked considerable media attention by revealing the story of a group of women quickly labeled "British Typhoid Marys." At least forty-three female typhoid carriers from London had been confined to the Long Grove mental asylum in Surrey, England, between 1907 and 1992. Researchers at the Surrey History Centre were able to save some of the institution's records, although most were destroyed when Long Grove was closed in 1992. Long Grove's "Typhoid Marys" were institutionalized because their status as typhoid carriers was considered a threat to the public health. Although they were apparently not insane when they were admitted to the asylum, by the time antibiotics transformed the treatment of typhoid fever, these patients were considered too fragile and mentally impaired for life in the outside world.

Every year, typhoid fever attacks some twenty million people and causes about five hundred thousand deaths. In the United States, about four hundred cases are reported each year, but the vast majority of these infections are acquired through international travel. American physicians are unlikely to be familiar with the disease, but it persists in the developing world, where drug-resistant forms of the typhoid bacillus are becoming increasingly common. *Salmonella typhi* is one of three species that belong to the *Salmonella* genus. All diseases caused by members of this group are known as salmonelloses, but only *Salmonella typhi* causes typhoid fever. The genomes of several distinct strains of this pathogen were sequenced in 2008 through the use of sophisticated new techniques. Researchers hope that decoding several different versions of the bacterial DNA sequence will lead to better methods of diagnosis, treatment, and ways of anticipating the distribution and evolution of the strains that cause typhoid fever. Researchers suspect that the microbe became a human pathogen between ten thousand and forty-three thousand years ago. Healthy carriers could have disseminated different strains of *Salmonella typhi* throughout the world. The genome of *Salmonella typhi* indicates that it has become well adapted to existence in human hosts and has lost many of the genes found in other members of the *Salmonella* group. Indeed, *Salmonella typhi* has no known reservoir outside of humans. The development of drug-resistant strains of *Salmonella typhi* indicates that providing effective treatment, especially in the case of chronic carriers, will become increasingly difficult. Public health experts hope that the ability to map and identify the genes that make specific strains of *Salmonella typhi* particularly virulent and most likely to produce chronic carriers will lead to more effective vaccination campaigns that could eventually eradicate typhoid.

SIX

❧❦❧

THE ART AND SCIENCE OF PREVENTING AND CONTROLLING EPIDEMIC DISEASES

SMALLPOX: INOCULATION, VACCINATION, AND ERADICATION

In addition to campaigning for safe drinking water and sewers, public health advocates generally agree that preventive vaccination is one of the greatest lifesaving measures in the history of medicine. Moreover, the global campaign for the eradication of smallpox demonstrates the benefits that can be achieved through international public health networks. The virus that causes smallpox in humans probably evolved from one of the pox viruses of wild or domesticated animals. Originally confined to Africa or Asia, the virus was eventually carried to Central Asia, China, Persia, and Europe as new patterns of human migration, warfare, and commerce developed. Smallpox probably made only sporadic incursions into Europe before the Middle Ages, but by the seventeenth century, smallpox was regarded as one of the unavoidable childhood diseases. Although doctors generally discussed diseases in terms of symptoms, such as fever, diarrhea, and skin lesions, Rhazes, a ninth-century Persian physician, urged physicians to distinguish between measles and smallpox. He believed that smallpox was the inevitable result of the fermentation of impurities in the blood that occurred as children matured. In seventeenth-century England, smallpox was so common that Thomas Sydenham, often referred to as the English Hippocrates, also assumed that this life-threatening eruptive fever was an unavoidable part of human maturation.

Smallpox virus generally spreads from person to person in the droplets expelled when victims cough, sneeze, or speak. The virus may also be transmitted by clothing, blankets, or shrouds contaminated with pus or scabs from smallpox vesicles. About two weeks after the virus enters the body, nonspecific symptoms, such as headache, coughing, back and muscle pain, fever, and fatigue, provide the first evidence of the presence of systemic infection. By the time the characteristic rash appears, the victim may have transmitted the virus to many others. Pus-filled blisters, which left permanent scars, usually developed in the mouth and on the face, arms, legs, and even on the palms of the hands and the soles of the feet. Victims of *Variola major* sometimes died of cardiovascular collapse, secondary infections, or internal and external bleeding. Septic poisoning, pneumonia, ugly scars, blindness, and deafness were not uncommon complications, but the worst form of the disease, known as black or hemorrhagic smallpox, was almost always fatal.

Both Rhazes and Sydenham believed that skillful medical care promoted healing and reduced the possibility of a fatal outcome. Incompetent treatment, however, could lead to confluent pustules, blindness, brain fever, and death. Patients who survived even a very mild case of smallpox achieved lifelong immunity from the disease. *Immunity*, like *virus*, is a Latin term that has acquired a specific meaning within the biomedical sciences. Originally, immunity referred to a special exemption from legal obligations such as the payment of taxes. In medicine, immunity refers to resistance to infection by specific pathogens. For most of human history, immunity could only be acquired by surviving an attack of a disease. Perhaps recognition of the fact that a mild case of smallpox conferred immunity as reliably as a severe attack led some people to attempt to acquire a mild case of this potentially life-threatening disease. Parents might deliberately expose their children to a person with a mild case of smallpox or to bedding that had been used by a person recovering from the disease. In Africa, Asia, India, and Turkey, some practitioners attempted to induce a mild case of smallpox by deliberately inserting material from smallpox pustules into a cut or scratch on the skin of a healthy individual. In China, children inhaled a powder made from the crusts of smallpox scabs. Until the eighteenth century, European physicians generally dismissed these practices as barbaric and superstitious.

The deliberate induction of smallpox was called ingrafting, inoculation, or variolation. (The term *inoculation* comes from the Latin *inoculare*, "to graft"; *variolation* comes from *variola*, the Latin name for smallpox.) Smallpox acquired by inoculation was usually mild, with few lesions and little scarring. Lady Mary Wortley Montagu, who observed the Turkish custom of taking the smallpox while living in Constantinople, where her husband served as ambassador, sent letters about the procedure to influential friends in England. Lady Mary's son was safely inoculated before she returned to England. To encourage others to adopt smallpox inoculation, Lady Mary arranged for her daughter to be inoculated during a smallpox epidemic in London. In response to clergymen and physicians who condemned the Turkish method as immoral and dangerous, in 1722, Lady Mary published an anonymous article in a London newspaper under the title "A Plain Account of the Inoculating of the Small Pox by a Turkey Merchant." The editor of *The Flying Post* did not reveal her identity, but he did attempt to tone down her outrage at the "Knavery and Ignorance of Physicians." Despite the skepticism of physicians and clergymen, many members of the aristocracy and upper classes adopted the procedure. Less incendiary accounts of smallpox inoculation, independently written by Emanuel Timoni and Jacob Pylarini, had been published in the *Philosophical Transactions of the Royal Society* in 1714. After these reports reached the British colonies in New England, the Reverend Cotton Mather and Zabdiel Boylston conducted a test of the procedure.

During a smallpox outbreak that struck Boston in 1721, Mather and Boylston inoculated almost three hundred people. Clergymen, doctors, and local officials denounced the experiment, but when the epidemic was over, Boylston's meticulous records demonstrated the value of inoculation. During the epidemic, the mortality rate for naturally acquired smallpox was about 14 percent. (Almost half of Boston's 12,000 inhabitants contracted the disease, and 844 died.) Of 280 people inoculated, only 6 had died, but some of these people might have contracted smallpox before inoculation. A 2 percent fatality rate for a modern vaccine would be totally unacceptable, but in comparison to naturally acquired smallpox, the benefits of inoculation clearly exceeded the risks. For parents who had experienced smallpox, weighing the risks and benefits of inoculation was a new and unprecedented responsibility. By the end of the eighteenth century, inoculation was widely accepted, despite the variable results reported by different inoculators. Inoculation had a limited impact on the overall incidence of smallpox, but it proved that medical intervention could modify the risk of death and disfigurement associated with naturally acquired smallpox. Inoculation did, however, become a fairly routine procedure, which made it possible for Edward Jenner to discover a related, but safer approach to preventing smallpox.

As practicing physician in rural Gloucestershire, Jenner was struck by the fact that some of the patients he inoculated seemed to be immune to smallpox, although they insisted they had never experienced the disease or previous inoculations. When he attempted to clarify this observation, he learned that local people believed that a mild disease known as cowpox provided protection from smallpox. Milkmaids and farmhands typically contracted cowpox from contact with pustules on the udders of infected cows. To test the relationship between cowpox and smallpox, Jenner inoculated healthy people with material taken from cowpox pustules. His experiments confirmed the hypothesis that cowpox did indeed protect people from both naturally transmitted smallpox and inoculated smallpox. From the Latin terms for *smallpox* and *cow*, Jenner created the term *Variola vaccinae*. To distinguish between the old practice of inoculation with smallpox matter and his new method, Jenner coined the term *vaccination.* In 1798, Jenner published the treatise that has become a landmark in the history of vaccinology: *An Inquiry into the Causes and Effects of the Variolae Vaccinae, a Disease Discovered in Some of the Western Counties of England, Particularly Gloucestershire, and Known by the Name of the Cow-Pox.*

Critics denounced vaccination as a disgusting and dangerous procedure, but despite some reluctance to transmitting a disease of animals to humans, tests conducted in prisons and orphanages indicated that the procedure was safe and effective. Advocates of Jennerian vaccination considered it the greatest discovery in the history of medicine. Vaccination quickly displaced inoculation throughout the world. On long voyages, vaccine was kept alive by a series of person-to-person transfers, generally using previously unvaccinated orphans. Vaccination was made compulsory in the United Kingdom in the 1850s. Public health leaders predicted that smallpox would disappear when all nations adopted compulsory vaccination. In America, Benjamin Waterhouse, a leading promoter of vaccination, sent some of his vaccine to Thomas Jefferson, who used it to vaccinate his entire household. In a letter to Jenner, written in 1806, Jefferson predicted that vaccination would totally eradicate smallpox in the not too distant future.

In contrast to the optimism of Jenner and his disciples, his critics continued to attack vaccination. Opponents of vaccination often warned that interfering with God's will and the laws of nature was immoral and dangerous. Deliberately introducing disease matter derived from an animal into a healthy person was denounced as disgusting and unnatural. Human-to-human transmission was attacked as an unsanitary procedure that might transmit syphilis and other diseases. Leaders of the antivaccination movement particularly objected to laws that established mandatory vaccination. Eminent critics of vaccination included the British philosopher Herbert Spencer, who said he disapproved of voluntary vaccination and absolutely detested compulsory measures. Alfred Russel Wallace, English naturalist and codiscoverer of natural selection, denounced mandatory vaccination as a crime against liberty, health, and humanity. The antivaccination movement was broad enough to encompass scientists, physicians, unorthodox healers, liberal individualists, members of various religious groups, and social reformers, who argued that vaccination allowed the state and wealthy individuals to ignore the social roots of disease, that is, poverty, overcrowding, and unsanitary conditions.

In response to the passage of compulsory vaccination laws, antivaccinators formed organizations that staged demonstrations, published pamphlets, and generated considerable public support. Antivaccine protests sometimes became violent when public health authorities attempted to enforce vaccination laws, isolate suspected smallpox cases, or imprison those who refused vaccination during epidemics. During a smallpox outbreak in Boston in 1901, the Anti-Compulsory Vaccination League led the opposition to vaccination. In Britain, antivaccinators claimed victory when the right to refuse vaccination was granted in 1907. Attempts to repeal the compulsory vaccination law of the state of Massachusetts led to a landmark legal case on the constitutionality of compulsory vaccination (*Johnson v. Massachusetts*). In 1905, the Supreme Court ruled in favor of the state. The Court said the state could pass laws requiring vaccination to protect the public from dangerous communicable diseases. Despite compulsory vaccination laws, during the first decades of the twentieth century, the rate of vaccination in the United States was the lowest among the industrialized nations. Enforcement of vaccination laws improved dramatically after World War II. By the 1970s, the risk of contracting smallpox within the United States became so small that the Public Health Service recommended ending routine vaccination.

THE GLOBAL ERADICATION OF SMALLPOX

By the 1960s, for most residents of the wealthy industrialized nations, the odds of suffering ill effects from vaccination became greater than the chance of encountering smallpox. In the United States, during this period, six to eight children died each year from vaccination-related complications. Nevertheless, as long as smallpox existed anywhere in the world, the threat of imported smallpox could not be ignored. The impact of such threats was demonstrated in 1971, when a Moslem cleric from Yugoslavia contracted smallpox during a pilgrimage to Iraq. After his return to Yugoslavia, 175 people contracted the disease, and 35 died. The outbreak was controlled when the government recognized a potential state of emergency and instituted mass vaccinations. For wealthy, industrialized countries, the worldwide eradication of smallpox offered a humane and economical solution to the threat posed by vaccination. The fact that scientists had never found an animal reservoir or human carrier state for smallpox made global eradication a realistic goal (see Figure 6.1).

In 1959, the World Health Organization (WHO) called for the eradication of smallpox. When the Smallpox Eradication Program was launched, smallpox was still endemic in thirty-three countries, and eleven were reporting sporadic or imported cases. According to WHO, in 1966, there were about one hundred million cases of smallpox worldwide, with about two million deaths, mainly in Bangladesh, Brazil, India, Indonesia, Nepal, Pakistan, and sub-Saharan Africa. Epidemiologists were generally skeptical about the likelihood of eradicating smallpox from the world's poorest nations, but the global program made remarkable progress. By 1974, smallpox was confined to parts of Pakistan, India, Bangladesh, Ethiopia, and Somalia. Three years later, smallpox cases were only reported in Ethiopia and Somalia. In 1977, the last case of smallpox acquired outside a laboratory setting was diagnosed in twenty-seven-year-old Ali Maow Maalin, who worked in a hospital in Somalia. Hospital officials failed to isolate Maalin when he first became ill because his illness was initially misdiagnosed as malaria and, later, as chicken pox. In 1980, after almost three years

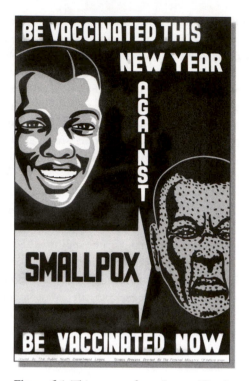

Figure 6.1 This poster from Lagos, Nigeria, promoted the worldwide smallpox eradication campaign. Credit: Public Health Image Library, Centers for Disease Control and Prevention, U.S. Department of Health and Human Services.

of anxious surveillance, WHO officially declared that the world was free of smallpox. Leaders of the eradication campaign and public health advocates proposed the next logical step, that is, using the lessons learned in the smallpox campaign to eradicate poliomyelitis, measles, diphtheria, whooping cough, and other preventable diseases.

In 1982, WHO recommended an end to routine vaccination and the destruction of all smallpox stocks within two years, except for samples that would be stored in designated laboratories in the United States and Russia. These collections of smallpox specimens are actually fairly large. The collection held at a secure facility in the United States contains about five hundred strains of the smallpox virus. The dangers posed by keeping smallpox virus in research laboratories were demonstrated in 1978, when Janet Parker, a photographer at the Birmingham University Medical School, died of smallpox. The virus apparently escaped via a network of air ducts from a laboratory that the university planned to close because it was considered too old and unsafe to be used for smallpox research. After the Birmingham episode, many researchers agreed to destroy their stocks of smallpox virus. Professional organizations, such as the American Society for Microbiology, the American Society for Virology, and the American Type Culture Collection, initially supported the destruction of all samples of the virus. For political and ethical, rather than scientific, reasons, many scientists agreed that all smallpox stocks should be destroyed. Destruction of the smallpox virus would remind the world that global cooperation had eradicated a terrible disease, which was widely seen as an inspirational message. Some scientists continued to argue that samples of the virus should be preserved because techniques not yet invented might eventually determine important information about host specificity, virulence factors, and the evolution of viruses that could lead to improved diagnostic tests and the development of safer vaccines and antiviral drugs. This prediction was apparently confirmed when the sequencing of different strains of the smallpox virus led to the discovery of very interesting genes. Comparative analyses of the genes of different viruses might lead to a better understanding of the infectivity, virulence, and natural history of viruses. The current consensus among scientists is that the genes of the smallpox virus and other disease-causing viruses should be preserved and studied.

Variola, the smallpox virus, is a member of the Orthopoxvirus family, which includes cowpox, camelpox, swinepox, monkeypox, and so forth. Based on the characteristics of the poxviruses and genomic sequencing, the poxviruses probably evolved from a common ancestral virus whose natural host was a rodent. Although smallpox has no known animal reservoir, recently discovered poxviruses have demonstrated the ability to jump from other animals to humans. Monkeypox virus, a close relative of smallpox, was first discovered in the 1950s in monkeys in Zaire, but squirrels, mice, and other small rodents are its natural hosts. Until the 1990s, when an outbreak of monkeypox occurred in central Africa, scientists thought the disease only rarely spread to humans. Hundreds of cases of monkeypox occurred in humans, and the mortality rate was about 10 percent. Monkeypox was not seen outside of Africa until 2003, when Gambian giant pouched rats from Ghana were shipped to pet stores in the United States. The virus was transmitted to other rodents, including prairie dogs that were sold as pets. Eventually, about one hundred cases of monkeypox were reported in the Midwest, even among people who had been vaccinated against smallpox as children.

Although the smallpox virus is a member of the Orthopoxvirus family, it is remarkably specific to humans. Several different strains of the virus, distinguished primarily by their virulence, have been isolated. Historical and epidemiological evidence suggests that *Variola major*, the more dangerous strain of the virus, evolved in South Asia. *Variola minor*, a less virulent form, was most common in Europe and North Africa. The smallpox virus is such an unusually large virus that it was probably seen, if not understood, by researchers using the light microscope in the 1880s.

Despite Jenner's speculations about the relationship between a disease of horses and cowpox, the origin of the vaccinia virus remains unclear. Smallpox, cowpox, and vaccinia viruses are all members of the genus *Orthopoxvirus*, but they are distinct species and cannot be transformed into each other. Horsepox was extinct by the time scientists could identify different viral species and subtypes. Today, vaccinia survives only in laboratories. The genome of the vaccinia virus was completely sequenced in 1990. Four years later, scientists completed the sequencing of the smallpox virus. In contrast to the poliovirus, which has about 12 genes, the smallpox virus has 187 genes. Virologists hope that genetic and immunological studies of smallpox, vaccinia, and other poxviruses will explain many aspects of the history of viral diseases, their host specificity, and their virulence.

With the threat of naturally occurring smallpox eliminated, fears have grown that the virus could be used as an agent of biological warfare. The smallpox virus has been called the ideal agent for bioterrorism because it is stable, easy to grow, easily dispersed, and produces a contagious, disfiguring, and potentially lethal disease. Military experts agree that smallpox would not be effective on the battlefield, but the threat of smallpox outbreaks would certainly cause fear and hysteria in the general population. A smallpox outbreak could have devastating consequences because routine vaccinations ended with the eradication of the disease. Therefore, almost all people born since 1980 have no immunity to the virus. A worst-case scenario suggests that a 30 percent mortality rate for what would be a so-called virgin soil smallpox epidemic might be an underestimate. Bioterrorists would presumably select the most deadly viral subtype or attempt to create a more virulent strain by following the steps used in 2001 by researchers who modified the mousepox virus. The altered virus infected and killed previously immunized mice. Theoretically, genetic engineering could also modify the smallpox virus, but so-called human missiles or smallpox martyrs infected with natural smallpox virus could trigger an outbreak by coughing and sneezing in airports, shopping malls, theaters, and so forth. In a confined space with recirculating air, the rate of infection could be very high.

Smallpox may have been used as an agent of biological warfare in eighteenth-century America. Many anecdotes suggest that Europeans attempted to infect Native Americans by giving them blankets that had been used by smallpox patients. Clues found in diaries, journals, and military correspondence suggest that British commanders attempted to use smallpox against American rebels during the Revolutionary War. Suspicions about such efforts might have stimulated George Washington's decision to have his entire army secretly inoculated at Valley Forge in 1777. British soldiers were inoculated when they were inducted into the army, but smallpox was a constant threat to the Continental Army. Washington, who contracted the disease at age nineteen, was well aware of the debilitating effects of smallpox.

Ironically, the vaccines that eradicated smallpox are now considered too dangerous for general use in the absence of an imminent threat. During the 1960s, routine vaccination apparently resulted in one or two deaths per million, but significant numbers of people experienced minor to severe complications. Experts estimate that if the United States returned to universal vaccination, there might be 180 deaths each year. People with HIV/AIDS, autoimmune diseases, organ transplant recipients, cancer patients, pregnant women, infants, and people with certain skin diseases could not be vaccinated or exposed to people who had recently been vaccinated. During a smallpox epidemic, those at a high risk of complications from vaccinia virus would presumably be most vulnerable to the smallpox virus, unless they were well protected by herd immunity. A population that has no memory of smallpox is unlikely to accept the risks associated with vaccination. Indeed, surveys conducted in 2003 indicated that many members of the Infectious Diseases Society of America would not accept a smallpox vaccination. In 2003, the Advisory Committee on Immunization Practices advised against mass smallpox vaccination programs in the United States in the absence of an imminent threat.

Attempts to create biological weapons are inherently dangerous to those working with pathogens and to people close to production and storage facilities. In 1971, a Soviet field test of weaponized smallpox caused an outbreak in Aralsk, a port city in Kazakhstan. Investigators believe that a ship came too close to an island where biological weapons were prepared and tested. An infected crew member brought the virus back to Aralsk and transmitted the disease to others. Ten people contracted the disease, three who had never been vaccinated died, and thousands of people were vaccinated. Ken Alibek (Kanatjan Kalibekov), a Soviet scientist who defected to the United States in 1992, later revealed many aspects of the germ warfare program of the former Union of Soviet Socialist Republics (USSR). In his widely read account of Soviet germ warfare research, *Biohazard*, Alibek suggested that samples of smallpox virus might have been sold or hidden by scientists who lost their jobs when the USSR collapsed. According to Alibek, when WHO announced the success of smallpox eradication, the Soviets increased their research on smallpox as a bioweapon. In 1997, prompted in part by Alibek's revelations, the Pentagon embarked on a major program to make new vaccines for the military.

ATTEMPTS TO ERADICATE DISEASES THROUGH UNIVERSAL IMMUNIZATION: MEASLES AND POLIOMYELITIS

In 1974, with the endorsement of the United Nations, WHO adopted the goal of universal vaccination to protect all children from six preventable infectious diseases— measles, poliomyelitis, diphtheria, whooping cough, tetanus, and tuberculosis—by

1990. During the 1980s, fewer than 20 to 40 percent of children in developing countries were vaccinated against these diseases, but global health leaders thought that the goal of universal immunization was accepted by almost all nations.

MEASLES

Encouraged by the success of the battle against smallpox, public health advocates called for the eradication of measles, another highly contagious disease spread by an airborne virus. WHO officials believed this was a realistic goal because safe and effective measles vaccines had been available since the 1960s and the virus apparently had no animal reservoir. As in the case of smallpox, eradication of measles would end the need for vaccination. The measles virus is closely related to the virus that causes rinderpest, a contagious disease of cattle, which suggests that an ancestral form of the virus made the jump from cattle to humans. Because measles is one of the most contagious human diseases, it can only be maintained in densely populated communities. When first introduced into an isolated population, the disease can be deadly to adults and children, but all the survivors will be immune. Only children born after the epidemic will be susceptible if outsiders reintroduce the virus.

Despite the widespread assumption that measles is a relatively minor childhood illness, characterized by a distinctive rash, the virus can result in pneumonia, blindness, encephalitis, convulsions, coma, and death. If the measles virus establishes a latent infection, it can be reactivated months or years later as subacute sclerosing panencephalitis, a deadly brain disease. Measles still kills about one million children every year, mostly in developing countries. Researchers have discovered that children with vitamin A deficiency are particularly likely to become blind or die as a result of measles infection. Moreover, because measles infection temporarily suppresses the immune system, these children are vulnerable to other infectious diseases.

In the early 1960s, measles killed about six million children each year. After the measles vaccine was introduced in 1963, the number of cases dropped dramatically in wealthy nations. In the United States, the number of cases fell from about five hundred thousand in 1962 to about fifteen hundred in 1983. By 1990, vaccination rates had decreased and the number of measles cases had risen to about thirty thousand. Public health experts believe that vaccination rates approaching 100 percent are required to control measles because the disease is so contagious. The relationship between declining vaccination rates and a resurgence in measles has been demonstrated in many countries, but WHO officials estimated that the global measles campaign had saved more than two million lives between 1999 and 2007. In some areas, children vaccinated for measles and polio may also receive deworming medicine, vitamin A, and insecticide-treated bed nets.

POLIOMYELITIS

Poliomyelitis—also known as infantile paralysis—was one of the six preventable diseases selected by WHO for universal childhood immunization. Before the introduction of polio vaccine, poliomyelitis was one of the most feared epidemic childhood diseases because it could lead to permanent paralysis or death when the virus attacked the nervous system. During the 1980s, when the disease still infected as many as five hundred thousand children each year, WHO officials called for the global eradication of polio by 2002.

Until recent times, paralytic polio was apparently quite rare, even in areas where polio infections were common among infants, but there is suggestive evidence of sporadic cases in ancient Egypt and Greece. Eighteenth- and nineteenth-century physicians, however, recognized an epidemic illness in children that was followed by permanent weakness of the muscles of the lower limbs. Several particularly severe outbreaks in Europe and the United States at the end of the nineteenth century suggest that the disease was occurring more frequently among older children and young adults. Epidemiologists concluded that when polio was one of the common gastrointestinal diseases of infancy, most adults had developed immunity. Infants who were exposed to the virus were probably protected by maternal antibodies acquired during gestation and breast-feeding.

The history of epidemic diseases demonstrates that modern sanitation profoundly affected the prevalence and incidence of intestinal infections, but the impact of changes in sanitation was not the same for all diseases. Because the poliovirus is found in human excrement, the threat of paralytic polio depended on prevailing standards of hygiene and sanitation. In communities that made significant improvements in sanitation and infant care, older children and young adults remained susceptible to the virus. The great majority of polio infections apparently produced very mild symptoms, but some cases resulted in permanent paralysis, respiratory failure, and death. Some polio patients eventually experience a condition known as postpolio syndrome, characterized by fatigue, loss of muscle tissue, joint pain, and respiratory problems. Thus, polio experts warn that even if polio is successfully eradicated, the problems created by prior infections could continue for decades.

Unsuccessful attempts to identify the pathogen that caused polio suggested that the disease might be caused by a filterable virus. In 1908, Karl Landsteiner demonstrated that cell-free, filtered preparations of spinal cord could transmit paralytic polio to monkeys. Virologists initially assumed that the poliovirus was primarily associated with the nervous system, but in 1948, John Enders, Thomas Weller, and Frederick Robbins demonstrated that it was possible to grow poliovirus in several kinds of human tissue. For establishing the techniques that were crucial to the development of vaccines for polio and other viral diseases, Enders, Weller, and Robbins were awarded the 1954 Nobel Prize in Medicine or Physiology. Producing a vaccine for polio was complicated by the discovery that there were three significant poliovirus subtypes. The existence of distinct strains of the virus explained the fact that although repeated attacks of polio were rare, they were not impossible. Immunity to one type did not establish immunity to others. By the 1950s, virologists had identified three major immunological groups of polioviruses.

Many virologists attempted to create a polio vaccine, but the killed virus vaccine developed by Jonas Salk was the first to win universal acceptance. In 1947, Salk obtained support from the National Foundation for Infantile Paralysis to study the poliovirus and develop a vaccine. Salk established a vaccine by inactivating the virus with formaldehyde and testing his preparations in monkeys to be sure that the virus was dead. To demonstrate that his vaccine was safe and effective, Salk vaccinated himself, his wife, and his three young children. When Salk presented his preliminary findings to a meeting of the National Foundation in 1953, there were immediate calls for large trials. Several pharmaceutical companies, including Parke-Davis, Eli Lilly, and Cutter Laboratories, competed to produce vaccine for clinical trials that enrolled more than four hundred thousand children. When the results were analyzed in 1955, officials at the National Foundation and other experts concluded that the Salk vaccine was safe and effective. The publicity that followed this announcement was overwhelming, and few Americans realized that scientists were still debating the merits of killed versus live polio vaccines.

The National Foundation operated the 1954 field trials, but the federal government had the power to license and regulate commercial polio vaccines. The National Foundation demanded that manufacturers produce eleven consecutive lots of vaccine that passed their safety tests, but the federal government did not call for or enforce the same rigorous standards. Producing large quantities of vaccine in industrial facilities creates problems that are different from those encountered by researches producing relatively small amounts of vaccine. In 1955, defective polio vaccine produced by Cutter Laboratories in Berkeley, California, caused about two hundred cases of permanent paralysis and ten deaths. What was later called the *Cutter Incident* led to improved production methods and stricter testing standards. But the Cutter Incident also set the stage for a liability system that led many pharmaceutical companies to abandon the development, testing, production, and marketing of vaccines.

Early attempts to prepare live, attenuated poliovirus vaccines were generally considered unsuccessful because some of those who had been vaccinated excreted live, virulent virus. Critics argued that live poliovirus vaccines were inherently dangerous because weakened viruses might mutate or revert to a virulent state. Albert Sabin argued that although a killed poliovirus vaccine was easier to develop than a live, attenuated vaccine, its effects might not be as long lasting. Moreover, a live vaccine could be administered by mouth, mimicking the normal mode of infection and inducing long-term, or even permanent, immunity. The Sabin vaccine was developed by serially culturing all three important strains of poliovirus in monkey kidney cells to produce strains that were no longer dangerous in monkeys and humans. Despite the advantages of Sabin's oral vaccine, the National Foundation for Infantile Paralysis was committed to the Salk vaccine and was unwilling to sponsor rival vaccines. WHO, however, continued to support tests of oral polio vaccines, which were less expensive and easier to administer.

After large and highly successful clinical trials in Mexico, Czechoslovakia, Singapore, and the USSR, the oral polio vaccine was widely adopted. Problems emerged as the number of people vaccinated increased and the number of naturally acquired cases decreased. Live attenuated polioviruses could infect and produce immunity in people who came in contact with vaccinated infants. This phenomenon, known as contact immunity, seemed to be a good way to raise the general level of immunization. When naturally acquired polio remained a significant threat, the transmission of the virus from those who had received the vaccine to others was seen as an advantage. If unvaccinated people were at risk of contracting natural poliovirus, the benefits of spreading attenuated virus probably outweighed the dangers. Where the risk of contracting natural poliovirus was negligible, the transmission of attenuated poliovirus was potentially dangerous. By the 1980s, in countries that were essentially polio-free, the risks associated with live polio vaccine became greater than the risk of contracting the disease. The Americas were officially certified as a polio-free region in 1994. Eight years later, Europe had also been certified as polio-free. The United States and other wealthy countries generally abandoned the use of live oral polio vaccines, but immunization with injectable inactivated polio vaccine is considered necessary as long as polio exists in any part of the world (see Figure 6.2).

As in the case of smallpox, public health experts determined that the most effective and equitable way to prevent adverse reactions to polio vaccine in wealthy countries was to adopt the goal of eradicating the disease throughout the world. In 1988, the World Health Assembly established the Global Polio Eradication Initiative and called for the global eradication of polio by 2002. Although the goals set by the World Health Assembly proved to be overly optimistic, the global campaign did lead to dramatic reductions in the incidence of polio throughout the world. In 1988, polio was still endemic in 125 countries, and the disease paralyzed about one thousand children each day. In 2001, about six hundred cases were reported from ten countries. In 2004, half as many cases of paralytic polio were reported, but the disease was still endemic in India, Pakistan, Afghanistan, Egypt, Niger, and Nigeria. Although many countries apparently achieved total eradication of all three types of poliovirus by 2000, the threat of imported cases remained, as demonstrated by the resurgence of

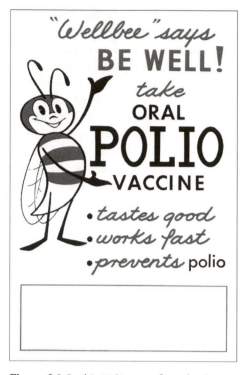

Figure 6.2 In this 1963 poster from the Centers for Disease Control and Prevention, "Wellbee," a symbol of American national public health programs, encouraged the public to adopt the Sabin oral polio vaccine. Credit: Global Health Odyssey Museum, Centers for Disease Control and Prevention, U.S. Department of Health and Human Services.

polio in Nigeria between 2000 and 2006 and the spread of the disease to neighboring countries. Increases in the number of paralytic polio cases in Nigeria were attributed to resistance to vaccination, primarily within the Muslim community. By 2005, hundreds of cases of paralytic polio in the region forced African countries that had been polio-free since 2000 to resume mass vaccination campaigns. Despite years of mass vaccination campaigns, polio remained a threat in India, Nigeria, Somalia, Niger, Afghanistan, Bangladesh, and Indonesia. In India, epidemiologists discovered that the oral polio vaccine was less effective in areas where diarrheal diseases were very common. By 2006, public health experts were questioning the feasibility of eradicating polio without a global commitment to improving the drinking water supplies and sanitary facilities of impoverished areas.

Although smallpox and polio can be prevented by vaccination and both viruses apparently have no natural animal reservoir or vectors, there are significant differences in the natural history of the two diseases. Unlike smallpox, polio is often a silent infection—not all who are infected show any significant symptoms—and infected individuals may continue to excrete poliovirus long after the acute phase of the disease is over. The small genome of the poliovirus, which has been sequenced and published on public databases, could be manipulated for many different purposes. In 2002, researchers in the growing field known as synthetic biology announced that they had synthesized a poliovirus that caused a paralytic disease in mice. Given the dangers of silent infections and the possibility that bioterrorists could create more virulent strains of poliovirus, a supposedly polio-free world could still contain hidden threats for unimmunized people. Critics of the polio eradication program question the assumption that routine immunization can be abandoned in polio-free countries. Several cases of polio in a small Amish community in Minnesota in 2005 confirmed warnings about the continued need for immunization.

Vaccines have had a greater impact on human health than any other single medical advance. As a result, adults who have never experienced the once universal childhood diseases tend to underestimate the dangers of these illnesses. In the United States alone, before vaccines became widely available, tens of thousands of children died every year of measles, whooping cough, and diphtheria. Each year, twenty thousand babies were born blind, deaf, or mentally retarded because their mothers had contracted rubella infections during pregnancy. Polio paralyzed thousands of children and killed hundreds. After the disintegration of the former Soviet Union, public health services, including routine vaccinations, were disrupted. Epidemiologists estimate that this resulted in some two hundred thousand cases of diphtheria and about five thousand deaths. Nevertheless, vaccines have also been associated with risks and adverse effects, some inherent in all medical interventions and some caused by errors of judgment, manufacture, and usage. The Cutter Incident was one of the most infamous disasters associated with the production of vaccines in America.

In 1955, shortly after the release of the Salk polio vaccine, defective vaccine produced by Cutter Laboratories of Berkeley, California, caused an epidemic of polio that affected thousands of people. Cutter vaccine, containing live polioviruses, was administered to about two hundred thousand people; about seventy thousand developed muscle weakness, two hundred were permanently paralyzed, and ten died. Reports of vaccine-associated deaths caused widespread panic and led to a temporary halt in vaccination and the establishment of stricter vaccine testing procedures. Investigators found that Cutter Laboratories made several mistakes in the production of polio vaccine and had failed to detect live virus in their final product. Cutter tested its vaccine on monkeys before children were inoculated and discarded bad lots, but the standard safety tests were not sensitive enough to detect small numbers of live viruses.

After the success of the 1954 polio field trial, the Laboratory of Biologics Control, a federal agency within the National Institutes of Health, was charged with licensing the polio vaccines produced by Eli Lilly, Parke-Davis, Pitman-Moore, Wyeth, and Cutter. Because of high demand, polio vaccines were licensed and rushed to market despite warnings by scientists at the Laboratory of Biologics Control. Soon after the Cutter vaccine was released, physicians began reporting cases of children who became paralyzed, usually in the injected arm. Even though scientists were quite certain that many lots of the Cutter vaccine contained live virus, taking action was difficult because the 1902 Biologics Control Act, which gave the federal government the power to regulate the shipment of sera, antitoxins, and vaccines for human diseases, did not give the agency the authority to force a manufacturer to stop selling a licensed vaccine.

When the Surgeon General asked Cutter to recall all lots of its polio vaccine, the company complied, but Cutter officials continued to argue that their vaccine had not caused paralytic polio. Naturally acquired polio was still a serious threat at the time, which made this argument plausible, but extremely unlikely, according to statistical evidence presented by epidemiologists at the Centers for Disease Control and Prevention (CDC). According to Alexander Langmuir's Epidemic Intelligence Service, the incidence of paralysis in children who received contaminated vaccine was about ten times greater than expected, based on the average incidence of paralysis in children for the preceding five years. Furthermore, the paralytic effect of the vaccine-caused virus was more severe than naturally acquired polio, presumably because virulent type 1 virus had been injected directly into muscle tissue.

Rather than admitting blame, Cutter officials argued that the science of virology and the difficulties of producing vaccine were irrelevant to companies that produced government-approved vaccines. As a manufacturer, Cutter claimed it was only responsible for following the guidelines established by the government. Many civil lawsuits against companies that had produced polio vaccine (Cutter, Wyeth, Eli Lilly, and Parke-Davis) were settled out of court, but the 1958 *Gottsdanker v. Cutter Laboratories* verdict became a landmark for future claims against pharmaceutical companies. Lawyers for a child paralyzed by Cutter vaccine argued that by selling "inactivated polio vaccine," Cutter became responsible for a 100 percent warranty that the vaccine would not cause polio. In his instructions to the jury, the judge essentially said that if the vaccine paralyzed the plaintiff, the jury must find Cutter guilty; that is, Cutter could not escape liability for damages by arguing that it had complied with established procedures. The jury found Cutter guilty and awarded $125,000 to the plaintiff, although members of the jury did not consider Cutter negligent. In an unsuccessful appeal, Cutter's lawyers warned that liability without fault would inhibit the development of new products. As a legal landmark, the Cutter verdict introduced the principle that a manufacturer could be found "not negligent" but still financially liable for the harm its product had done. The Cutter decision also raised questions about who would bear the burden for injuries from vaccines: pharmaceutical companies, the government, insurance companies, the injured parties, or the public as a whole?

Critics of the lawsuits and trial decisions that found Cutter liable warned that this precedent would inhibit the development and marketing of vaccines. Vaccines benefit the world as a whole, but they account for a very small part of the profits of large pharmaceutical companies and a very large part of their liability issues. According to a study released by the CDC in 2007, death rates in the United States for thirteen diseases that can be prevented by childhood vaccines fell to their lowest point in 2006. Since the introduction of routine vaccination in the United States, many previously deadly childhood diseases, including smallpox, diphtheria, polio, measles, and rubella, have essentially disappeared, and others have decreased dramatically. Children are usually vaccinated against diphtheria, pertussis, tetanus, hepatitis B, polio, bacterial pneumonia, hemophilus influenza, measles, mumps, and rubella, but other vaccines are becoming available.

Rubella vaccine is usually administered as part of the MMR vaccine (measles, mumps, rubella). By the end of the twentieth century, wherever rubella vaccine was widely used, this once-universal disease essentially disappeared. However, because the disease remains endemic in many developing countries, the virus is still a threat to all unprotected children and pregnant women. Rubella, which is also known as German or three-day measles, is a high contagious disease that leads to a characteristic rash, mild respiratory symptoms, and lifelong immunity. Because of the rash and the brief duration of the illness in children, rubella was originally thought of as a mild form of measles, but by the end of the nineteenth century, it was officially recognized as a distinct disease. Adult women sometimes experience serious complications when infected, but the major danger is to a fetus in the first trimester of pregnancy. The relationship between rubella and birth defects was first recognized in the 1940s when Sir Norman Gregg, an Australian ophthalmologist, drew attention to the high frequency of congenital cataracts in babies born to women who had contracted rubella during their pregnancy. Major outbreaks of rubella in the 1960s confirmed the relationship between the disease and a group of birth defects, collectively known as congenital rubella syndrome (CRS): cataracts, blindness, heart defects, deafness, and mental retardation. The isolation of the rubella virus in 1961, and the surge in cases of CRS, stimulated the development and widespread use of live attenuated rubella vaccines. Herpesvirus and cytomegalovirus (CMV) are also known to cause serious birth defects. CMV infections acquired during fetal development or at birth may cause microencephaly, encephalitis, seizures, deafness, mental retardation, or death. Researchers suspect that other obscure viral and bacterial infections might play a role in fetal damage and infant mortality.

ANTIVACCINATIONISTS AND VACCINE RESISTERS

Antivaccination protests began with the introduction of smallpox inoculation and grew more focused in response to attempts to mandate universal smallpox vaccination. From the beginning, leaders of the antivaccine movement questioned the validity of statistics used to demonstrate the safety and effectiveness of smallpox vaccination. During the 1960s, the value of preventive vaccines was generally appreciated because the danger of polio, measles, rubella, mumps, diphtheria, pertussis (whooping cough), and even smallpox was understood. By the 1990s, public health experts noted a shift in the socioeconomic groups most likely to avoid mandatory vaccines. Before the 1990s, incomplete vaccination was most common among poor, uninsured children, but after the 1994 Vaccines for Children Program minimized the economic obstacles, wealthy and middle-class families were more likely to avoid immunizations than impoverished families. Infectious disease experts have tried to warn the public that modern antivaccinationism has become a significant threat to the public health.

The antivaccination activism and hostility to compulsory immunization associated with Jennerian vaccination never entirely disappeared, but the modern backlash against routine immunization began in the 1970s with reports from Great Britain that claimed that pertussis vaccine caused permanent brain damage. Pertussis, better known as whooping cough, is a bacterial infection caused by *Bordetella pertussis*, which produces toxins that attack the cells lining the respiratory tract. Infants, the elderly, and people with a weakened immune system are most likely to experience life-threatening complications such as hemorrhages, fractured ribs, hernias, pneumonia, convulsions, encephalitis, spastic paralysis, mental retardation, and other neurological disorders. Before the introduction of the pertussis vaccine in the 1940s, whooping cough was one of the leading causes of death in young children in the United States. The combined pertussis, diphtheria, and tetanus (DPT) vaccine was considered a major advance in vaccinology, but the vaccine was associated with a high incidence of side effects. According to antivaccination activists, the pertussis components of the vaccine caused epilepsy, mental retardation, learning disorders, Reye's syndrome, sudden infant death syndrome (SIDS), and other adverse reactions. Despite the introduction of an improved DPT vaccine in the 1990s, the vaccine remained the major focus of antivaccination activity. In the United States, hundreds of lawsuits were filed against manufacturers. In response, pharmaceutical companies raised the price of the vaccine or withdrew from the market. Outbreaks of pertussis increased in many countries as immunization rates fell. In England, immunization rates dropped from 80 to 30 percent. Deaths occurred among the tens of thousands of children hospitalized by the disease. Statistical studies demonstrating that there was no increase in the incidence of neurological conditions in vaccinated children had no effect on antivaccine activists. Epidemiological studies, according to antivaccine activists, fail to discover a subset of the population that is particularly susceptible to vaccine-induced injuries.

With growing distrust of authority—including government, science, and the pharmaceutical industry—skepticism about the safety of vaccines increased in the last decades of the twentieth century. Antivaccine groups claim that vaccines are unnatural and inherently dangerous toxins that are responsible for life-threatening diseases and disabilities. Vaccines have been blamed for many disorders, including autism, learning disabilities, multiple sclerosis, and a form of paralysis known as Guillain-Barré syndrome. Pediatricians note that convincing people that the benefits of vaccination clearly outweigh the risks has become increasingly difficult. Growing resistance to vaccines can be seen as a consequence of the success of vaccinations and the common but false assumption that all infectious diseases can be cured by antibiotics. Vaccines have been so successful that by 2000, most people in wealthy, industrialized nations had no direct knowledge of poliomyelitis, diphtheria, pertussis, measles, mumps, or rubella. Therefore, they generally underestimate the danger of infectious diseases and overestimate the risks of vaccination. Although all medical interventions may cause adverse effects in some people, the side effects associated with vaccination are rare and generally much less serious than the effects of the disease.

Many stories of adverse effects that are blamed on vaccination are actually examples of the *post hoc ergo propter hoc* logical fallacy: the unwarranted assumption that an event that follows a prior action was caused by that prior action. According to the dictates of science and logic, the components of a vaccine do not necessarily cause all adverse events that occur days, months, or years after vaccination. As indicated by Koch's postulates, proving causality is a difficult process. Nevertheless, the influence of the antivaccination movement has been growing since the 1990s, resulting in increased demands for exemptions to mandatory immunizations for school-age children. Despite mandatory immunization rules for most school systems, obtaining exemptions is not very difficult in the United States. Every state allows medical exemptions for children who are immunocompromised or allergic to vaccines, almost all states allow exemptions based on religious beliefs, and many allow exemptions for philosophical or personal beliefs. Religious exemptions have led to outbreaks of polio, measles, and rubella in Amish, Mennonite, and Christian Science communities. Some churches have been established as a way of securing donations from parents seeking certificates that guarantee religious exemptions. Demands for exemptions are particularly high in certain parts of Oregon, Washington, and California. Where such trends become entrenched, outbreaks of measles, mumps, pertussis, and other preventable diseases endanger unvaccinated babies and children as well as those who are susceptible because of their age or medical problems. Some parents who reject vaccination as dangerous and unnatural advocate a return to the ancient folk practice of deliberately exposing children to "natural" cases of childhood illnesses to build immunity, forgetting how natural it was for children to die of diseases that can be prevented with vaccines. As Benjamin Franklin warned parents, there is no way of predicting the severity or outcome of a disease that has been contracted in the natural way. Vaccine resistance is not, of course, limited to the wealthy, industrialized nations. The resurgence of polio in Nigeria and India, in areas where Muslim critics of vaccination claimed that polio vaccine caused sterility in girls, demonstrated that many factors can affect parental attitudes toward vaccines.

In 1986, the United States created the National Vaccine Injury Compensation Program, as part of the National Childhood Vaccine Injury Act. The purpose of the program was to encourage manufacturers to continue production of vaccines despite the threat of lawsuits. Scientists, epidemiologists, statisticians, and other experts were asked to evaluate and review scientific evidence and present their findings to a special vaccine court. People could not sue manufacturers without going through the federal vaccine court, but if the court agreed that a child had been injured by a vaccine, the program would provide compensation for medical expenses and damages. Pharmaceutical companies claim that the system does not provide sufficient protection and inhibits the availability and development of vaccines for adults. Critics of the program argue that the compensation program intensifies suspicion and fear of vaccines, without educating the public about the risks and benefits of vaccination.

In the 1990s, the principal targets of antivaccine litigation were the MMR vaccine and thimerosal (a mercury-based preservative used in some vaccines), based on allegations that the vaccine caused autism. Autism, a neurological disorder that causes problems with behavior, communication, and the ability to have normal social interactions, is said to affect 1 in 150 children. Between 1999 and 2007, the parents of about five thousand children with autism filed claims in vaccine court. MMR has been in widespread use in the United States since the early 1970s, and since 1988 in the United Kingdom. Large, well-controlled studies that have followed thousands of children for twelve or more years after immunization with the MMR vaccine have not found any linkage between autism and the vaccine, with or without thimerosal. The removal of thimerosal from childhood vaccines in 2001 had no apparent effect on autism rates. Major medical studies indicate that the alleged relationship between autism and MMR, with or without thimerosal, is coincidental, rather than causal. Children are routinely vaccinated at the age when autism is first recognized. The debate about thimerosal may be replaced by a case presented in 2008, which argued that the "stress" of vaccination caused or aggravated a mitochondrial disorder, resulting in so-called mitochondrial autism.

Epidemiological studies that find no causal relationship between MMR and autism have been largely ignored by the popular media and have had very little impact on the public perception that vaccines are dangerous. Popular media reports generally disregarded scientific studies and emphasized sensational stories linking the vaccine to autism. The press gave particular attention to an article published in the prestigious medical journal *The Lancet* in 1998, by British researcher Andrew Wakefield. Despite the fact that his study included only twelve children and had no control group, media reports proclaimed that Wakefield's work proved that MMR causes autism and inflammatory bowel disease. Close scrutiny of Wakefield's work by scientists and investigative reporters found serious discrepancies in the *Lancet* paper as well as a very lucrative business relationship between Wakefield and lawyers representing the families of autistic children in lawsuits against vaccine manufacturers. When critics suggested that a conflict of interest raised serious questions about Wakefield's objectivity and credibility, Wakefield argued that objectivity was not relevant to the *Lancet* paper because it was a clinical report, rather than a scientific paper. Media reports, however, focused on the alleged causal relationship between MMR and autism. Fears generated by the media storm promoting Wakefield's claims were blamed for a precipitous decline in immunization rates, followed by dramatic increases in cases of measles and mumps.

When evaluating the safety and efficacy of vaccines, the balance between risks and benefits may be very different in wealthy and poor countries. Preventive vaccines are desperately needed in the developing world, where the burden of infectious disease is very high and medical resources are limited. However, vaccines that are highly effective in wealthy countries may not be as effective in impoverished areas, as demonstrated by problems with the polio vaccine and the rotavirus vaccine. Rotavirus, which causes diarrhea in infants and young children, is so common that almost all children are exposed to the virus by age five. Most cases are mild, but diarrhea and vomiting can lead to severe dehydration and death. Although intravenous rehydration is almost always effective, the disease kills more than six hundred thousand children each year. A rotavirus vaccine introduced in 1998 was withdrawn one year later because it was associated with intussusception, a life-threatening blockage of the intestines. This condition, which occurs spontaneously for unknown reasons, was reported in one in ten thousand vaccinated children. For poor countries, the benefits of the vaccine would have outweighed the slight risk, but manufacturers could not market a vaccine that was ruled unsafe in the United States. When a new oral rotavirus vaccine was approved in 2006, large clinical trials suggested that the rate of intussusception was about the same in children who got the vaccine and those who got a placebo. Within a year, questions were being raised about the safety of the vaccine, even though epidemiological data indicated that the number of cases of intussusception in children who received the vaccine was significantly lower than the expected number of spontaneous cases.

Most antivaccine activity has focused on childhood vaccines, but attempts to mandate immunization of specific groups of adults have also been controversial. In response to the threat of bioterrorism, policy makers called for mandatory immunization of members of the armed forces and first responders against pathogens that might be used as weapons. The vaccines available for smallpox and anthrax, the diseases most likely to be used as bioweapons, are very controversial because of potential adverse effects. In 1998, in response to warnings that Iraq and other nations had produced biological weapons, the U.S. Department of Defense launched its Anthrax Vaccine Immunization Program. Antivaccine groups mobilized against the vaccination program, claiming that it caused Gulf War syndrome and other medical problems. In 2002, the Pentagon agreed to vaccinate only troops with the highest risk of exposure to anthrax, but many soldiers refused to be vaccinated.

CANCER VIRUSES AND VACCINES

Since the introduction of Jenner's cowpox vaccine, almost all vaccines have been developed though trial and error. Vaccinologists are now hopeful that progress in molecular biology, genomics, and immunology will lead to the design of vaccines for diseases like malaria, tuberculosis, and HIV/AIDS, which have resisted conventional vaccines. Studies of the more subtle, chronic effects of pathogenic microbes may also lead to the development of vaccines that will prevent, cure, or alleviate chronic infections, autoimmune disorders, allergies, and certain kinds of cancer.

Evidence of a causal link between cancer and viruses had been established by Francis Peyton Rous in 1910. It was not until 1966 that Rous finally received the Nobel Prize in Medicine or Physiology, which acknowledged his contributions to the study of animal tumor viruses and stimulated hope that vaccines might prevent human cancers. The first licensed vaccine against a cancer caused by a virus was developed by Maurice R. Hilleman to prevent a contagious, often fatal disease that poultry farmers called *range paralysis*, or Marek's disease. Viral infection resulted in damage to the nerves of the leg, leading to paralysis, and tumors of the skin, heart, kidneys, liver, ovaries, and spleen. The herpesvirus that causes Marek's disease affected about 20 percent of all chickens grown in the United States and killed about 30 percent of the affected birds. Although little known outside the world of vaccinology, Hilleman is credited with major contributions to the development of vaccines for measles, mumps, hepatitis A, hepatitis B, chicken pox, meningitis, pneumonia, and *Haemophilus influenzae* bacteria. Hilleman's vaccine for Marek's disease can be thought of as proof of the concept that it is possible to establish vaccines that can prevent cancers caused by viruses. The hepatitis B vaccine, licensed in 1981, can be thought of as the first vaccine to prevent a human cancer, a form of liver cancer associated with the hepatitis B virus. A more complex and controversial cancer vaccine, designed to prevent cervical cancer caused by certain strains of the human papilloma virus (HPV), was awarded approval by the U.S. Food and Drug Administration (FDA) in 2006.

In 1932, Richard Shope identified a virus as the cause of a bizarre kind of tumor found in the semilegendary creatures known as jackalopes—rabbits with large warts or tumors that looked like horns. Shope proved that he could transmit these rabbit fibromas to healthy laboratory rabbits by injecting them with cell-free extracts of the tumors. The rabbit papilloma virus is a member of a large family of viruses that cause warts, genital warts, cervical cancer, and other disorders in humans. Identification of HPV and recognition of the role that HPV plays in the development of human cancers was the culmination of centuries of observation, speculation, and research. A paper published by Italian physician Domenico Antonio Rigoni-Stern in 1842 on the prevalence of various diseases, including cervical cancer and breast cancer, has been cited as one of the first attempts to find differences among the groups of women who succumbed to these diseases. Because married women were more likely to die of cervical cancer than nuns, and nuns were more likely to die of breast cancer than married women, doctors suggested that cervical cancer might be related to a woman's sexual history.

Epidemiological studies indicated that about half of all women with cervical cancer had a history of genital herpes. Searching for other possible viral agents that might be linked to cervical cancer, Harald zur Hausen found suggestive evidence that HPVs associated with genital warts might be linked to cervical cancer. Zur Hausen and his coworkers found two previously unknown strains of HPV, HPV16 and HPV18, in about 70 percent of cervical cancer biopsies. By the mid-1980s, zur Hausen was seeking support for the development of a vaccine to prevent cancers induced by HPV. Virologists eventually identified more than one hundred different strains of the papilloma virus. About forty HPV strains are sexually transmitted and capable of causing genital warts, but HPV16 and HPV18 seem to be responsible for the vast majority of cancers of the cervix, vagina, penis, anus, and rectum.

In the United States, HPV has become the most common sexually transmitted infection. Epidemiologists estimate that at least 50 percent of sexually active men and women contract genital HPV, but many people have no symptoms. Only a small percentage of HPV-infected women develop cervical cancer, but 470,000 new cases and 240,000 deaths occur each year. About 80 percent of all cervical cancer deaths occur in developing countries. In the United States, the Papanicolaou test (Pap smear), named for George N. Papanicolaou, has been used since the 1950s to detect precancerous lesions. New tests that detect specific HPV markers are under development. Despite the emphasis on early detection, about four thousand American women die of cervical cancer every year, and thousands undergo painful medical procedures to remove precancers and early cancers caused by HPV.

Pharmaceutical companies had developed several experimental HPV vaccines by 2006, when Gardasil, Merck's HPV vaccine, was approved for use in the United States. Gardasil targets four strains of HPV that collectively cause about 70 to 90 percent of all cervical cancers and genital warts. Because the same strains of HPV cause both cervical and anal cancer, officials in Australia and the European Union approved Gardasil for boys aged nine to fifteen. Excitement about a vaccine that could prevent cancer was initially very high, but recommendations that all girls receive Gardasil before entering the sixth grade made the HPV vaccine exceptionally controversial.

Gardasil sparked debates about the economic, political, and cultural impact of preventive immunizations. Opponents of Gardasil included antivaccinationists, groups that distrusted the drug industry, and religious and cultural conservatives who objected to discussing the relationship between HPV and sexual activity with preteen girls. Critics argued that public health officials could not assert a compelling reason for mandatory HPV immunizations because the virus was not transmitted during normal school activities. Religious fundamentalists called mandatory vaccinations for HPV an intrusion into private family issues. Abstinence-only advocates argued that the vaccine would encourage promiscuity. Those who welcomed a vaccine that could prevent specific cancers were concerned about securing equal access to a very expensive vaccine and the financial burden it would entail for parents, government agencies, and international public health programs.

INSECT AND ARTHROPOD VECTORS OF DISEASE

Public health measures that attempted to prevent epidemic diseases by isolating the sick or eliminating noxious air and contaminated water had little or no impact on diseases transmitted by insect and arthropod vectors. Ancient writers had speculated about the role of insects in the transmission of disease, but scientific proof was not established until the late nineteenth century. Some of the most devastating epidemic diseases in human history are transmitted by mosquitoes, fleas, ticks, and mites. In many diseases associated with these vectors, human beings are the accidental victims of pathogenic viruses, bacteria, protozoans, and parasitic worms that have a natural reservoir in reptiles, birds, and mammals. By the 1920s, more than two hundred diseases had been linked to insect and arthropod vectors.

Credit for establishing the relationship between mosquito vectors and human diseases is traditionally attributed to Patrick Manson and Ronald Ross. In 1880, Patrick Manson demonstrated the role of the mosquito in transmitting elephantiasis (filariasis) and other diseases caused by parasitic worms. In the case of elephantiasis, tiny filarial worms damage the lymphatic system, causing gross enlargement of the legs and scrotum. According to Manson's "mosquito theory," these insects served as intermediate hosts and carriers of the parasites that cause tropical diseases. After studying Manson's work, Ronald Ross demonstrated that the malaria parasite, which Charles-Louis-Alphonse Laveran had discovered in human red blood cells, was transmitted by Anopheles mosquitoes. These discoveries suggested that if the causative agents for specific diseases were transmitted by insects or arthropods, the geographical distribution of fleas, mosquitoes, lice, bugs, sand flies, ticks, and so forth, would determine the distribution of the disease.

YELLOW FEVER

Since the early twentieth century, yellow fever has generally been confined to developing countries, but it was one of the most feared epidemic diseases of eighteenth-century America. Epidemics occurred in Philadelphia, New Orleans, Savannah, Mobile, Charleston, and the islands of the Caribbean. Indeed, yellow fever, malaria, and the African slave trade played a large role in shaping the population of the Caribbean. Epidemic yellow fever killed many European settlers and forced others to leave the islands. Many Europeans erroneously concluded that Africans were essentially immune to yellow fever. Whether or not yellow fever was present in pre-Columbian America is uncertain, but immunological and entomological studies suggest that the virus was brought to the Americas from Africa. *Aedes aegypti*, the mosquito that is the best vector of the yellow fever virus, might have been brought to the Americas as a result of the African slave trade.

Yellow fever begins with fever, chills, headache, severe pains in the back and limbs, sore throat, nausea, and vomiting. Determining the fatality rate is difficult because mild cases are often ignored or mistaken for malaria. Studies of yellow fever in Africa suggest that about 15 to 20 percent of those who contract the virus experience jaundice, high fever, delirium, kidney failure, and hemorrhaging from the mouth, nose, and eyes. About 20 to 50 percent of those with the severe form of the disease become comatose and die. Like the onset of jaundice, the "black vomit," which reveals bleeding into the stomach, was considered an ominous sign. In northern regions, yellow fever epidemics always appeared during the summer and vanished with the return of cold weather. The devastating 1793 epidemic in Philadelphia, then America's cultural, social, and political center, was particularly striking. When winter finally brought an end to the outbreak, about 10 to 15 percent of the approximately forty thousand residents of Philadelphia had died of the disease. Benjamin Rush, the new republic's most prominent physician, attributed the epidemic to local conditions, including the morbid vapors released by rotting materials on the city's wharf. His critics insisted that the disease had been imported from the West Indies and called for the imposition of strict quarantine regulations. Nevertheless, yellow fever did not seem to be transmitted by a contagion because people who took care of the sick did not necessarily become ill.

Yellow fever became a disease of special interest to the United States as a result of the Spanish American War of 1898 and the subsequent occupation of Cuba. Because of the threat to the American army in 1900, the Surgeon General sent a team of doctors, headed by Walter Reed, to discover the cause and means of transmission of yellow fever. Members of the Yellow Fever Commission met with Cuban physician Juan Carlos Finlay, who had assembled suggestive evidence that the disease was transmitted by the bite of the female Culex mosquito (now known as *Aedes aegypti*). Serving as their own guinea pigs, Reed's colleagues proved that yellow fever was not transmitted by fomites or miasma. Only infected mosquitoes, or blood from a patient, transmitted the disease. The infectious agent could not be identified under the microscope, but filtered blood serum could transmit the disease. Blood serum that had been heated did not transmit the disease, which suggested that the causative agent was a filterable virus, rather than a toxin. The causative agent was only present in the blood of victims during the first three to six days of infection. Mosquitoes could not transmit the virus for a ten-day period after biting an infected person, but after this incubation period, they remained infective for the rest of their lives.

The realization that mosquitoes transmitted yellow fever established a new focus for public health campaigns. In many cities, mosquito control was so effective that public health workers predicted that yellow fever would soon be extinct. Unfortunately, the discovery of so-called jungle yellow fever among wild primates in South America and Africa effectively ended all hope of eradicating the virus. While the threat of urban epidemics could generally be minimized, the only way to fully protect individuals at risk was to establish a preventive vaccine. The first safe and effective yellow fever vaccine was developed in the 1930s by Max Theiler, who won the 1951 Nobel Prize in Medicine or Physiology for demonstrating that yellow fever was caused by a virus. Unfortunately, the vaccine has always been too expensive for routine use in areas threatened by yellow fever. Thus, public health workers continued to focus on eliminating insect vectors and unsanitary conditions to control the disease. Researchers hope that studies of the viral genome may lead to better diagnostic tests, vaccines, and treatments as well as an understanding of the evolutionary relationship between the yellow fever virus and other RNA viruses.

According to WHO, yellow fever still causes about thirty thousand deaths each year, and the disease seems to be reemerging in areas where it was generally under control. Public health experts warn that simultaneous outbreaks in densely populated African cities would rapidly deplete the entire international stockpile of vaccine. Vaccination campaigns from 1940 to 1960 dramatically reduced the incidence of yellow fever. Those who were vaccinated probably acquired lifelong immunity, but those who were born after these programs ended were vulnerable when the disease returned in the 1990s. Modern cities provide many havens for *Aedes aegypti*, and the virus found a new population lacking natural or vaccine-induced immunity. In 2007, WHO, the Global Alliance for Vaccines and Immunization, and other agencies launched a major initiative to vaccinate millions of people in West Africa.

MALARIA

Malaria has often been called the most devastating disease in history. Hiding among the undifferentiated "fevers" found in every part of the world, malaria has caused more misery and taken more lives than any other disease. Malaria can be chronic, endemic, debilitating, and deadly. Symptoms of malaria may include headache, thirst, fever, shivering, nausea, delirium, and convulsions, but in particular, malaria involves episodes of fevers and chills that alternate with periods of apparent remission. Ancient physicians paid close attention to the timing of the patient's symptoms and divided febrile illnesses into intermittent and continuous fevers. Humans are vulnerable to several forms of malaria that differ in severity, from the most common form, known as benign tertian malaria, to the deadly malignant tertian malaria. Physicians generally described three types of malaria, which were referred to as benign tertian (fevers every third day), benign quartan (fevers every fourth day), and malignant tertian (almost continuous fever). Unlike many other infectious diseases, recovering from one attack of malaria does not provide immunity against further attacks.

Malaria is caused by obligate intracellular protozoan parasites of the genus *Plasmodium*. More than one hundred species of *Plasmodium* are known, but only four species cause human malaria: *Plasmodium falciparum*, *Plasmodium vivax*, *Plasmodium malariae*, and *Plasmodium ovale*. Other strains of the malaria parasite are known to infect apes, monkeys, rodents, birds, and reptiles. By differentiating the four species of human malarial parasites, scientists were able to associate the traditional clinical forms of the disease with their specific causative agents. *P. falciparum*, which causes malignant tertian malaria, is found in tropical regions. As its descriptive name suggests, the disease is very often fatal because of damage to the heart, kidneys, respiratory system, and central nervous system. Benign tertian, or relapsing, malaria, in which the fever recurs every third day, is associated with both *P. vivax* and *P. ovale*. Vivax malaria, which is common in subtropical and temperate regions, is very persistent and difficult to cure because latent parasites can remain in the liver for months or even years. Although vivax malaria is rarely fatal, it can result in severe complications, including deadly cerebral malaria. *P. ovale*, the least common malarial species, is usually found in Africa. Benign quartan malaria, in which fever recurs every fourth day, is caused by *P. malariae* and occurs only in subtropical areas. Pregnant women with malaria are at particular risk of complications because the parasites readily colonize the placenta, leading to severe infections in both the mother and the fetus. In areas where malaria is endemic, it is a major cause of stillbirths, low birth weight, and infant death.

Although today malaria is thought of as a tropical disease, malarial fevers were previously endemic in much of Europe and the Americas, as far north as Canada and Scandinavia. Throughout history, natural and social forces have affected the distribution of the disease, sometimes allowing malaria to become endemic in some

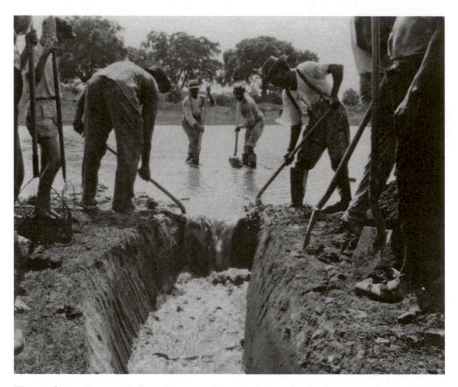

Figure 6.3 A photograph from the 1920s shows workers in the southern United States digging a drainage ditch to promote mosquito control. Eliminating standing water reduced the breeding ground for the *Anopheles* mosquitoes that spread malaria and other diseases. Credit: Public Health Image Library, Centers for Disease Control and Prevention, U.S. Department of Health and Human Services.

areas and sometimes eliminating the environmental factors that allow the disease to persist. Malaria has been a significant force in human evolution and in determining the success or failure of settlements and colonial ventures throughout the world. War, land development, changes in the distribution and flow of water, failing public health systems, globalization, and climate change can create conditions that favor the malaria parasite and its mosquito vector. The ancient Greeks and Romans attributed malaria to the noxious vapors thought to arise from swamps, but the basis of the relationship between malaria and the mosquitoes that thrived in marshy areas was not discovered until the end of the nineteenth century. Anopheline mosquitoes are essential to the complex life cycle of malaria parasites, both as vectors and as hosts in which *Plasmodia* complete part of their growth cycle. Female mosquitoes acquire malaria parasites by taking a blood meal from an infected human carrier. Infected mosquitoes carry the parasites in their salivary glands and transmit them to new victims when they take another blood meal (see Figure 6.3).

Human evolution, as revealed by the selection of genes that provide some protection from malaria, testifies to the antiquity and pervasiveness of malaria. Genes that offered a selective advantage when malaria was a major threat also created a burden in the form of genetic diseases such as sickle cell anemia and thalassemia. Sickle cell disease is the result of a mutation in the hemoglobin gene that changes the shape and properties of the hemoglobin molecule. Red blood cells carrying the altered hemoglobin can assume an abnormal sickle shape. If these cells are infected by malaria parasites, they may be destroyed by the spleen before the parasites are able to reproduce and attack new blood cells. In areas where malaria is highly prevalent, individuals who have inherited genes for both sickle cell hemoglobin and normal hemoglobin are apparently more likely to survive and reproduce. Unfortunately, individuals who inherit the sickle cell gene from both parents develop sickle cell anemia and were unlikely to survive to adolescence. Malaria was such a strong selective force throughout human history that in some populations, the frequency of the sickle cell gene was as high as 10 percent. Several other forms of mutated hemoglobin are found in Africa and Southeast Asia, where malaria was highly endemic.

Cinchona, the first effective remedy for malaria, has been called one of the most valuable drugs in human history. Europeans did not learn about the medical virtues of cinchona until the 1630s, but Peruvian Indians had traditionally used a preparation derived from the bark of the cinchona tree as a remedy for fevers. During the seventeenth century, European physicians discovered that when carefully prepared and administered, cinchona (also known as Peruvian bark, Jesuits' bark, or devil's bark) provided a specific remedy for malaria. In 1820, chemists identified quinine as the active ingredient in cinchona. Quinine made it possible for Europeans to survive in malarial regions and was a significant factor in the establishment of European colonial rule, especially in Africa.

Since the introduction of quinine, researchers have identified many chemicals that can kill malaria parasites, but very few of these potential remedies were both safe and effective. Many once powerful antimalaria drugs lost their effectiveness because of indiscriminate and inappropriate use. Chloroquine, a synthetic derivative of quinine, was developed in the 1940s, but drug-resistant *Plasmodia* strains began to appear in the 1960s, and by 2000, chloroquine was virtually useless. Artemisinin, the most valuable new antimalaria drug, was isolated from a traditional Chinese medicinal plant known as sweet wormwood (*Artemisia annua*) in the 1960s. When taken alone, artemisinin quickly reduces fevers, but it usually takes at least seven days to rid the body of malaria parasites. Malariologists say artemisinin should be used only in combination with other drugs to reduce the chance that resistance to any one drug will develop.

Ever since the introduction of cinchona, victims of malaria have been plagued by quacks and charlatans selling counterfeit drugs. In many areas, investigators have found that more than half of the antimalaria drugs sold in local markets were coun-terfeit. Epidemiologists estimate that a fifth of the one million annual deaths from malaria could be prevented if all the antimalaria medicines in the marketplace were genuine. Given the toll taken by malaria, public health workers would like to see drug counterfeiting treated as a form of manslaughter.

During the first half of the twentieth century, the conquest of malaria seemed to be a real possibility. In the 1950s, WHO endorsed malaria eradication programs that relied on chloroquine and the insecticide dichlorodiphenyltrichloroethane (DDT). DDT, which repels and kills mosquitoes, was considered the most effective weapon in the battle against malaria and other mosquito-borne diseases. Much of the credit for the virtual eradication of malaria in the United States, Europe, Latin America, and many parts of India and Asia has been attributed to DDT. Public health advocates warned that the eradication of malaria in rich countries was a disaster for people with malaria in poor countries. Geopolitical and economic factors, along with the emergence of chloroquine-resistant parasites, pesticide-resistant mosquitoes, and the fear of DDT that followed the publication of Rachel Carson's *Silent Spring* (1962), led to the resurgence of malaria. By the 1980s, the hope that malaria could be eradicated throughout the world had been abandoned. Adopting control, rather than eradication, as a more reasonable goal, in 1998, WHO officials endorsed plans for reducing the global burden of malaria cases by 50 percent. Unfortunately, within five years, malaria experts concluded that achieving even this modest goal was not feasible. Indeed, faced with the possibility that the number of malaria cases would double, WHO endorsed limited, carefully targeted use of DDT as a mosquito repellent on the inner walls of houses in malarial regions.

One to three million people die of malaria each year; hundreds of millions of people suffer from persistent, debilitating attacks of the disease; and two billion people are at risk of infection. Studies of the epidemiology of AIDS and malaria confirmed the suspicion that people with HIV/AIDS are particularly susceptible to malaria. Moreover, people with HIV/AIDS are more likely to transmit the virus to others if they contract malaria. Therefore, protecting people with HIV/AIDS from malaria would help limit the notoriously rapid spread of HIV in areas where the two diseases are so prevalent. Globally, malaria is responsible for almost 90 percent of all deaths from vector-borne diseases. In Africa, malaria is one of the major killers of young children.

Advances in molecular biology, such as the successful determination of the com-plete genome of *Plasmodium falciparum*, the deadliest malaria species, and that of the mosquito *Anopheles gambiae*, may lead to the development of preventive vaccines, new antimalaria drugs, insect repellents, and mosquito traps. Identifying genes that are essential to the malaria parasite but have no human counterparts could establish safe targets for drugs. Skeptics predicted that the excitement generated by malaria genomics in 2002 would be counterproductive because resources would be diverted from more pragmatic control programs. Molecular biology has raised hopes for the eventual development of effective vaccines and new drugs, but simple measures, such as bed nets and mosquito repellants, could have an immediate effect on the toll taken by malaria and other mosquito-borne diseases. Many exciting experimental malaria vaccines have been created and tested, but so far, they have all been unsuccessful.

RESURGENCE OF MOSQUITO-BORNE DISEASES

The Americas were essentially free of *Aedes aegypti* by the 1960s, but within twenty years, the mosquito population rebounded, as control measures were relaxed or even abandoned. During the same period, global commerce, travel, development, habitat destruction, war, migration, and the neglect of public health services facilitated the dissemination of pathogens and their vectors. Although people in wealthy countries apparently had little interest in malaria and yellow fever, the emergence of urban outbreaks of West Nile fever in the 1990s caused an immediate resurgence of interest in mosquito-borne diseases. West Nile fever demonstrated just how quickly a new viral disease could spread to previously unaffected areas. Within a few years of the first outbreak in the United States, West Nile fever was considered a significant public health threat. Epidemiologists warned that West Nile fever might be just the first of many old and new mosquito-borne viral diseases making their way into new regions. In the absence of preventive vaccines, eliminating mosquitoes would be the only way to control such diseases. Critics of previous bans on DDT argued that governments should consider the dangers posed by the resurgence of mosquito-borne diseases and make DDT available for mosquito control.

Dengue fever is another viral infection transmitted by the *Aedes aegypti* mosquito and, like malaria, is most often found in tropical regions. *Aedes aegypti* was identified as the vector of the disease in 1906, and one year later, researchers suggested that the causative agent was a filterable virus. In addition to high fever, rash, and vomiting, dengue causes joint and muscle pains so intense that the disease was called *breakbone fever* when major epidemics were first identified in North America, Asia, Africa, and North America. Although many cases of dengue fever are mild, dengue hemorrhagic fever (DHF) and dengue shock syndrome (DSS) lead to internal bleeding, shock, and death. WHO estimates that there may be fifty to one hundred million cases of dengue infection worldwide every year, including more than five hundred thousand reported cases of DHF/DSS. Dengue fever has become endemic in more than one hundred countries in Africa, Asia, the eastern Mediterranean, the Caribbean islands, and the Americas. Since 2005, Singapore, Indonesia, Malaysia, and other Southeast Asian countries have experienced a serious resurgence of dengue fever, and the virus seems to be spreading to new areas. The most significant factor in the rapid emergence of dengue as a global public health threat seems to be the explosive growth of densely populated cities that lack appropriate water, sewer, and waste management systems. Rapidly growing urban areas bring more people into contact with *Aedes aegypti* and all four subtypes of the dengue virus. International commerce carries mosquitoes to all parts of the world, and infected humans can carry subtypes of the dengue virus to new regions before their illness is diagnosed.

Attempts to establish a safe and effective vaccine for dengue fever have been complicated by the fact that there are four major viral subtypes. Immunity to one type does not provide immunity to the other types. People who have survived an attack by one strain are more likely to suffer DHF if they become infected by a different strain. To prevent DHF/DSS, a dengue vaccine would have to produce immunity to all four subtypes of the dengue virus simultaneously. More people are now at risk of DHF/DSS because dengue fever viral subtypes are losing their previous geographic isolation. With the threat of dengue fever increasing and the lack of progress in developing preventive vaccines, scientists are exploring innovative approaches such as the possibility of using *Wolbachia* bacteria to kill the mosquito vector. Like viruses, *Wolbachia* are obligate intracellular microbes and cannot be cultured in vitro. Although they are closely related to the rickettsia and ehrlichia, *Wolbachia* bacteria seem to be harmless to mammals. However, their ability to parasitize many kinds of insects might prove useful in controlling the mosquitoes that transmit dengue fever and other human diseases. At present, mosquito control remains the only viable means of preventing dengue epidemics.

NEGLECTED DISEASES AND THEIR VECTORS

WHO established special programs to support research on malaria, leishmaniasis, schistosomiasis, trypanosomiasis, filariasis, and other diseases that are largely confined to the world's most impoverished nations. Although many of these diseases are virtually unknown in wealthy, industrialized countries, their persistence in the global germ pool can affect travelers and military personnel, as demonstrated in 2003 by the diagnosis of visceral leishmaniasis in American soldiers returning from Iraq and Afghanistan. Leishmaniasis, also known as black fever or kala-azar, is caused by protozoan parasites belonging to the genus *Leishmania* that live in vertebrate hosts and are transmitted by tiny sand flies. Variations in the clinical pattern of disease range from localized skin lesions to the deadly form known as visceral leishmaniasis. Public health battles against visceral leishmaniasis usually involve spraying houses with insecticide and killing infected dogs, but this approach has not been very successful. In the 1960s, preliminary trials indicated that paromomycin was effective in treating leishmaniasis, but pharmaceutical companies have little incentive to develop and market drugs for tropical diseases. Paromomycin has been classified as an orphan drug.

Although the disease is a persistent burden in endemic areas, molecular biologists have been successful in analyzing the genome and proteome of *Leishmania*.

In addition to flying insects, such as mosquitoes and sand flies, many important diseases of humans and animals are transmitted by ticks, mites, and other bloodsucking arthropods. During the 1890s, the role of ticks as disease vectors was demonstrated for a disease of cattle, generally known as Texas cattle fever, and a disease of humans, known as Rocky Mountain spotted fever. Texas cattle fever often attacked and killed northern cattle after they were pastured in fields that had been used by southern cattle. Cattle ranchers thought that Texas fever was caused by a bloodsucking tick but could not explain why southern cattle remained healthy despite their continuous exposure to ticks. In 1893, Theobald Smith and Frederick Kilborne published a landmark account of the role of the cattle tick as the vector for *Babesia bigemina*. In addition to suggesting simple ways to prevent Texas fever, Smith also provided valuable insights into the nature of immunity. Southern cattle were almost invariably exposed to *Babesia bigemina* while they were still protected by antibodies produced by their mothers. This resulted in a mild infection that allowed them to develop active immunity. In contrast, cattle that contracted the infection as adults were severely affected.

An unusual group of bacteria, known as the *Rickettsiaceae*, typically survive and multiply only within living cells and are typically transmitted by arthropod vectors. Diseases caused by the rickettsia include Rocky Mountain spotted fever, typhus fever, scrub typhus, Q fever, trench fever, and rickettsial pox. Rocky Mountain spotted fever was first described in 1899. In 1906, Howard Taylor Ricketts proved that wood ticks serve as the vector of this disease. Three years later, Ricketts published a preliminary report of an unusual microorganism found in blood smears from victims of the disease, but he was unable to culture the microbe in the laboratory. Ricketts also discovered the microbe that causes typhus fever and showed that typhus fever and Rocky Mountain spotted fever were different diseases. In 1915, Stanislaus Prowazek and fellow researcher Henrique da Rocha-Lima contracted typhus while investigating a typhus outbreak among Russian soldiers in a German prison camp. Da Rocha-Lima recovered and isolated the causative agent, which he called *Rickettsia prowazekii*, in honor of Prowazek and Ricketts, who both died of typhus while investigating the disease. The causative agent of Rocky Mountain spotted fever was given the name *Rickettsia rickettsii*.

Charles Nicolle, director of the Pasteur Institute in Tunis, demonstrated in 1920 that typhus fever is transmitted by the body louse *Pediculus corporis*. Lice from infected people could transmit the disease to monkeys. Recognition of the role of the louse had an immediate impact on the management of hospital patients. Systematic delousing campaigns became an important focus of public health work, particularly during World War I. For his work on typhus, Nicolle was awarded the Nobel Prize in Medicine or Physiology in 1928. Typhus remains a problem today in various parts of the world, as do the body lice that transmit the disease. All of the usual human body lice—body, head, and pubic lice—can transmit *Rickettsia prowazekii* from person to person. Rats, mice, flying squirrels, and other rodents are the usual reservoirs of the rickettsia. A related rickettsial disease known as murine typhus, caused by *Rickettsia typhi*, is generally transmitted by fleas. The disease is known throughout the world, but it is a particular problem in rat-infested cities and ports. In some parts of the United States, opossums and cats serve as the major reservoir.

Tick-transmitted diseases have received considerable attention since the recognition of Lyme disease. Allen C. Steere, epidemiologist and rheumatologist, began studying Lyme disease in 1975 and is generally credited with identifying the disease. Patient groups, however, believe that Polly Murray should be remembered for her role in calling attention to an unusual cluster of cases of juvenile rheumatoid arthritis in and around Lyme, Connecticut. Steer suspected an insect vector because symptoms generally began in summer or fall. *Ixodes scapularis*, a tiny tick that usually lives on deer and field mice, was identified as the vector of Lyme disease as well as ehrlichiosis and babesiosis. Epidemiological investigations indicate that Lyme disease is the most common tick-borne disease in the United States. *Borrelia burdoferi*, a spirochete that was discovered in 1982 by Willy Burgdorfer, causes the disease.

Lymerix, a preventive vaccine for Lyme disease, was granted FDA approval in 1999, but the National Vaccine Advisory Committee recommended that the vaccine only be used for people at high risk of contracting the disease. Shortly after the vaccine reached the marketplace, people who claimed that the vaccine itself caused arthritis and other symptoms of Lyme disease filed lawsuits. When people who had been vaccinated were compared to a control group, statisticians found no difference in chronic arthritis, muscle pain, headaches, memory loss, paralysis, fatigue, and so forth. Nevertheless, because of the lawsuits, the vaccine was withdrawn from the market in 2002. Controversy surrounding Lyme disease provides a remarkable example of the problem of diagnosing and treating diseases with complex clinical patterns. Patient advocacy groups believe that Lyme disease can become a chronic condition associated with serious but ill-defined symptoms that require long-term treatment with powerful antibiotics. Steere and other scientists reject the concept of chronic Lyme disease and consider such treatments useless and dangerous.

GLOBAL HEALTH: NEGLECTED TROPICAL DISEASES

Epidemiologists estimate that about half of the 2.7 billion people living in poverty suffer from one or more debilitating tropical diseases. Many of these diseases are targets of global health programs coordinated by WHO and the Global Network for Neglected Tropical Diseases: Buruli ulcer, Chagas' disease, cholera and endemic

diarrheal disease, dengue fever, dracunculiasis (guinea worm disease), endemic treponematoses, human African trypanosomiasis (sleeping sickness), leishmaniasis, leprosy, lymphatic filariasis (elephantiasis), onchocerciasis (river blindness), schistosomiasis, soil-transmitted helminthiasis, and trachoma. These diseases are virtually
unknown in the United States and other wealthy nations, but they kill and maim
hundreds of thousands of people around the world every year.

Some of the tropical diseases imported to the Americas from Africa as a consequence of the slave trade included malaria, yaws, leprosy, guinea worm, filariasis,
ascariasis, tapeworm, hookworm, and typanosomiasis. When the slave trade ended,
African diseases that could not survive in the Americas essentially disappeared. For
example, African sleeping sickness, which is caused by *Trypanosoma gambiense*, could
not adapt to the Americas without its vector, the tsetse fly. In contrast, the filarial
roundworm, *Wunchereria bancrofti*, which causes elephantiasis, became endemic in
parts of the South, where appropriate mosquitoes served as vectors. Filariasis was
particularly common in Charleston, South Carolina, and Barbados in the West Indies. Recognition of the relationship between the disease and the mosquito vector
led to intensive mosquito control programs in the 1920s. According to WHO, about
120 million people in eighty countries are infested with filarial worms. Lymphatic
filariasis is not curable, but the disease could be eradicated by using deworming drugs
to prevent transmission. Deworming drugs do not reverse the damage to infected
individuals or kill adult worms, but they can break the cycle of transmission. WHO
called for global eradication by 2020, but that goal seems overly optimistic.

Many of the diseases that affect impoverished areas are caused by worms or other
parasites. By definition, parasites are creatures that live on or in another organism at
the expense of the host. This definition could apply to all microbial forms of life, but
after the establishment of scientific germ theory, the term *parasite* was very rarely used
in reference to viruses, bacteria, and fungi. Microbiology and parasitology gradually
separated from each other as it became apparent that the infectious diseases of most
concern to Europeans and North Americans were caused by bacteria and viruses.
Tropical medicine and parasitology were seen as problems of poor and backward
countries and became peripheral to biomedical science. Nineteenth-century evolutionary biologists often described parasites as degenerate life-forms, but they were
difficult to study in the laboratory because of their complex life cycles and specific
host requirements. Actually, parasites are generally quite complex and extremely successful. To cope with the challenge of adapting to different hosts and environments,
parasites have apparently developed a variety of mechanisms for manipulating their
hosts into behaviors that make transmission of the parasite to the next host more
likely.

Some epidemiologists argue that given the volume of international travel and
commerce, no pathogen or parasite need remain localized. In a rapidly changing,

interconnected world, neglected tropical diseases can become a threat to wealthy countries, as demonstrated by Chagas' disease and dengue fever. Chagas' disease is named for Brazilian doctor Carlos Chagas, who identified a new trypanosome in 1908 while studying a disease referred to as American trypanosomiasis. The new trypanosome was named *Trypanosoma cruzi* in honor of Oswaldo Cruz for his work on the epidemic diseases of Brazil. Chagas' disease seemed to be transmitted by a South American bug known as the kissing bug, assassin bug, or barbeiro. This bloodsucking insect lives inside houses and prefers to bite people on the face as they sleep, leaving parasite-laden feces at the site of the bite. Almost a century after the identification of Chagas' disease and the bug involved in its transmission, researchers discovered that the disease could also be transmitted by contaminated food. Endemic in Mexico, Central America, and South America, the disease infects about twenty million people and causes about fifty thousand deaths each year. The disease can remain dormant for many years, but damage to the heart, intestines, and nervous system can cause sudden death. Modern medical practices—blood transfusions and organ transplants—can transmit the disease. In the United States, the first known cases of transmission through donated blood occurred in 1988. In 2006, the FDA approved a test for Chagas' disease that can be used to protect the blood supply.

Bartonellosis, or Carrión's disease, found only in certain parts of South America, is transmitted by the bite of a sand fly. Traditionally known as *verruga peruana* or Oroya fever, the disease was apparently known to the Incas. Verruga peruana, the chronic form of the disease, is characterized by lumpy, wartlike skin eruptions. In some victims, the disease appears as Oroya fever, an acute, life-threatening systemic infection. In 1885, medical student Daniel Alcides Carrión demonstrated the fundamental identity of verruga and Oroya fever by having himself inoculated with blood from a verruga patient. This heroic and fatal experiment proved that the acute disease called Oroya fever and the chronic condition called verruga peruana are two stages of the same disease. The causative bacterial agent, *Bartonella bacilliformis*, was discovered by Alberto Barton in 1905.

Dracunculiasis, commonly known as guinea worm disease, is a threat to people who come in contact with water containing the larvae of the guinea worm, *Dracunculus medinensis*. Calcified examples of these roundworms have been found in Egyptian mummies from the New Kingdom period (fifteenth century BCE). People contract the disease by drinking water contaminated by tiny arthropods known as copepods, or water fleas, that have eaten worm larvae. Once inside the stomach, the worms are liberated from the water fleas and migrate through the body. After mating, the male guinea worm dies, but the female may remain in the body for a year or more and reach a length of two to three feet. When the mature female worm is ready to leave the body, typically through the skin of the lower limbs, a painful swelling develops at the site where the worm will emerge. Attempts to remove the worm more rapidly can cause it to break, leaving parts inside the body that calcify and cause permanent deformities. During this period, people often attempt to ease the burning and itching sensations by soaking their legs in water, which allows larvae to enter the local water system. A procedure as simple as straining drinking water to remove copepods could prevent almost all cases of guinea worm disease, even in areas that lack proper sanitation and safe drinking water.

In the 1980s, when the number of cases of dracunculiasis was estimated at about three and a half million, international health workers launched a campaign to eradicate the disease. By the end of the twentieth century, the number of cases was cut to about sixty-five thousand, but the disease remained endemic in thirteen countries. About 80 percent of the world's reported guinea worm cases occur in southern Sudan, where control efforts for a host of preventable infectious diseases—onchocerciasis (river blindness), trachoma, leishmaniasis, malaria, sleeping sickness, cholera, and nonspecific diarrheal diseases—were disrupted by civil war. The Dracunculiasis Eradication Program still hopes to establish global eradication of guinea worm disease, even if the original target of 2009 cannot be met.

Trachoma, a preventable cause of blindness, is virtually unknown in the United States and Europe today, but it is still endemic in parts of Africa, Latin America, and Asia. WHO estimates that seventy million people suffer from trachoma. *Chlamydia trachomatis*, the microorganism that causes trachoma, thrives among people living in crowded, unsanitary conditions. Controlling trachoma depends on fairly simple hygienic measures to prevent transmission and medical interventions to treat early infections.

Europeans first became familiar with African sleeping sickness in the eighteenth century as a deadly condition of humans and cattle in a region known as the fly belt of Africa. Victims of African sleeping sickness may suffer violent hallucinations and coma before dying. In the 1880s, trypanosomes, which had been discovered in the 1840s, were found in the blood of horses, mules, and camels with a fatal disease known as surra. The disease was transmitted by a biting fly, but it could be transferred to healthy animals by inoculating them with blood from an affected animal. In the 1890s, British colonial farmers found it impossible to raise European cattle in Africa because of a disease known locally as nagana. David Bruce discovered that the disease was caused by a trypanosome that was transmitted by the tsetse fly. *Trypanosoma brucei* was commonly found in wild animals such as buffalo, wildebeest, and bushbuck. The causative agent for African sleeping sickness, *Trypanosoma gambiense*, was discovered in 1901. Like nagana, the disease was spread by tsetse flies. WHO estimates that about 150,000 people contract African sleeping sickness each year, but the distribution of the tsetse fly and the parasite put some 50 million people at risk. The drugs available to treat sleeping sickness are generally very difficult to use and often quite toxic to the patient, but eflornithine, a drug discovered in 1980, is so effective that its administration sometimes revives comatose patients. Eflornithine was originally developed as a cancer drug, but when the drug proved unsuccessful in cancer therapy, the manufacturer stopped production. In 2000, Sanofi-Aventis began exploring the possibility of marketing eflornitine as Vaniqa, a topical cream to prevent the growth of facial hair in women. Facing adverse publicity about selling eflornitine as an expensive cosmetic formulation while victims of African sleeping sickness were dying without treatment, Sanofi-Aventis agreed to produce the drug for distribution by WHO and Doctors Without Borders.

GLOBAL WARMING AND PUBLIC HEALTH

Some researchers believe that climate change could expand the range of the tropical diseases that are now largely confined to developing countries. Diseases transmitted by insects and arthropods would be affected because both temperature and water can be limiting factors for the survival and reproduction of vectors and pathogens. Particular concerns include well-known diseases transmitted by contaminated water supplies, such as schistosomiasis, and diseases transmitted by mosquitoes, such as malaria and dengue fever. But once obscure diseases, previously confined to isolated areas, may become threats to vast new areas. Warmer temperatures and changes in precipitation as well as the water levels of ponds, lakes, rivers, and oceans will presumably increase the threat of many diseases transmitted by contaminated water or by insect vectors. Malaria, dengue fever, yellow fever, and other diseases transmitted by mosquitoes may increase their geographical range because temperature affects the distribution of mosquitoes, the frequency of mosquito bites, and the development of the pathogen. The complexity of the interactions among the factors that affect the pattern of infectious diseases makes it difficult to predict the effects of climate change on human health. Nevertheless, although epidemiologists acknowledge a large measure of uncertainty, there are many reasons to expect that global warming will be a major factor in the global distribution of infectious diseases in the future.

SEVEN

EMERGING INFECTIOUS DISEASES

MICROBIOLOGY AND CHANGING PATTERNS OF DISEASE

The early twentieth century has been called the golden era for microbiology and public health because overall improvements in health, as measured by increases in life expectancy, decreases in infant mortality, and successful management of many epidemic diseases, seemed to validate sanitary projects inspired by the modern germ theory of disease. As the fear of infectious, epidemic diseases decreased and cardio-vascular diseases, cancers, and other chronic, degenerative diseases became the major threats in wealthy, industrialized nations, the value of traditional public health work was no longer obvious. By the 1960s, many physicians were convinced that antibiotics would eliminate the threat of bacterial diseases and that vaccines would control viral diseases. Indeed, Sir Macfarlane Burnet, who won the Nobel Prize in Medicine or Physiology in 1960 for his work on the immune system, said that the infectious diseases were essentially disappearing as a challenge to the biomedical community. Despite his interest in the ecology of disease, Burnet thought that the future study of infectious diseases would be very limited and quite dull. His predictions reflected the prevailing assumption that the war against the epidemic diseases of the past had been won, at least for residents of wealthy, industrialized nations. Optimists even predicted the imminent conquest of infectious disease on a global scale. In 1978, representatives of 134 countries and 67 international organizations attending the International Conference on Primary Health Care adopted the motto "Health for All." Five years later, the General Assembly of the United Nations approved a resolution endorsing a Global Strategy for Health for All by the Year 2000.

Historical studies of changing patterns of disease and life expectancy provided support for optimism about the possibility of improving health throughout the world. Although the major causes of morbidity and mortality vary with time and place, between 1800 and 2000, all parts of the world apparently experienced a dramatic change in life expectancy. The most striking aspect of this global epidemiological transition was an increase in life expectancy at birth from about thirty years in 1800 to a global average of sixty-seven years in 2000. Statisticians predicted that by 2030, infectious diseases would account for only 30 percent of all deaths globally. The vast majority of deaths would be caused by heart disease, stroke, and cancers in the elderly. By the end of the twentieth century, however, the rapid evolution of multidrug-resistant microbes and the emergence of new diseases, such as AIDS, had effectively discredited optimistic predictions about the conquest of infectious diseases. Old diseases, some on the brink of eradication, had returned and spread into new areas. Moreover, infectious diseases were still the major killers in the developing world.

EMERGING DISEASES

The first International Conference on Emerging Infectious Diseases was held in 1998, almost two decades after the emergence of AIDS demonstrated that totally unanticipated threats could rapidly become major pandemics. Since that meeting, epidemiologists have emphasized the importance of developing long-term programs to monitor and react to emerging and reemerging infectious diseases. In a general sense, emerging infectious diseases can be defined as illnesses that were generally unknown or sporadically affected very small numbers of people in isolated areas but have rather suddenly become more much common and widespread. Newly discovered diseases may simply be new names for old diseases that were previously hidden among the undifferentiated fevers and diarrheal diseases of rural areas and isolated villages. However, thinking about emerging infectious agents in terms of three general categories is useful because understanding the factors that trigger an increase in incidence and geographical range is critical in planning effective global preventive or control strategies; that is, emerging diseases may be thought of in terms of the emergence of diseases that have never before affected human beings, the reemergence or resurgence of diseases that had virtually disappeared or were effectively under control, and diseases that are deliberately emerging because of acts of bioterrorism that use pathogens as biological weapons. The anthrax letters of 2001 provide an instructive example of the deliberate use of a naturally occurring pathogen, but microbes genetically engineered for increased virulence or drug resistance would also belong to this category (see Chapter 8).

By the 1990s, public health experts generally agreed that new and previously obscure infectious diseases were appearing at an unprecedented rate in regions that were previously unaffected, causing epidemics among people who were unfamiliar with them. Microbiologists discovered that some emerging infectious diseases were caused by pathogens that were able to jump from their traditional animal reservoirs to human populations. This phenomenon certainly occurred sporadically many times in the past, but in the modern world, once a microbe spreads from animals to humans, many factors, including rapid transportation and standard medical or surgical practices, may actually contribute to its dissemination. Inadequate sterilization of medical equipment and the reuse of disposable syringes are common in many developing countries and have contributed to the spread of HIV/AIDS and other diseases. In other cases, such as Legionnaires' disease, sporadic cases of a newly recognized disease were misdiagnosed until the isolation of the causative agent provided a new means of differential diagnosis. After the causative agent was identified, researchers realized that common features of modern buildings, such as air-conditioning systems, provided a new ecological niche for previously obscure microbes.

LEGIONELLOSIS: LEGIONNAIRES' DISEASE AND PONTIAC FEVER

Improved diagnostic techniques and heightened surveillance add to the catalog of human diseases by redefining previously localized diseases and vague categories such as "fevers of unknown origin" and undifferentiated pneumonias. On the basis of clinical symptoms alone, it is very difficult to differentiate respiratory illnesses, but knowing whether the symptoms are caused by viruses, bacteria, or molds is important to treating the sick and preventing the spread of the disease. The importance of making such distinctions was demonstrated in 1976 during a widely publicized outbreak of a disease that became known as Legionnaires' disease. At the time, public health officials were very concerned about the possibility of a major influenza pandemic and initially thought that the outbreak might be caused by the swine flu virus. Of the thousands of members of the American Legion celebrating the American Bicentennial at the Bellevue Stratford Hotel in Philadelphia, Pennsylvania, more than two hundred experienced an unusually lethal form of pneumonia, and thirty-four died. After an intensive search for the cause of the outbreak, in January 1977, researchers identified the causative agent and named it *Legionella pneumophilia*. Because Legionnaires' disease is a bacterial pneumonia, rather than a viral disease, it responds to treatment with appropriate antibiotics. The epidemic was attributed to bacteria growing in the cooling tower of the Bellevue Stratford Hotel's air-conditioning system.

Although Legionnaires' disease was first recognized in 1976, once the causative agent was discovered, epidemiologists identified *Legionella pneumophilia* as the cause of previously unidentified pneumonia-like outbreaks throughout the world. Further studies indicated that *Legionella pneumophilia* caused two distinct clinical patterns: the deadly pneumonia known as Legionnaires' disease and a mild, flulike illness called Pontiac fever. Legionnaires' disease and Pontiac fever are sometimes referred to as legionellosis. People contract legionellosis by aspirating aerosolized water droplets containing *Legionella pneumophilia* directly into their lungs. Legionella bacteria are found in lakes, rivers, hot springs, and soil at low levels, but the air-conditioning and water-storage systems of modern buildings have created new niches in which these bacteria thrive and multiply. Legionella bacteria can also survive by forming biofilms inside pipes, faucets, and showerheads. People are, therefore, most likely to inhale large numbers of *Legionella pneumophilia* while indoors. Most cases have been traced to bacterial contamination of the water in air-conditioning systems, water heaters, medical respiratory equipment, whirlpool baths, showers, humidifiers, ice-making machines, and even the water sprayed over fruits and vegetables in grocery stores. People have also contracted legionellosis from hot tubs, swimming pools, and decorative fountains. An estimated eight thousand to eighteen thousand cases of legionellosis occur each year in the United States, but many cases are not diagnosed or reported. Outbreaks of Legionnaires' disease have been reported throughout the world, often in older hotels, cruise ships, hospitals, nursing homes, schools, and prisons. During various outbreaks, the fatality rate of Legionnaires' disease has been estimated at 5 to 30 percent (see Figure 7.1).

EMERGING DISEASES AND THE GLOBAL GERM POOL

At the beginning of the twenty-first century, researchers listed 175 pathogenic agents known to cause emerging infectious diseases; the vast majority of these diseases were transmitted from the animals that have been their traditional hosts. The pathological agents included viruses, bacteria, protozoa, parasitic worms, and fungi. Diseases that have emerged since the 1970s include Legionnaires' disease, HIV/AIDS, Ebola fever, hantavirus pulmonary syndrome, West Nile fever, SARS, and mad cow disease.

Until the introduction of modern means of transportation and international networks, the dissemination of localized diseases of humans and animals was a slow, unpredictable, and rare event. Improvements in transportation and communication during the nineteenth and twentieth centuries revolutionized the interchange of

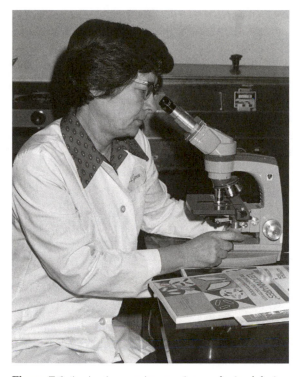

Figure 7.1 A scientist examines specimens obtained during an outbreak of a pneumonia-like disease in 1980 to confirm a diagnosis of Legionnaires' disease. The causative agent of Legionnaires' disease, *Legionella pneumophilia*, had been identified in 1977. Credit: Public Health Image Library, Centers for Disease Control and Prevention, U.S. Department of Health and Human Services.

people, animals, microbes, and information throughout the world, but the airplane made it possible to carry pathogens and their vectors to any part of the world within hours. Indeed, it is useful to think of the airplane as an extremely large mosquito that can serve as a global vector of a multitude of exotic diseases. Modern commerce and transportation create a global germ pool as well as a global village. Infectious agents become part of the worldwide movement of people and commodities that is accelerated by warfare, migration, trade, tourism, air travel, and so forth. Globalization of trade and transportation, which is removing many of the ancient physical barriers to the movement of people, animals, and pathogens, will have a profound impact on future patterns of infectious diseases among humans and animals, both domesticated and wild. Changes in population density and human behaviors also influence the distribution of potential pathogens and the emergence of new diseases. The high population density of modern cities favors the rapid transmission of infectious disease agents. People moving into formerly wild areas are likely to displace or come into contact with wild animals that serve as reservoirs for potential pathogens. Modern institutions—such as hospitals, clinics, nursing homes, prisons, schools, and day care centers—bring large numbers of strangers into close contact and serve as incubators and amplifiers for infectious diseases.

More than twelve thousand years ago, when all human beings lived as hunters and gatherers, their population density was too small to sustain most epidemic diseases. They could, however, acquire infectious agents when they butchered and ate wild animals. When humans domesticated animals, they acquired a more reliable source of food and other goods, but they also changed their exposure to the microbes carried by animals. Since the Neolithic Age, humans have typically lived in close proximity to domesticated or semidomesticated animals. Epidemic diseases that were probably the result of the domestication of animals include tuberculosis from goats and cows, whooping cough (pertussis) from pigs, glanders from horses, measles from cattle (bovine rinderpest virus), typhoid fever from chickens, and influenza from ducks.

Ancient people apparently kept various species of animals as companions and pets, but the practice of keeping pets inside the home has become increasingly popular. Bites by dogs and cats are a source of many serious injuries, infections, and diseases. Cats are known to harbor diseases that are dangerous to humans such as cat scratch disease, toxocariasis, and toxoplasmosis. Cats that catch plague-infected rodents have been known to transmit *Yersinia pestis* to humans. Toxoplasmosis is a particular danger to pregnant women and their infants and to people with suppressed immune systems, especially people with AIDS. Pet birds can spread salmonellosis, giardiasis, influenza, Newcastle disease, and psittacosis (parrot fever). Rather like our ancestors in the Neolithic era, modern humans are entering into intimate new relationships with animals, as dogs, cats, and canaries are joined by exotic species from every corner of the world. Exotic animals sold as pets include creatures ranging from African pouch rats and hedgehogs to iguanas and prairie dogs. Throughout the world, rodents provide a major reservoir for pathogenic microbes. Depending on their country of origin and their exposure to other animals, pets have been the source of salmonella, rabies, monkey pox, tularemia, and so forth. Even city children without pets have been exposed to the microbes carried by typical farm animals and more exotic creatures during visits to zoos, especially petting zoos.

FOOD POISONING AND FOOD-BORNE DISEASE

Changes in the way human beings have obtained and prepared their food through-out history have obviously affected patterns of food-borne disease. Paleolithic hunters and scavengers must have contracted various parasites and microbes by butchering dead animals, through contact with animal excreta and eating meat. When animals were domesticated, humans could contract pathogens through close contact with live animals and from drinking milk or blood. Modern methods of food production, preservation, and preparation generally reduce the risk of exposure to food-borne pathogens, but many people are willing and eager to consume sushi, sashimi, raw milk, and unpasteurized juices. Fish are known to carry many kinds of parasites, and raw shellfish can transmit hepatitis A and Norwalk-type viruses. Unpasteurized milk can transmit *Listeria monocytogenes*, a bacterium widely found in soil and water that causes a life-threatening disease known as listeriosis. Healthy farm animals can carry the bacteria, and vegetables can be contaminated by soil or manure used as fertilizer. *Listeria monocytogenes* can survive moderate heat, salt, acidity, and freezing and can even multiply in the refrigerator. Listeriosis has been linked to many different food products, from hotdogs to bean sprouts, and is especially dangerous to pregnant women, infants, the elderly, diabetics, and people with a weakened immune system. Since listeriosis was recognized as a threat in the United States in the 1980s, more virulent strains have been detected. According to the Centers for Disease Control and Prevention (CDC), about twenty-five hundred people become seriously ill with listeriosis each year, and five hundred people die. Botulism, a rare, life-threatening paralytic illness, is usually caused by eating improperly canned foods that contain a powerful toxin produced by *Clostridium botulinum*, an anaerobic bacterium. Today, most people are more familiar with the cosmetic use of this toxin as Botox than as a particularly deadly form of food poisoning. The word *botulism* comes from the Latin *botulus*, for "sausage," a common source of the disease in nineteenth-century Europe. The toxin can also be found in fat from marine mammals, which is a good incubator for *Clostridium botulinum*. Outbreaks of botulism among Native Alaskans have been traced to the consumption of raw blubber from beached whales. The toxin has also been blamed for mass deaths of birds that were poisoned when they consumed fish and weeds contaminated by *Clostridium botulinum*.

Changing methods of beef preparation and distribution have been blamed for the emergence of a deadly form of food poisoning caused by *Escherichia coli* O157:H7 that was first identified in the 1980s. The genus *Escherichia* is named after Theodor Escherich, a pediatrician who was particularly interested in using bacteriology to improve the health of infants and young children. In 1884, while examining stool samples under his microscope, Escherich discovered a bacterium that is always present in the feces of normal individuals. In 1919, the bacterium was named *Escherichia coli* in his honor. Sanitary engineers realized that monitoring the levels of *Escherichia coli* provided a warning that raw sewage containing feces was present in the water supply.

Most strains of *Escherichia coli* are harmless, or even beneficial, members of the normal intestinal microbial community, but some strains cause chronic urinary disease or deadly intestinal infections. *Escherichia coli* O157:H7, which was first identified in the 1980s as the cause of food poisoning contracted at several fast-food restaurants, produces a toxin that can cause severe bloody diarrhea (hemorrhagic colitis), anemia, and kidney damage. In some cases, kidney failure leads to a fatal condition known as hemolytic uremic syndrome (destruction of red blood cells and kidney failure). The toxin is most dangerous in children, the elderly, and people with weakened immune systems. Antibiotics are generally ineffective because the deadly toxin has usually been released into the bloodstream before the infection is diagnosed. By 1998, the CDC estimated that *E. coli* O157:H7 caused about forty thousand cases of food poisoning per year. Later reports suggested that the number of cases per year was actually much higher, but mild cases were probably not reported. In addition to ground beef, food poisoning caused by *E. coli* O157:H7 was also attributed to contaminated fruits and vegetables, raw milk, unpasteurized cheese, swimming pools, petting zoos, and even a gourmet brand of unpasteurized apple juice. Increases in the number of *E. coli* O157:H7 cases suggest poor sanitation at meat-processing plants and the contamination of groundwater by manure discharged by infected cattle at feedlots, which allows the bacteria to become associated with produce growing on neighboring farms. Since the 1990s, slaughterhouses and meat-processing plants have added new procedures to prevent the distribution of contaminated beef, but *E. coli* O157:H7 remains a threat to the food supply.

The CDC estimates that each year, five thousand people die and seventy-six million become ill from food poisoning. Since the 1990s, sources of food-borne illnesses have been as varied as beef, poultry, seafood, eggs, canned chili sauce, snack foods, baby carrots, spinach, raspberries, cantaloupes, tomatoes, green onions, cucumbers, and unpasteurized apple and orange juices. Meat, chicken, and eggs are the usual suspects when outbreaks of bacterial food poisoning occur, but *Escherichia coli* O157:H7 and *Salmonella* are also associated with produce, that is, spinach, lettuce, and various fruits and vegetables. The bacteria probably come from groundwater contaminated with animal feces. In the past, outbreaks were typically localized, but as centralized processing of vegetables and meats replaced localized markets, food-borne pathogens achieved nationwide distribution. Cross-contamination and attempts to wash fruits and vegetables before shipping provide another opportunity for the redistribution of pathogens.

THE EMERGENCE OF THE AIDS PANDEMIC

The effectiveness of the first antibiotics encouraged people to believe that all infectious diseases could be cured by these so-called miracle drugs. Although antibiotics have saved countless lives, they have no effect on viral diseases. Vaccines made it possible to control some viral diseases, but no vaccines are available for AIDS, SARS, West Nile fever, Ebola fever, Lassa fever, and other deadly viral diseases that have been recognized since the 1970s. With the emergence of the AIDS pandemic, the limitations of medical therapies for viral diseases became obvious, amplified by the difficulty of treating normally benign or self-limited infections in patients with a severely impaired immune system. The AIDS epidemic transformed common bacteria and fungi into deadly opportunistic infections and challenged assumptions about the genesis of cancers and the relationship between pathogens and the immune system.

The first warning of the future AIDS pandemic appeared on June 4, 1981, in *Morbidity and Mortality Weekly Report*, a weekly newsletter published by the CDC that described five unusual cases of pneumonia that had recently been diagnosed in Los Angeles, California. All the patients were previously healthy homosexual men suffering from *Pneumocystis carinii* pneumonia, a rare fungal infection usually seen only in adults undergoing intensive chemotherapy or in severely malnourished children. By 1982, similar cases were reported in New York, Florida, and Texas, often complicated by Kaposi's sarcoma, a rare cancer typically found in elderly men. The mysterious phenomenon, which became known as acquired immune deficiency syndrome (AIDS), was characterized by the appearance of pneumonia caused by *Pneumocystis carinii*, a variety of opportunistic infections, and Kaposi's sarcoma. In AIDS patients, these conditions progressed rapidly and were almost invariably fatal. The disoriented behavior in AIDS patients was originally attributed to depression caused by awareness of their fatal illness, but autopsies of AIDS patients demonstrated that pathogens never before found in brain tissues had attacked the central nervous system. Once diagnosed with AIDS, most patients survived for only a year or two. By the end of 1988, almost fifty thousand Americans had died of AIDS. Within five years of the first reports of AIDS, the U.S. Public Health Service estimated that more than one million Americans were infected with the virus that causes the disease. Confronting AIDS was made more difficult in the 1980s by the political climate embodied in the Reagan administration, which did not want to acknowledge the threat of HIV/AIDS, primarily because the disease was initially associated with gay men.

The appearance of AIDS in very different populations, including gay men, intravenous drug users, immigrants from Africa and the Caribbean, hemophiliacs, blood transfusion recipients, the sexual partners of people in these risk groups, and infants born to women with the disease, indicated that AIDS was probably caused by a previously unknown infectious agent. Epidemiological and clinical studies suggested that the disease was transmitted by sexual intercourse, contaminated needles, blood transfusions, and blood plasma and blood products, including the clotting factor used to treat hemophilia.

Identifying an infectious agent that destroyed the immune system and left the body vulnerable to other microbes represented an unprecedented challenge. Clinical evidence indicated that AIDS had a long, variable incubation period of months or years before symptoms appeared. Moreover, the primary defect, the damage to the immune system, allowed mildly pathogenic microbes to proliferate, which confused the search for the specific causal agent. The discovery of the virus now known as human immunodeficiency virus (HIV) by Luc Montagnier's group at the Pasteur Institute and by Robert Gallo and his colleagues at the U.S. National Institutes of Health in 1984 was marked by rancorous controversy within the biomedical community and wildly inaccurate accusations of fraud and misconduct in the popular press. After many painstaking investigations, the evidence assembled from laboratory notebooks, interviews, and published reports supports the view that Montagnier was the first to identify the virus and that Gallo was the first to prove that HIV caused AIDS; that is, Montagnier was apparently the first to report the discovery of the AIDS virus, but Gallo's work was critical to establishing the fact that HIV is the specific cause of AIDS. Moreover, techniques previously developed by Gallo made it possible to grow HIV in the laboratory. The identification of the virus that causes AIDS led to the development of a test that could detect HIV in blood, thus preventing the dissemination of HIV through blood transfusions, organ transplants, and the blood products essential to hemophiliacs. After a bitter priority dispute, Gallo and Montagnier reluctantly accepted the status of codiscoverers of HIV, largely as a result of a political solution devised by U.S. president Ronald Reagan and French prime minister Jacques Chirac as a means of resolving patent rights disputes for HIV blood tests. In 1986, the names previously used by Montagnier and Gallo (LAV and HTLV-III, respectively) for the AIDS virus were dropped and the term HIV was eventually universally adopted. The idea that a condition as complex as AIDS could be caused by a specific virus remained controversial long after the discovery of HIV. Indeed, various HIV/AIDS "denialists" have attracted international attention that AIDS researchers consider very harmful to efforts to contain the AIDS pandemic, prevent transmission of the virus, and treat those already infected.

Scientists discovered two major types of HIV, called HIV-1 and HIV-2. HIV-1 is the type found throughout most of the world; HIV-2 is found mostly in western Africa. A virus very similar to HIV, which was found in African primates in 1985, was called simian immunodeficiency virus (SIV). In general, subtypes of the virus do not cause disease in their host species, but they may be very dangerous when transmitted to another species. Studies of subtypes of HIV and SIV support the hypothesis that AIDS began in Africa, but the specific sequence of events that transformed a viral infection of African primates into a deadly virus capable of human-to-human transmission is still uncertain. Nevertheless, some observers have called HIV the revenge of the African jungle because of evidence that HIV evolved from a SIV that jumped the species barrier.

Soon after the discovery of the first cluster of AIDS cases, bizarre speculations about the disease began to appear. Attempts to explain the origin of the AIDS pandemic led to many very peculiar and controversial theories, including some that have little to do with virology and epidemiology. Religious fanatics claimed that the AIDS virus was created as a way of punishing immoral sexual conduct because antibiotics made it possible to cure syphilis and gonorrhea. Conspiracy theorists attributed the creation of HIV to a secret genetic engineering or biowarfare project that created a disease that was being used to kill homosexuals and drug addicts. American conspiracy theorists claimed that HIV was created by Soviet scientists as a biological weapon. The Soviets circulated the same kind of theory, but attributed the creation of the AIDS virus to American scientists. These theories clearly demonstrate the suspicion and fear that permeated international relationships, but they do not explain how a disease with the long incubation and variable progression of AIDS would function as an agent of biological warfare. Nor do such theories explain how the AIDS virus could have been deliberately created in the 1950s when the knowledge and techniques that made genetic engineering possible did not yet exist. Another version of this theory— sometimes called the *designer virus theory*—suggests that HIV was deliberately created by combining two retroviruses, the human T cell leukemia virus (HTLV) and the visna virus of sheep. Although both viruses cause deadly, progressive illness, the genetic sequences of HIV do not match those of HTLV or the visna virus. When sequence data ruled out this theory, its advocates insisted that the original genetically engineered AIDS virus was genetically unstable and rapidly evolved from the parental strains.

The high prevalence of AIDS in Africa led to claims that HIV had been created by the West as a tool of genocide. After the discovery of SIV in African primates, some journalists attributed the spread of HIV to polio vaccine tests conducted in Africa in the 1950s. In 1992, reports of what was called the *polio vaccine scandal* reached the public, primarily through an article by Tom Curtis in *Rolling Stone*. British journalist Edward Hooper also expounded the polio-AIDS hypothesis in his book *The River: A Journey to the Source of HIV and AIDS* (1999). According to Curtis and Hooper, green monkey tissue used in developing Hilary Koprowski's polio vaccine carried SIV. If some recipients of the oral vaccine had ulcers or cuts in their mouths, SIV could have entered the bloodstream directly. Earlier versions of the polio vaccine story were put forth in the 1980s by the National Antivivisection Society, a British animal rights advocacy group. Virologists have discounted this theory for several reasons, including doubts that an oral vaccine would have been as effective as injections as a means of transmitting SIV or HIV. Koprowski's vaccine was also used in Poland, Yugoslavia, Switzerland, and other countries, without any indication that it led to any reports of AIDS-like illnesses. Moreover, the poliovirus used in Koprowski's vaccine was grown on tissue from Asian macaques, not chimpanzees or African green monkeys. (SIV does not infect Asian macaques.) Scientists who analyzed old samples of Koprowski's vaccine found no evidence of HIV or SIV.

In the 1950s, when various polio vaccines were being tested, very little was known about the viruses carried by monkeys and other primates, and nothing was known about retroviruses. During the 1960s, scientists discovered a simian virus called SV40 in polio vaccines cultured in monkey tissues and instituted new techniques for the preparation of live polio vaccines. However, SV40 is very different from SIV and HIV and could not have triggered the AIDS epidemic. Genomic and immunological studies of various subtypes of SIV and HIV also provide evidence that the polio vaccine was not linked to the emergence of the AIDS pandemic. The virus that caused the AIDS pandemic is now known as HIV-1. This subtype is found in central Africa and is not closely related to the monkey virus that allegedly contaminated Koprowski's polio vaccines. The SIV isolated from the sooty mangabey, an African monkey, is closely related to HIV-2. Mangabeys were never used for polio vaccine preparations. HIV-2 was generally found only in West Africa, in areas about three thousand miles from the central African countries where tests of Koprowski's vaccine began in 1957. If Koprowski's polio vaccine trials in Africa triggered the AIDS pandemic, no cases of AIDS could have occurred before 1957. However, researchers have discovered evidence of Europeans who spent time in Africa before dying of AIDS-like illnesses in the 1940s and 1950s. Most of the evidence is circumstantial because of the lack of blood or tissue samples, but in a few cases, well-preserved samples of blood serum from people who died in the 1960s have tested positive for AIDS. Given the incubation period for AIDS, some of these people must have contracted the virus before the vaccine trials began. Another medically related theory suggests that malaria researchers injected human volunteers with blood from chimps, mangabeys, and macaques. Although the history of medicine provides many examples of scientists who experimented on themselves and others in attempts to identify the causative agents of infectious diseases, if such experiments caused SIV to become HIV, these research programs should have been followed by clusters of AIDS-like cases.

A more likely scenario for the origin of AIDS is that humans acquired the ancestral virus by hunting, butchering, and eating various apes and monkeys. The transition from SIV to HIV probably began when the virus was transmitted to a hunter who was bitten or injured while capturing and butchering an infected monkey. HIV-2 is close to the SIV of sooty mangabeys, and the original focus of HIV-2 infection in West Africa is located where mangabeys live and are killed and eaten. A virus similar to HIV-1 has been isolated from chimpanzees in central Africa, suggesting that chimpanzees might have been a natural reservoir of the virus that was responsible for the AIDS pandemic. Although there is little or no evidence that HIV was established in humans before the 1960s, it is possible that early cases of AIDS in Africa were rare and that deaths from the complications of AIDS would have been attributed to common, undifferentiated "fevers." People who became extremely sick because of HIV and other infections were unlikely to live long enough to transmit the virus to many other people. Indeed, AIDS was not recognized as a diagnostic entity until unusual clusters of deaths in previously healthy American men occurred in California. Before the identification of HIV/AIDS, isolated deaths associated with the virus would have been attributed to common opportunistic infections, especially fevers and diarrheal diseases.

AIDS researchers suggest that although AIDS was not recognized until the 1980s, the virus was probably circulating for several decades in Africa, where deaths from the undifferentiated fevers and diarrheal diseases that were so unusual in Western nations were not uncommon. Sporadic human deaths caused by the complications of AIDS in rural areas and isolated villages would have gone unnoticed, but the incidence of AIDS might have increased as a result of development and modernization. Economic development included urbanization, deforestation, migration of rural people to towns and cities, road construction through previously isolated areas, long-distance trucking, increased travel and tourism, prostitution, and so forth. People who lived in cities could still come in contact with SIV through the bush meat trade, that is, by purchasing, preparing, and eating the meat of apes and monkeys. High rates of SIV infection have been detected in primate meat sold in various bush meat markets in Africa. Obviously, the expansion of international markets for bush meat and exotic pets could lead to the transmission of other previously unknown animal viruses to humans.

In 2008, studies of tissue samples taken from a lymph node biopsy of a woman who died in 1960 in what is now the Democratic Republic of Congo confirmed suspicions that HIV had emerged by the early twentieth century. Previously, scientists had identified HIV in a tissue sample from 1959, but they suspected that there might be other samples of preserved human tissue in various hospital laboratories that would provide a more complete picture of the early history of the AIDS pandemic. Comparisons of the genetic sequence of HIV in tissue samples from 1959, 1960, and the 1970s are providing important insights into the emergence and molecular evolution of the virus. Although the biological prehistory of the HIV/AIDS pandemic remains uncertain, researchers speculate that the ancestral virus may have jumped from chimpanzees to humans sporadically. Historical studies of the growth of large cities, colonialism, and commerce in the late nineteenth and early twentieth centuries in areas where HIV first emerged could hold the key to determining the factors that accelerated the transmission of a once rare virus to large numbers of new victims.

For example, modern medical practices, compromised by the lack of sufficient funding and resources, might have amplified and accelerated the transmission of HIV within Africa and throughout the rest of the world. Hospitals and clinics, in particular, can serve as incubators and amplifiers of the virus because the use and reuse of medical equipment for injections, blood transfusions, vaccinations, and surgical procedures would provide unprecedented opportunities for transmission of the virus.

Medical workers and missionaries who cared for patients with fevers, diarrheal diseases, and other complications associated with AIDS could have contracted the virus and transported it to other parts of the world. It was not uncommon for Europeans to return to their country of origin in poor health, suffering from nonspecific Africa fevers. In general, poor health and a high burden of infectious diseases, including malaria, makes HIV more transmissible. Researchers think that individuals who are HIV-positive are at increased risk for malaria and that malaria infection promotes the replication of HIV. Thus, simultaneous infection with AIDS and malaria might have promoted the explosive growth of the AIDS epidemic in Africa. Once HIV became established in humans, inadequate sterilization techniques in clinics, hospitals, and mass-vaccination campaigns throughout the world could transmit HIV. During the 1980s, changes in human behavior—increased travel, changing sexual customs, intravenous drug abuse, blood transfusions, and the use of pooled blood to produce special products such as clotting factors for hemophiliacs—accelerated the spread of HIV.

Studies of the AIDS epidemic in China provide a troubling but compelling example of how the medical marketplace can amplify the spread of HIV and how attempts to ignore and conceal the problem can create further tragedy. By 2001, reports of AIDS devastating remote villages in China reached international public health experts. However, Chinese officials continued to underestimate the prevalence of HIV, despite evidence that more than a million people had contracted HIV from a blood product program in Henan Province alone. In some villages, the majority of all adults had HIV/AIDS. Companies marketing biological products, such as gamma globulin and clotting factors, had established blood plasma collection centers in Chinese villages. In many cases, plasma was separated from pooled blood, and the remaining pooled blood cells were reinfused into donors so that they could donate plasma more frequently. Under these conditions, if one donor was infected with HIV or hepatitis, many others could contract the disease. In 2006, government officials finally acknowledged that unsanitary practices in the collection of blood and the use of tainted blood and blood products in hospitals were major factors in the AIDS epidemic in China.

Epidemiologists may sometimes overlook customs and traditions that transmit pathogens to infants, children, and adults when they search for the origins of epidemics in unfamiliar cultures. For example, traditional mourning rituals, such as washing the body of relatives (even if they died of a very dangerous disease) or consuming the brains of victims of kuru, have been known to transmit the Ebola virus and prions, respectively. During coming-of-age ceremonies, healing rituals, and childbirth, traditional healers in many societies may carry out scarification, circumcision, infibulation, or the cutting of the umbilical cord with unsterilized blades. When these rituals involve groups of people, rather than individuals, the same blades are typically used on all participants. Such practices inevitably involve cross-contamination and favor the transmission of pathogens. Not surprisingly, in some parts of Africa, many traditional healers are HIV-positive because of their frequent contact with blood and body fluids. In Africa, HIV-positive mothers may feel compelled to participate in public ceremonies in which they are expected to breast-feed their infants. Lactating women in small villages or polygamous households may share the task of nursing the infants. All of these practices are very dangerous in areas where a large percentage of the population is infected with HIV. In some cultures, babies are exposed to HIV through food pre-chewed by an infected parent or caretaker. Three cases involving this form of transmission were documented in the United States in the 1990s, but pre-chewed food is not uncommon in developing countries. Virologists generally assumed that the concentration of HIV in saliva was too low to allow transmission, but if the individual chewing the food has open sores or scratches in the mouth, saliva could be mixed with enough blood to allow transmission of the virus. Having confirmed the transmission of HIV from caregivers to infants through pre-chewed food, researchers suggested that this previously overlooked custom might also transmit other pathogens, including hepatitis B virus and *Helicobacter pylori*.

Epidemiological studies indicate that some traditional practices, such as male circumcision, may reduce the risk of contracting AIDS. Statistical studies indicated that the incidence of AIDS was higher in areas of Africa where men were not circumcised and lower in areas where the procedure was common, but many scientists were skeptical about the significance of this correlation. Controlled studies in Kenya, South Africa, and Uganda in 2006 provided convincing evidence that male circumcision reduced the risk of HIV infection by 50 to 60 percent. AIDS specialists note that a vaccine providing greater than 50 percent protection would have created a great deal of excitement. In 2007, the World Health Organization (WHO) endorsed male circumcision as part of its African anti-AIDS programs.

Despite the evidence that HIV is the causative agent of AIDS, groups known as *AIDS denialists* continue to assert that HIV does not cause AIDS, or, more generally, that AIDS is a diagnostic myth, rather than a true disease. Some scientists and journalists have supported the proposition that HIV does not cause AIDS. Peter Duesberg, a well-known molecular biologist, has been a leading advocate of the proposition that HIV does not cause AIDS. In 1987, Duesberg published a paper in *Cancer Research* that denied a causal relationship between AIDS and HIV, which Duesberg described as one of many essentially harmless retroviruses that replicate in human beings. According to Duesberg, AIDS is not an infectious disease caused by a virus, but a collection of variable symptoms caused by lifestyle issues, such as using recreational drugs and taking medical drugs, such as azidothymidine (AZT). His arguments ignore the fact that even before HIV was discovered, the CDC had evidence that blood from donors with AIDS transmitted the disease to male and female recipients, young and old, with no history of drug abuse. Another argument put forth by Duesberg was that AIDS, the diagnostic entity associated with homosexual men in the United States, did not exist in Africa because the kinds of opportunistic infections that originally defined AIDS in America were different from the kinds of infections associated with the condition identified as AIDS in Africa.

Although Duesberg claimed that his views were being censored by publishers and the scientific community, his arguments have been published and analyzed in prominent journals, including *Cancer Research, Science, Nature,* and *The Lancet.* In several books, including *Inventing the AIDS Virus* (1995) and *Inventing the AIDS Epidemic* (1994), Duesberg explained his ideas and disparaged his critics. He also formed the Group for the Scientific Reappraisal of the HIV-AIDS Hypothesis, which included 1993 Nobel laureate Kary Mullis, inventor of the polymerase chain reaction (PCR), to send letters to various science journals expressing opposition to the concept that AIDS is a disease caused by HIV. Outside of the AIDS denialist network, scientists are convinced that studies of the relationship between HIV and AIDS in every population group in every part of the world unequivocally prove that HIV causes AIDS. Former AIDS denialists and skeptics have publicly expressed their conviction that the evidence that HIV causes AIDS and that antiretroviral therapy saves lives is now indisputable. Unfortunately, questions about the cause of AIDS raised by prominent scientists before HIV was discovered are still cited in AIDS denialist literature as proof that HIV does not cause AIDS.

In 1985, the first AIDS conference, held in Atlanta, Georgia, attracted about two thousand scientists. By 2002, when the Fourteenth International AIDS Conference was held, more than twenty million people had died of AIDS. Since AIDS was recognized as a global catastrophe, the International AIDS Conferences have served as a forum for the exchange of information among scientists, people with HIV, AIDS activists, social workers, economists, lawyers, policy makers, and pharmaceutical companies. The conferences have also provided a focus for protests against politicians, the pharmaceutical industry, and the biomedical community by AIDS activists frustrated by the lack of effective remedies and preventive vaccines. Some of the conferences have been held in countries where the AIDS epidemic was particularly devastating, health care facilities were limited, and research laboratories were essentially nonexistent. In 2006, at the Sixteenth International AIDS Conference, the United Nations AIDS Program (Unaids) and WHO reported that the number of people living with AIDS had climbed to almost forty million. During the period from the 1990s to 2006, AIDS had caused about 2.8 million deaths every year. Epidemiologists predicted that unless prevention programs were greatly expanded, AIDS might claim almost seventy million more lives by 2020, more than triple the number who died in the first twenty years of the epidemic. Based on the analysis of data from more than one hundred countries, demographers estimated that close to 120 million people could die of AIDS from 2006 to 2030.

By 2000, AIDS experts generally agreed that combinations of drugs, known as medical cocktails, had revolutionized the treatment of HIV/AIDS. International public health advocates urged all nations to support universal access to antiviral drug treatment and comprehensive prevention programs. When the AIDS epidemic began, antiviral drugs—unlike antibacterial agents—were virtually nonexistent, but antiviral drug development was stimulated by the emergence of AIDS. By 1987, AZT, the first drug that seemed to slow the progression of AIDS, was generally available. AZT targets reverse transcriptase, the enzyme that HIV needs to make a DNA copy of its genome. However, AZT was associated with many adverse reactions and it was not effective in advanced disease. At the 1996 International AIDS Conference, researchers were able to report that a complex and expensive regimen of new antiretroviral drugs, called *protease inhibitors*, in combination with older drugs increased the life expectancy of AIDS patients. The effectiveness of antiviral drug cocktails helped convince some skeptics that HIV was the causative agent of AIDS. Transforming HIV/AIDS from a death sentence to a very costly chronic disease produced new questions, complications, and challenges, as patients survived decades of chronic AIDS, AIDS drugs, and the aging process.

Despite evidence that antiviral therapy could improve and extend the lives of people with HIV/AIDS, only a small fraction of the people who need antiviral therapy get appropriate treatment. The United Nations called for universal access to AIDS treatment by 2010, but this goal was generally regarded as overly optimistic. Improved life expectancy for people with HIV/AIDS has decreased interest in funding universal access to treatment and prevention programs. Wealthy nations, where antiviral drugs have largely transformed HIV/AIDS into a chronic condition that can be managed by antiretroviral therapy, are no longer driven by the sense of urgency that AIDS originally inspired. Unfortunately, successful development of treatment options for HIV/AIDS was not accompanied by success in developing safe and effective preventive vaccines.

According to a 2006 report by Unaids, the AIDS pandemic continues to grow, even in countries that had previously demonstrated significant success in containing the disease. Determining the number of deaths caused by AIDS is complicated by the fact that in some countries, such as South Africa, HIV/AIDS is a major factor in deaths attributed to malaria, tuberculosis, and other diseases. Dramatic increases in the death rates for adult age groups from 1997 to 2005 in South Africa suggested a surge in HIV/AIDS cases, but because of government policies, South African doctors generally do not designate AIDS as the cause of death. South Africa's president Thabo Mbeki's skepticism about the relationship between HIV and AIDS became widely known in 2000, when the Thirteenth International AIDS Conference was held in Durban, South Africa. Mbeki and health minister Dr. Manto Tshabalala-Msimang famously argued that traditional African remedies, such as lemons, beetroot, and garlic, were more effective than antiviral drugs in preventing and curing the diseases that Western doctors attributed to HIV/AIDS. To promote the views of Duesberg and other AIDS denialists, Mbeki convened his own Presidential Advisory Panel on HIV and AIDS. Like Duesberg, Tshabalala-Msimang and Mbeki insisted that Western antiviral drugs were dangerous poisons. Therefore, the South African government refused to give antiviral drugs to HIV-positive pregnant women, an approach that prevents the transmission of the virus to newborn babies. Two years later, the Treatment Action Campaign, an AIDS advocacy group, and the South African courts forced the government to reverse this policy. In response to global attention, by 2006, South Africa's government agreed to increase the distribution of antiretroviral drugs.

In 2007, the United Nations issued a report lowering its estimate of the number of people living with HIV/AIDS from about forty million to thirty-three million. Nevertheless, about two and a half million people become infected with HIV each year, and more than two million people die of AIDS annually. Globally, AIDS has become the fourth leading cause of death. Without a preventive vaccine, the number of people with HIV/AIDS will continue to increase, as antiretroviral drugs become more effective and more accessible.

In 1984, when the AIDS virus was discovered, federal health officials optimistically predicted that a vaccine would be produced within three years. More than twenty years later, the attempt to establish an AIDS vaccine was considered a failure, and many scientists wondered whether the nature of the virus made it impossible to create a preventive vaccine. Twenty-four year later, in his presidential address at the 2008 meeting of the American Association for the Advancement of Science, David Baltimore acknowledged that scientists were no closer to a preventive vaccine for HIV/AIDS than they were in the early 1980s, when the pandemic began. Advocates and critics of HIV vaccine research considered Baltimore's assessment of advances and failures very significant because of his leadership in the field since the discovery of HIV. Indeed, the discovery of the enzyme known as reverse transcriptase, for which Baltimore shared the 1975 Nobel Prize in Medicine or Physiology with Howard Temin, was fundamental to the work that made it possible to identify and analyze HIV. Baltimore served as the first chair of the National Institutes of Health's (NIH) AIDS Vaccine Research Committee.

In 1986, the Institute of Medicine and the National Academy of Sciences funded a study of the virus, the disease, and its history in order to suggest a national strategy for coping with the emerging epidemic. Finding a vaccine was one of the key recommendations of the report, titled *Confronting AIDS: Directions for Public Health, Health Care, and Research*. During the 1980s, scientists had not yet realized that HIV would be such a difficult target for a preventive vaccine. Ten years after the publication of *Confronting AIDS*, Baltimore became the chairman of an NIH-sponsored committee attempting to energize the ten-year search for an AIDS vaccine. Once again, the establishment of a safe and effective AIDS vaccine seemed to be at least ten years away.

When the search for an AIDS vaccine began, scientists tried conventional techniques to create either a killed vaccine or a live attenuated vaccine. Advances in molecular biology led to attempts to create subunit vaccines, that is, vaccines containing only parts of the virus, usually surface proteins that normally stimulate the immune system. This approach worked for the hepatitis B virus, but not for HIV, an insidious stealth virus that has the ability to camouflage and conceal its critical antigens from the immune system, while hiding in many different types of cells and tissues. Even if the immune system detects viral antigens, HIV's high rate of mutation outpaces the body's defense mechanisms. Despite pressure to accelerate the development of a preventive vaccine, the ability of HIV to elude and destroy the immune system and its high mutation rate have confounded efforts to establish a safe and effective AIDS vaccine.

Public health experts and virologists generally agree that vaccines are the only, or at least the most effective, way to control and eradicate epidemic viral diseases. However, pessimism about the prospects of developing an AIDS vaccine increased in 2007 when yet another AIDS vaccine trial was terminated. One potential AIDS vaccine actually seemed to increase vulnerability to HIV infection, at least in some recipients. On the other hand, some tests of SIV vaccines in nonhuman primates were more successful than preliminary trials of similar human HIV vaccines. After so many fruitless attempts to establish an effective AIDS vaccine, some scientists are calling for a new balance between applied research and basic research, although HIV has probably been the object of more scientific research than any other pathogen. The benefits of basic research are obvious in terms of the unprecedented development of antiviral drugs to treat AIDS. Because of antiretroviral drugs, the life expectancy for people with AIDS has increased, but the HIV/AIDS pandemic has not subsided.

Critics of ongoing HIV/AIDS research efforts, such as the AIDS Healthcare Foundation (AHF), argue that after so much evidence that the quest for an AIDS vaccine has been a failure, funding for AIDS vaccine research should be directed to prevention and treatment programs for AIDS and cures for other diseases. The AHF, founded in California in 1987 to care for dying AIDS patients, evolved into a global organization dedicated to AIDS treatment, prevention, and advocacy.

Despite disappointments and failures, interest in an AIDS vaccine remains high, according to the International AIDS Vaccine Initiative. Optimism is generally justified by studies of several categories of individuals who do not progress to AIDS despite exposure to HIV. First, there are rare individuals known as *elite controllers* or long-term nonprogressors who have been infected but remain healthy for many years. Second, some individuals (usually sex workers) have been repeatedly exposed to HIV but have not become infected. Third, some HIV-infected individuals develop antibodies that are capable of neutralizing a broad range of HIV strains. Researchers hope to find out how the immune systems of these unusual individuals resist or control the virus. By studying their immune responses, scientists might learn how to design an effective AIDS vaccine or find ways of stimulating the production of more effective antibodies. Nevertheless, there is no evidence that anyone with an established HIV infection has spontaneously eradicated the virus, which is the usual response to viruses like smallpox, measles, and influenza.

Like David Baltimore, Anthony Fauci has been at the forefront of HIV/AIDS work since the first cases were detected. Since he agreed to serve as director of the U.S. National Institute of Allergy and Infectious Diseases in 1984, Fauci has become widely known for his research and his ability to communicate with the public about the threat of infectious diseases and bioterrorism. In addition to stimulating the expansion of AIDS research at the NIH, Fauci has also worked with AIDS activists and advocates to improve communication and advance treatment and testing programs. Although Fauci has been cautious in his predictions about the development of an AIDS vaccine, he is adamant about the need for a preventive vaccine. Some AIDS activists argue that research funds should be dedicated to testing and treatment, rather than further attempts to create a vaccine. Offering an historical context, Fauci has urged critics to remember that it took many decades to create safe and effective vaccines for relatively simple viral diseases like measles and pertussis (whooping cough).

In view of the history of the HIV/AIDS pandemic, Fauci has suggested that it might be necessary to accept a partially effective AIDS vaccine. Many existing vaccines are not 100 percent effective, but if a majority of a population is immunized, the dissemination of a pathogen will be inhibited. A less than perfect vaccine could, therefore, be a valuable component of a preventive strategy to ease the terrible burden of disease that is overwhelming poor countries devastated by AIDS. Because of the complicated social and economic factors that operate in different countries and communities, no simple solution is likely to control the global AIDS pandemic but public health advocates insist that, in the long run, preventive vaccines are the most effective and least expensive way to control AIDS and other life-threatening viral diseases.

VIRAL HEMORRHAGIC FEVERS

As the pace of discovery of new viruses seemed to accelerate, experts on emerging diseases suggested that learning to cope with unfamiliar diseases might become the new status quo. Not all newly emerging pathogens will have the ability to become global threats, but the factors that transform localized outbreaks into potential pandemics are not always obvious. Many of the emerging diseases detected since the 1960s are caused by pathogens previously confined to the jungles of Africa, the rain forests of South America, and other previously isolated areas. The most deadly of the newly emerging diseases, generally known as hemorrhagic viral fevers, may be capable of spreading to new areas. It is difficult to diagnose specific viral hemorrhagic fevers on the basis of symptoms alone. Without specific diagnostic tests, at least in the early stages and in mild cases, these diseases are often mistaken for other febrile illnesses such as malaria.

In 1967, a deadly unknown disease attacked more than thirty people associated with two research institutes, one in Marburg, Germany, and one in Belgrade, Yugoslavia. Seven people died. Those who contracted the disease experienced high fever, diarrhea, bloody vomit and feces, and, in some cases, bleeding from essentially all body orifices. All of the initial victims, including technicians making polio vaccine, had direct contact with monkeys or monkey blood, organs, or tissue cultures. The disease also spread to six people who had contact with the first group of patients. Eventually, the causative agent, now known as the Marburg virus, was identified as a virus carried by monkeys imported from Uganda. The Marburg virus is a member of the *Filoviridae* family, which consists of RNA viruses with a threadlike structure. The Marburg virus was the first of several deadly filoviruses to be identified by the end of the twentieth century, but the mortality rate for Marburg fever has been difficult to measure because cases have been very sporadic.

After the virus was identified, Marburg fever outbreaks were identified in South Africa, Kenya, the Democratic Republic of Congo, and Angola. In the Democratic Republic of Congo, among 154 cases recorded between 1998 and 2000, there were 128 deaths. One case of an unidentified hemorrhagic fever in a hospital in Angola in 2004 might have been the source of an outbreak of Marburg fever that eventually killed three hundred people. Although monkeys were thought to be the normal host of the virus, in 2007, researchers found the Marburg virus in cave-dwelling fruit bats. All of the infected bats appeared healthy, which suggests that the bat-infested lead and gold mines in western Uganda provide the natural reservoir for the virus.

Ebola hemorrhagic fever was first identified in 1976 after outbreaks in the Democratic Republic of Congo and Sudan. The virus was named for the Ebola River Valley in the Congo. Since the 1990s, Ebola fever outbreaks have also occurred in Gabon, Uganda, and Ivory Coast. In 1995, a major outbreak of Ebola in Kikwit, Democratic Republic of Congo, killed about 250 people. By 2007, WHO had documented about 1850 cases with more than 1200 deaths since the Ebola virus was discovered. Ebola virus has also killed thousands of chimpanzees and gorillas in African wildlife sanctuaries and national parks. During some outbreaks, the mortality rate for gorillas seemed to be as high as 90 to 95 percent. As in human populations, the disease seems to be transmitted from its natural host species, perhaps through contaminated food, and by ape-to-ape transmission within social groups.

Like the Marburg virus, the Ebola virus is a member of the *Filoviridae* family; both viruses are transmitted by blood and body fluids. Since the first Ebola fever virus was discovered, several distinct subgroups have been identified and their genomes sequenced, which should help explain differences in virulence and transmission. Determining the mortality rate for Ebola fever has been difficult, but during various outbreaks, case fatality rates have ranged from 50 to 90 percent. Initially, patients experience fever, headache, vomiting, diarrhea, and internal and external bleeding, which usually progresses to bleeding from the nose, mouth, and anus, followed by death from shock or organ failure. The first known outbreak was traced to a hospitalized patient who was originally thought to have malaria. The virus was apparently transmitted to nurses and doctors who had taken care of the patient and to other patients by means of contaminated instruments. A second wave of cases occurred among people who participated in traditional burial rites that involve washing and touching the body of a dead relative. In most outbreaks, clinics and hospitals have served as incubators and amplifiers for the virus because of the lack of resources, from sterile needles and syringes to the disposable gloves, masks, and gowns needed for rigorous infection control procedures.

Several Ebola virus subgroups have been found in apes and monkeys, which suggests that people might have contracted the virus by handling meat, blood, and organs from infected chimpanzees, gorillas, monkeys, antelopes, and porcupines. In isolated areas, infected individuals probably died too quickly to transmit the virus to many other people. The incubation period for the disease is short and the onset of serious symptoms is so sudden that victims are unlikely to travel or come into direct contact with many people before they die. Family members who care for the patient and prepare the body for burial are, however, at risk. In more densely populated areas, where victims of Ebola are likely to be hospitalized, the virus has the unprecedented opportunity to infect unrelated people, that is, hospital staff members who come in contact with infected blood and bodily fluids and other patients who are infected by means of contaminated medical and surgical instruments.

A strain of the virus known as Ebola Reston was discovered in 1989 when monkeys that had been shipped from the Philippines to the Hazleton Research Products' Primate Quarantine Unit in Reston, Virginia, began dying of an unknown disease. Veterinarians suspected that the deaths were caused by simian hemorrhagic fever, but tissue samples examined at the United States Army Medical Research Institute of Infectious Diseases (USAMRIID) revealed the presence of the Ebola virus. Under the electron microscope, Ebola Reston is essentially identical to the subtypes that cause disease in humans. Although Ebola Reston is very deadly in monkeys, it does not cause illness in humans. However, antibodies to the virus have been detected in some people who worked with infected monkeys or tissue from infected animals. So far, only the Ebola Reston virus seems to be capable of spreading through the air. The Ebola strains that are deadly in humans have not developed the capacity for airborne transmission. Richard Preston's book *The Hot Zone*, which describes the Reston outbreak, and the 1995 film *Outbreak*, a fictionalized version of an Ebolalike virus, provoked intense interest in Ebola and other emerging diseases.

The natural reservoir of the Ebola virus is uncertain, despite tests conducted on various mammals, birds, reptiles, amphibians, and arthropods from affected areas in Africa. At the time of the Reston, Virginia, outbreak among monkeys imported from the Philippines, researchers were unable to conduct field studies in the Philippines because of a civil war in the area where the monkeys were originally collected. As in the case of the Marburg virus, fruit bats are considered the most likely hosts. In regions where outbreaks of Ebola have occurred, people are known to eat bats. Several species of bats harbor the Ebola virus without becoming sick, even when they are experimentally infected. Bats also seem to be the natural reservoir for the Nipah virus, Hendra virus, and lyssaviruses. Other rodents, typically mice and rats, serve as the natural reservoir for many other emerging viruses, including the Lassa fever virus and the hantaviruses.

People usually contract the Lassa fever virus when they come in contact with mouse excrement, either by inhalation or by consuming contaminated foods. The virus can also be transmitted from person to person via airborne viral particles and contact with blood and body fluids. After the Lassa fever virus was described in 1969 in Lassa, Nigeria, researchers discovered that the disease was endemic to several countries in West Africa. The vast majority of infections seem to be mild or asymptomatic, but almost 20 percent of patients sick enough to be hospitalized die of the disease.

Ancient Chinese texts suggest the existence of hemorrhagic fevers that might have been caused by hantaviruses, but this family of diseases was apparently unknown to Western doctors until the 1950s. After hantavirus fever outbreaks in Korea, Japan, Russia, and Europe, at least twenty members of the hantavirus family were discovered.

The hantaviruses are named for the Hantan River in Korea, where a disease previously known as Korean hemorrhagic fever virus was identified during the Korean War. Diseases caused by the hantaviruses are now known as hemorrhagic fevers with renal syndrome (HFRS). Hantaviruses that cause HFRS have been found in China, Korea, Russia, Europe, and North and South America. In 1993, a new hantavirus was identified as the cause of an outbreak of hantavirus cardiopulmonary syndrome (HCPS, or HPS) that killed at least thirty people in the Four Corners region, where New Mexico, Colorado, Utah, and Arizona meet. The virus has been called the *sin nombre* (nameless) virus. Victims of the disease contracted the virus by inhaling dust particles containing viruses excreted by deer mice, which were unusually abundant that year. Since the disease was recognized, hundreds of cases have been reported from California to the East Coast and Florida. The mortality rate seems to be about 50 percent.

Changes in the geographic distribution of fruit bats may be responsible for the emergence and dispersal of a significant number of viruses new to humans such as Hendra virus, Nipah virus, Ross River virus, Barmah Forest virus, and Chikungunya virus. The Hendra virus (named after a suburb of Brisbane, Australia) and the Nipah virus (named for a village in Malaysia) were first discovered in the 1990s. During the 1990s, the Hendra virus suddenly appeared among pigs, horses, and humans in Australia. Originally known as equine morbillivirus, the Hendra virus is a single-stranded RNA virus that is closely related to the Nipah virus. Infection with Hendra virus can result in encephalitis, convulsions, coma, and death. Epidemiological studies indicated that people contracted the infection through direct contact with tissues or secretions of horses that were ill and later died. Australian fruit bats apparently provide the natural reservoir for Hendra virus.

Once known as the Hendra-like virus, the Nipah virus was identified after people contracted a severe form of encephalitis after coming in contact with infected Malaysian pigs. Symptoms exhibited by sick pigs included coughing, seizures, and high fevers. In pigs, the disease seemed to be highly contagious and often lethal. People who came in contact with infected pigs became ill with fever, headache, drowsiness, disorientation, seizures, respiratory problems, and coma. The fatality rate among people hospitalized during the outbreak was about 40 percent. The disease did not seem to spread readily from person to person because nurses and doctors who cared for the sick did not contract the disease. Tissues from infected people and pigs revealed the presence of a previously unknown virus that closely resembled the Hendra virus. Scientists think that fruit bats, which carry the virus, were driven out of their normal habitat by the destruction of the rain forests. Displaced bats spread the virus to pigs, but Nipah virus can also infect horses, dogs, cats, and people.

Malaysian authorities ended the outbreak by destroying about half of Malaysia's 2.4 million pigs. These control measures were devastating to affected workers and farmers. Although Nipah virus is virtually unknown outside of Malaysia and Singapore, scientists consider it one of many emerging viruses likely to invade new areas as a consequence of changing patterns of animal husbandry and commercial relationships. Once the Nipah virus and its natural host had been identified, scientists were able to identify outbreaks in other countries, including Bangladesh. Fruit bats are widely distributed throughout Australia, Malaysia, Indonesia, the Philippines, and some Pacific islands. If modified strains of Nipah or Hendra virus become highly contagious and escape from their present geographic regions, they could cause catastrophic pandemics and pose a threat to domesticated animals.

Rift Valley fever is caused by a virus found in cattle and other hoofed mammals, primarily in sub-Saharan Africa and Egypt. The virus is transmitted to humans by the bite of a mosquito; by exposure to blood, raw milk, or other fluids from infected animals; or by milking, slaughtering, and butchering infected animals. In humans, the virus can cause hemorrhagic fever, brain infection, and death. The disease is especially dangerous in pregnant animals and women in the third trimester of pregnancy. The disease was described in livestock in Kenya in the early part of the twentieth century, and the virus was identified in the 1930s. Rift Valley fever outbreaks typically occur in sub-Saharan Africa, but outbreaks have occurred in Egypt, Saudi Arabia, Yemen, Kenya, Somalia, South Mauritania, and Madagascar. The virus has been isolated from livestock, wild animals, bats, and sand flies as well as mosquitoes, but the natural reservoir of the virus and the factors that trigger large outbreaks are still obscure. The mosquitoes that carry Rift Valley fever virus are widely distributed and will take a blood meal from cattle, sheep, goats, horses, and chickens as well as humans.

Predicting new outbreaks of Rift Valley fever and other rare, emerging viral diseases is highly speculative, but following the prevalence and feeding behavior of insect vectors is an important component of disease surveillance and early warning systems. Moreover, attempts to identify the natural reservoir and vectors for one emerging pathogen may lead to the discovery of other viruses. For example, in the 1960s, during a study of dengue fever in Malaysia and Indonesia, researchers investigated the ecology of mosquitoes carrying the dengue fever virus; they collected mosquitoes from different habitats and took blood samples from animals and humans. In addition to tracking the distribution of dengue fever viruses, virologists collected information about other viruses, including Zika, Japanese encephalitis, Chikungunya virus, and several still unidentified arthropod-borne viruses (arboviruses). At least eighty different arboviruses are known to cause diseases in humans.

Dengue fever is considered one of the most dangerous mosquito-borne epidemic diseases. Many aspects of the immunological response to repeated dengue fever attacks remain unclear, but confusion between dengue fever and little-known diseases caused by other arboviruses might account for part of the problem. For example, the disease caused by the Zika virus resembles a mild attack of dengue fever. Like the dengue fever virus, the Zika virus is transmitted by mosquitoes. Although the Zika virus is not well known, it has been found in many widely separated areas and in very different environments. First discovered in the 1940s in monkeys in the Zika forest of Uganda, the virus was only associated with a few sporadic human cases in Africa and Southeast Asia until 2007, when an outbreak occurred in Micronesia and spread to Guam.

Chikungunya fever, another emerging viral disease, also resembles a mild attack of dengue fever. The Chikungunya virus was identified in Tanzania (southeastern Africa) in the 1950s, but its natural reservoir is uncertain. Until 2006, when a major outbreak struck India, Madagascar, and Réunion, Chikungunya fever was considered a rare tropical disease. Sporadic outbreaks had previously been detected in Asia and Africa, but the 2006 epidemic caused more than one million cases and many deaths in India.

Epidemiologists concluded that the disease spread from Kenya to Réunion and other islands off the east coast of Africa, infecting more than ten thousand people within two years. Travelers with Chikungunya fever carried the virus from India and Réunion to Europe and North America, but public health authorities did not expect the virus to find appropriate vectors outside its original geographical zone. An outbreak of Chikungunya fever in Italy in 2007 challenged that belief and demonstrated that tropical arboviruses were spreading into new areas and finding suitable vectors. Many infectious disease experts believe that this pattern has been accelerated by global warming as well as international trade and travel. Although the Chikungunya virus is usually transmitted by *Aedes aegpti*, *Aedes albopictus*, the tiger mosquito, can also serve as a vector. Tiger mosquitoes reached southern Italy in shipments of tires during the 1990s, and their range apparently expanded northward with rising temperatures.

Epidemiologists suggest that the appearance of Chikungunya fever in Europe may be a preview of new patterns of infectious disease made possible by climate change and globalization. If so, then other emerging tropical diseases might become a persistent threat to northern countries. West Nile virus, which first appeared in New York City in 1999, demonstrated how easily emerging viruses could spread from continent to continent and become established in new regions. At least sixty people in the New York area contracted West Nile fever, and seven died of encephalitis. By 2001, West Nile virus could be found in various species of mosquitoes, birds, and mammals all across the United States. The dispersal of West Nile fever in North America presented a rare opportunity for scientists to chart this phenomenon. West Nile fever also shows how newly emerging diseases attract more attention and generate more anxiety than diseases considered ordinary. For example, although St. Louis encephalitis has a much higher case fatality rate than West Nile, it receives very little media attention. West Nile fever was first identified in the West Nile district of Uganda in 1937. During an outbreak in Egypt in the 1950s, scientists detected the virus in birds and mosquitoes. Before its first appearance in North American, the virus was found in Africa, the Middle East, parts of Europe, western Russia, southwestern Asia, and Australia.

Researchers say West Nile may be just one example of an infectious disease whose incidence and geographic range have expanded because of human activities affecting the mosquitoes, birds, rodents, and other animals that help spread the infection. Warm winters and summer droughts punctuated by torrential rains favor the mosquitoes involved in the spread of West Nile virus as well as the rate of maturation of viruses within mosquitoes. The destruction of wilderness, with its specialized niches, favors the extinction of native creatures and the multiplication of opportunistic creatures like rats and crows. Crows are important to West Nile virus because they are capable of spreading it to mosquitoes that also bite people.

INTERNATIONAL TRAVEL AND SARS

The expansion of the international trade in exotic animals, often taken from wild, previously isolated areas, whether for foods or as pets, has created many opportunities for the emergence of new diseases. Once a microbe spreads from animals to humans, many factors in modern life can contribute to its further dissemination. Diseases directly transmitted via the respiratory route are particularly likely to be disseminated by international air travel, as demonstrated by the rapid dispersal of a previously unknown disease that was described as severe acute respiratory syndrome (SARS) in 2003. The first cases of the disease apparently occurred in southern China by 2002. After the disease reached Hong Kong and Singapore, airline passengers carried the SARS virus to thirty countries on five continents. By the middle of 2003, SARS had infected more than eight thousand people and caused about nine hundred deaths. Initially, scientists suspected that the SARS virus might be related to the measles virus, but under the electron microscope, the virus resembled the coronaviruses that cause the common cold. Further work confirmed the fact that SARS was caused by a previously unknown coronavirus. Attempts to identify the natural reservoir of the virus led to the discovery of the SARS virus in Himalayan palm civets, catlike animals sold in live food markets in Chinese cities. Although the SARS virus can also infect rats, mice, ferrets, cats, foxes, and monkeys, the Chinese horseshoe bat seems to be the natural animal reservoir.

SARS demonstrated how quickly a few imported cases of an unknown disease could trigger a widespread epidemic. An investigation of the SARS outbreak in Toronto, Canada, blamed poor hospital infection-control procedures for turning one case imported from Hong Kong into an outbreak that killed more than forty people, including one doctor and two nurses, and caused about four hundred cases of SARS in Ontario Province. Almost half of the sick were health care workers. Public health authorities concluded that quarantines imposed in some affected countries helped stop a potentially catastrophic pandemic.

INFLUENZA: THE LAST GREAT PLAGUE

Before the appearance of AIDS, SARS, and other newly emerging infectious diseases, many scientists were calling influenza the "last great plague." Often dismissed as a commonplace annual nuisance, influenza is a highly contagious viral disease that causes deadly pandemics when novel forms of the virus appear. Viruses cause many exotic and life-threatening diseases, but in any given year, about 80 percent of the acute illnesses that occur in the United States are respiratory infections caused by cold and flu viruses. In an ordinary year, influenza viruses infect an estimated 30 to 120 million people worldwide. Influenza and its complications kill about a million people each year, including about thirty-six thousand in America, mainly the elderly and those with weakened immune systems. However, because respiratory illnesses may be misdiagnosed, many deaths ascribed to influenza and its complications are probably caused by other pathogens. On the other hand, influenza in young children is often misdiagnosed as asthma or pneumonia (see Figure 7.2).

Descriptions of major outbreaks of influenza have appeared in the literature since the term was introduced in Italy in the fifteenth century, but the disease associated with this term appears to be quite ancient. Pandemic influenza apparently originated in Asia and then spread to Africa and Europe. Influenza epidemics typically occur during the coldest months of the year in temperate zones, but the disease is not seasonal or common in the tropics. Attempting to determine the factors that lead to seasonal outbreaks, scientists determined that influenza virus transmission varies with air temperature and relative humidity. Influenza viruses spread most efficiently not by direct contact, but through respiratory droplets, which are most stable in cold, dry air. Cold viruses, in contrast, are usually spread by direct contact with infected people or contaminated surfaces.

Of the three influenza pandemics that occurred in the twentieth century, the worst was the 1918 pandemic that coincided with World War I. Some researchers suggest that the virus was already circulating by 1916, but wartime secrecy may have obscured evidence of the initial outbreaks and other aspects of the pandemic. Influenza epidemics generally originate in China, but the 1918 pandemic might have begun on the pig farms of Haskill County, Kansas. In the United States, the first known victims were soldiers at an army camp in Kansas. The virus quickly spread among soldiers in America and Europe. Eventually, the highly contagious and deadly influenza virus spread to almost every part of the world, adding to the turmoil caused by the war. Presumably, the 1918 influenza spread so rapidly because the entire global population had little or no immunity to the virus. Despite the origins of the pandemic, after the disease spread to Europe, it became widely known as the Spanish flu.

In 1918, British researchers trying to identify the pathogen that causes influenza discovered that ferrets made a good experimental animal because infected ferrets transmit the disease, whereas infected mice do not. Bacteria-free filtrates from human victims sickened healthy ferrets, and the disease could be transmitted from sick to healthy ferrets. Thus, the influenza virus was one of the pathogens originally classified as a filterable, invisible virus. At the time, however, the medical community was uncertain about the relationship between annual, localized outbreaks of influenza and catastrophic global pandemics of a disease that clinically resembled influenza. Many futile therapies were prescribed, such as vaccines against other diseases, quinine, codeine, morphine, heroin, and even bleeding. Attempts to stop the disease included the use of gauze masks, bans on shaking hands, and the killing of stray dogs, which were thought to be spreading the disease.

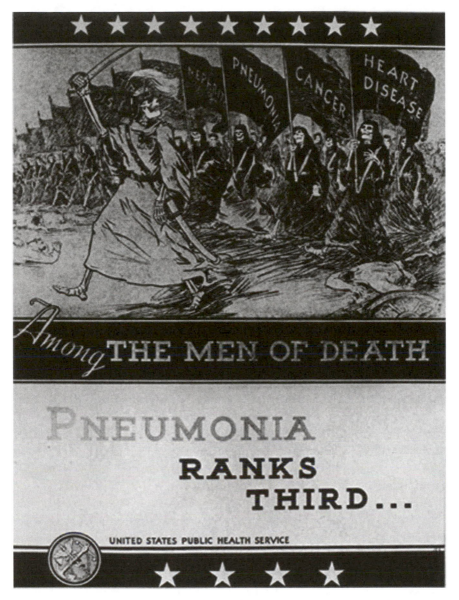

Figure 7.2 A poster used by the U.S. Public Health Service in the 1930s to educate Americans about the danger of contagious respiratory diseases such as pneumonia, which was one of the leading causes of death at the time. Credit: National Library of Medicine, National Institutes of Health, U.S. Public Health Service.

Epidemiologists consider the influenza pandemic of 1918 to 1919 one of the single deadliest infectious disease outbreaks in human history. Demographers estimate that at least 20 percent of the global population became infected. The overall case fatality rate was estimated at 2.5 percent. In contrast, the case fatality rate during ordinary flu outbreaks is usually about 0.1 percent. Although considerable uncertainty remains about the total number of victims in various parts of the world, early estimates indicated that the pandemic caused twenty to forty million deaths worldwide. Recent calculations suggest that the death toll might have been as high as fifty to one hundred million. In the United States, more than 25 million people, about one-quarter of the population, became infected, and about 675,000 died. In some parts of Alaska and the Pacific islands, more than half the population died. Scholars continue to revise estimates of the scope, impact, and number of deaths caused by the pandemic. Surviving records probably understate the scope of the pandemic because of underreporting and inaccurate diagnoses. Many countries lacked the capacity or willingness to measure and record the impact of the epidemic. Although precision is impossible, there is little doubt that the 1918 pandemic was one of the deadliest in recorded history.

In many ways, the 1918 pandemic followed the pattern of other influenza epidemics, but the virus was very highly transmissible, and the morbidity and mortality rates were unusually high. In most communities, 25 to 30 percent of the population contracted the disease, and many cases quickly progressed to fatal pneumonia. The unusually high fatality rate, especially among previously healthy people between fifteen and forty-five years of age, was one of the most striking aspects of the pandemic. Death was usually the result of severe, complicated infections of the respiratory tract. Many previously healthy adults, whether they were soldiers or civilians, sickened and died within twenty-four hours, suffocated by the buildup of fluid in their lungs. Among elderly patients, the death rate during the 1918 pandemic was relatively low.

Some influenza viruses are particularly dangerous because they are able to invade cells deep in the lungs as well as the cells of the upper respiratory tract that are attacked by common seasonal flu viruses. This was clearly one of the deadly characteristics of the 1918 influenza virus. When examining the lungs of influenza victims, pathologists found severe and unusual damage, including extensive hemorrhaging, the accumulation of fluid, and the destruction of tissues deep within the lungs. In addition to the traits that allowed the virus to invade lung tissues, the virus seems to have triggered a massive, but ultimately counterproductive response by the immune system. Although pathologists could not explain why the virus was more virulent in healthy young adults, scientists now think that it was primarily the very active immune response launched by young adults that contributed to the destruction of the delicate architecture of their lung tissues.

Scientists were unable to identify the agent that causes influenza until the 1930s, but since then, the virus has been studied in great detail. In 1933, virologists isolated and cultured the human influenza virus, a spherically shaped virus with a spiky surface primarily made up of proteins known as hemagglutinin (H) and neuraminidase (N). The genetic material of the virus consists of eight single-stranded RNA segments. Variants of the influenza virus present different combinations of hemagglutinin and neuraminidase as surface antigens. Hemagglutinin sticks to receptors on the surface of host cells, primarily those in the respiratory tract, so that the virus can enter the cells and multiply. Neuraminidase is an enzyme that helps new virus particles burst out of the host cell by disrupting the membrane. The newly released viruses can then repeat the process in other host cells. Hemagglutinin is the viral antigen that is most important in stimulating the host's immune system to produce antibodies that interfere with binding between the virus and host cell receptors, thereby preventing reinfection with previously encountered viruses. Influenza pandemics are, therefore, correlated with major changes in the gene for hemagglutinin. Reassortment of the genes coding for hemagglutinin and neuraminidase can produce many distinct influenza virus subtypes.

Gradual changes in the surface proteins of the influenza virus are responsible for the yearly recurrence of influenza epidemics. Genetic modifications allow new strains of the virus to evade antibodies evoked by the viruses that caused previous epidemics. In the early 1950s, Maurice R. Hilleman, eminent virologist and vaccinologist, described a pattern of genetic changes that characterize the evolution of the influenza virus. The minor changes that occur over time are known as *drift*. Major changes in the prevailing viral subtype, which are known as *shifts*, are likely to be followed by unusually extensive epidemics or even pandemics. Minor changes in the prevailing strains of influenza virus appear almost every year, but every ten or so years, major modifications occur that produce novel viral strains. When major changes occur, the entire human population is susceptible, and if the virus is highly contagious, the new virus can trigger a serious pandemic. A pandemic is most likely to occur with the emergence of an influenza virus with a novel hemagglutinin protein and the ability to spread from person to person.

The origin of the great pandemic influenza viruses is unclear, but scientists suspect a combination of mutational events and the exchange of genetic material between viruses associated with different host species, including domesticated animals and migratory birds. Therefore, epidemiologists are attempting to monitor animal influenza viruses throughout the world to anticipate potentially devastating pandemics. The severity of a pandemic depends on the virulence and contagiousness of the virus and the immune status of the population—that is, what portion of all people have antibodies to the viral antigens because of previous infections. Although scientists know that new strains of viruses emerge through reassortment and mutation, they have not yet been able to predict how and when new pandemic influenza strains will emerge or the virulence of novel strains.

If the genome of the 1918 influenza virus could be analyzed, scientists might be able to answer many questions about the most catastrophic pandemic in history. As the techniques of molecular biology improved, scientists realized that it might be possible to transform speculation about that possibility into reality. By recovering fragments of the 1918 influenza virus from preserved human tissue and analyzing its genetic material, scientists have come close to determining the factors that made it so deadly. In the 1990s, fragments of the 1918 influenza virus were recovered from preserved tissue samples of two American soldiers who had died of influenza and from the lungs of an Inuit woman who had been buried near a remote settlement in Alaska. From this fragmentary material, Jeffery Taubenberger and his coworkers at the Armed Forces Institute of Pathology (AFIP) were able to copy, amplify, and sequence the genome of the 1918 influenza virus. These studies have made it possible to reconstruct the virus and test hypotheses about its origin and its unusual virulence.

Jeffery Taubenberger and his colleagues in the Department of Molecular Pathology pioneered sensitive techniques for retrieving genetic material from the institute's remarkable collection of biological samples that dated back to the Civil War. Based on the success of these studies, Taubenberger decided to look for the 1918 virus in samples of preserved lung tissue. When Taubenberger's group recovered a tiny fragment of the viral genome, they used PCR technology to amplify their material. A preliminary account of this work was published in *Science* in 1997. Despite significant progress toward the task of assembling viral genes, Taubenberger needed more material to complete the sequence of the viral genome. Pathologist Johan Hultin discovered another source of viral material. In the 1950s, Hultin had unsuccessfully attempted to recover viable influenza virus from bodies buried in a mass grave in the Alaskan permafrost. After learning about Taubenberger's work, Hultin returned to Alaska, and this time, he was able to obtain well-preserved samples of lung tissue.

It took Taubenberger's team almost ten years to decipher the entire genome of the 1918 influenza virus. In 2005, the genetic sequence that defined the deadly 1918 influenza virus was published and added to a rapidly growing database of genomes that scientists could analyze. Once the entire genetic sequence was known, scientists were able to reconstruct the 1918 influenza virus. Experiments designed to recreate the 1918 virus and test its virulence in mice were carried out in a high-biosecurity laboratory. Defending the decision to recreate the 1918 flu virus, Terrence Tumpey, a microbiologist at the Influenza Branch of the CDC, argued that it was an essential step toward determining what made the virus so exceptionally deadly and contagious. Indeed, deciphering the genome of the 1918 influenza virus and then recreating it has been compared to constructing a virtual time machine. Comparing the genome of the 1918 virus to more recent strains has provided key insights into the origins and virulence of pandemic influenza viruses. The combination of rapid spread and severe illness suggests that the influenza strain that emerged in the fall of 1918 was both antigenically novel and well adapted to multiplying rapidly in human lung tissues. Genomic analysis suggests that the ancestral form of the 1918 virus was avian, but how the virus made its way from birds to humans is unclear. Scientists hope to solve this puzzle by finding samples of the avian viruses from the 1910s. To determine how the 1918 virus made the jump from birds to humans, Taubenberger is hoping to find traces of influenza viruses in preserved specimens in natural history museums.

Comparisons of the genetic sequences of different strains of the influenza virus could provide insights into how these viruses adapt to new host species, the factors that determine their virulence in different host species, and how pandemic strains emerge. Understanding the genetic modifications that lead to virulence and contagiousness could be valuable in predicting potentially pandemic strains and designing strategies to prevent pandemics. Analysis of the genes of the 1918 influenza virus indicates that different pathways can lead to novel viruses capable of causing serious epidemics. Studies of other influenza viruses suggest that the pandemics in 1957 and 1968 were caused by human flu viruses that acquired genes from bird flu viruses. The 1918 virus did not acquire its virulence by combining avian and mammalian genes. Its sequence indicates that it was an avian virus that acquired several mutations that made it highly virulent and highly contagious among human beings. This suggests that with a few unpredictable mutations, other common avian flu viruses could become very dangerous to humans without first combining with a human flu virus. Nevertheless, predicting the outcome of mutations and genetic reassortment is difficult because the potential virulence of a novel virus is the product of complex interactions between the host and the virus.

THE SWINE FLU DILEMMA

The difficulty of planning for a flu pandemic was demonstrated in 1976 when epidemiologists saw troubling signs of a virulent new strain of influenza. The campaign to begin mass vaccinations was triggered by several particularly virulent cases of influenza among soldiers at Fort Dix, New Jersey. Virologists isolated a new influenza virus that became known as *swine flu* from a soldier who died of influenza complicated by pneumonia. These early findings immediately conjured up fears that another pandemic like that of 1918 might occur. Epidemiologists, public health experts, and reporters warned that swine flu might be as contagious and deadly as the virus responsible for the 1918 influenza pandemic. Media reports generated widespread fear, bordering on hysteria.

In response to growing fears of a pandemic, President Gerald R. Ford supported a campaign to immunize all Americans. Some medical experts urged a more conservative course, that is, stockpiling vaccine and initiating mass immunizations *if* an epidemic seemed imminent. Manufacturing a safe and effective vaccine for the new virus proved to be more difficult than anticipated. To encourage pharmaceutical firms to create and market a swine flu vaccine, the federal government agreed to assume responsibility for adverse effects of vaccination. After three elderly people vaccinated at one clinic died, many states decided to terminate their immunization campaigns, despite the fact that investigators concluded that the deaths were not vaccine related. Fear of the vaccine soon exceeded fear of the disease because of media reports about a rare paralytic disease known as Guillain-Barré syndrome in people who had been vaccinated. Among the forty-eight million Americans vaccinated, there were about five hundred cases of Guillain-Barré syndrome. Statisticians raised questions about whether or not the vaccine had caused some or all of these cases, but the credibility of the immunization campaign was effectively destroyed. The ambitious plan to prevent a deadly pandemic had been transformed into what the media referred to as the swine flu fiasco.

Influenza expert Edwin D. Kilbourne asserted that it was better to have a vaccine without an epidemic than an epidemic without a vaccine, but the failure of the inoculation program had serious repercussions for public health programs dealing with infectious diseases and preventive vaccines. The swine flu vaccine program demonstrated how rumors of vaccine-related complications and fatalities could generate a media frenzy that eclipsed rational discussions of risks and benefits. Public health officials pointed out that some degree of risk is invariably associated with all medical interventions. Moreover, when large numbers of people are vaccinated, some unrelated deaths and illnesses will inevitably occur in that population. In a litigious modern society, such events inevitably lead to lawsuits. Instead of a pandemic of swine flu, which never materialized, the government confronted an epidemic of lawsuits filed by people who claimed that the vaccine had caused Guillain-Barré syndrome, multiple sclerosis, heart attacks, strokes, rheumatoid arthritis, impotence, fainting spells, and other adverse effects. Later research suggested that even the association between vaccine and Guillain-Barré syndrome was spurious.

Even if a virus as deadly and contagious as the 1918 influenza virus appeared in the twenty-first century, the impact of a potential pandemic would probably be mitigated by preventive vaccines, antiviral drugs, and improvements in the management of symptoms and complications. Nevertheless, experts predict that an influenza pandemic in the not too distant future could kill millions of people. The CDC's worst case predictions suggest that a pandemic comparable to that of 1918 could infect one-third of the population, incapacitate 40 percent of the workforce, and cause two million American deaths. Without a preventive vaccine, hospitals would be overwhelmed by the burden of caring for large numbers of critically sick patients. In contrast to the status of medicine in 1918, however, the sick would probably benefit from antiviral drugs, antibiotics for secondary bacterial pneumonia, and mechanical ventilators. Modern therapies and supportive technologies should, theoretically, reduce the death toll, but most experts believe that even the wealthiest nations would not be adequately prepared for a serious pandemic. Vaccine production would almost certainly be too little and too late, despite international influenza monitoring systems. Although medical interventions could mitigate the impact of a deadly new influenza virus in areas with appropriate resources, modern transportation would provide unprecedented opportunities to disseminate the virus throughout the world before infected individuals were aware of their illness. Airline travel has a significant effect on the spread of influenza, but the establishment and enforcement of flight restrictions and international quarantine measures would be difficult. Restrictions on air travel and other quarantine measures would certainly have major economic and social repercussions that would be as unwelcome as medieval quarantine rules, and they might be just as useless.

BIRD FLU IN THE TWENTY-FIRST CENTURY

When a deadly new strain of avian flu, identified as A(H5N1), appeared in 2003, epidemiologists raised concerns about the possibility that the virus might become the cause of the next influenza pandemic. Despite efforts to contain the virus by killing chickens, ducks, turkeys, and wild birds, outbreaks of the H5N1 flu occurred in China, Vietnam, Cambodia, Indonesia, Thailand, Egypt, Nigeria, and Turkey. Genetic tests suggest that the H5N1 avian flu originated in Guangdong Province in southern China, known as the birthplace of previous epidemic influenza strains as well as SARS. Epidemiologists suggest that the system of fish farming in southern China plays a critical role in the generation of novel influenza viruses. Aquatic birds are the natural reservoir of influenza viruses, and traditional Chinese fish farms bring together ducks, fish, pigs, humans, and their assorted microbial companions. If several strains of virus infect one animal, the opportunity for genetic recombination is greatly increased. Wild ducks and other aquatic birds that visit traditional fishponds have been called the "Typhoid Marys" of influenza viruses. Infected birds remain healthy and capable of flying long distances, while the viruses multiply in their intestines. As epidemiologists often point out, dead birds do not fly. When wild birds migrate, they excrete influenza viruses into lakes and marshes, where other birds acquire them. Avian flu viruses are also spread through the international trade in baby chicks, which has effectively transformed the domestic chicken into an international migratory bird.

H5N1 avian flu virus was clearly highly lethal to humans, but almost all cases involved close and prolonged contact with infected chickens. The disease was rarely, if ever, transmitted from person to person. The majority of human deaths were in Indonesia, Vietnam, Egypt, China, and Thailand. About 60 percent of people diagnosed with avian flu died. At autopsy, their lungs were as severely damaged as those of victims of the 1918 influenza virus. According to WHO, at least 357 people throughout the world contracted bird flu between 2003 and 2008; of those infected, 224 died, but because of inadequate reporting, the true number is probably much higher. In countries where outbreaks of H5N1 were detected, public health officials called for killing poultry, vaccinating people, and prescribing antiviral drugs. The goal of this strategy is to avoid the exchange of genes between human and avian flu viruses that could occur in people with mixed infections. A contagious strain could develop from H5N1 flu through a series of mutations or reassortment with human flu viruses. Highly contagious human flu viruses infect cells in the upper respiratory tract and are efficiently spread by coughing and sneezing, but avian H5N1 binds to receptors on cells in the deepest branches of the human respiratory tract. Because influenza viruses are always undergoing mutation and reassortment, virologists and public health officials consider it essential to monitor the spread of H5N1 and other influenza viruses.

In 2005, WHO called avian flu the world's greatest public health threat. Predictions of the death toll from an avian flu pandemic ranged from a low of 2 million to a high of 360 million, but epidemiologists generally agreed that it is impossible to know how deadly an avian flu pandemic would be if the virus were to acquire the ability to spread from person to person. Although public health authorities and physicians could do very little to control or treat influenza in 1918, by the end of the twentieth century, improvements in medical technology and the development of antiviral drugs offered the possibility of mitigating the impact of a potentially catastrophic pandemic. Controlling a major pandemic would, however, require international cooperation and the mobilization of resources that are unavailable in poor countries and generally neglected in wealthy nations.

EIGHT

❦

BIOLOGICAL WEAPONS AND BIOTERRORISM

Long before the development of microbiology in the late nineteenth century, human beings had attempted to enlist deadly diseases and toxins as weapons of warfare and conquest. The means used were nonspecific and perhaps ineffective, ranging from begging the gods to send plagues, contaminating wells with animal carcasses, or luring enemy troops into malarial swamps. Many allegations have been made that Europeans deliberately used smallpox as a weapon against Native Americans. Advances in science and technology led to the identification of dangerous pathogens and toxins, techniques that could produce large quantities of such agents, and methods for weaponizing and disseminating biological agents. Biological warfare allegations have been powerful components of propaganda wars, at least in part because of the difficulty, until recent times, of determining whether outbreaks of disease were natural consequences of warfare and social chaos or the result of deliberate biological attacks. The infectious agents that are most frequently considered as potential biological weapons include those that cause diseases that are very deadly (anthrax, smallpox, plague, tularemia, viral hemorrhagic fevers, and botulism) and agents that incapacitate but are not necessarily fatal.

Horror at the use of chemical warfare during World War I led to the 1925 Geneva Protocol for the Prohibition of the Use in War of Asphyxiating, Poisonous or Other Gases, and of Bacteriological Methods of Warfare. Many of the nations that signed the Geneva Protocol continued to conduct biological weapons research programs.

In 1969, a resurgence of concern about the dangers of biological warfare led to a proposal that the United Nations investigate means of prohibiting the development, production, and stockpiling of biological weapons. Analyses of the potential consequences of biological warfare led to the 1972 Convention on the Prohibition of the Development, Production, and Stockpiling of Bacteriological (Biological) and Toxic Weapons and on Their Destruction. Although the Biological Weapons Convention gained many signatories, it was largely unenforceable and probably had very little effect on secret research and development.

The development of a major biological weapons program in the United States, from 1942 to 1969, largely originated in response to warnings that Germany might use biological weapons against Great Britain during World War II. During the 1940s and 1950s, facilities for the production of various pathogens, including anthrax and brucellosis, were built in several states, including Arkansas, Indiana, Mississippi, Maryland, and Utah. Camp Detrick (later Fort Detrick), Maryland, became known as a major center of biological weapons research and development. Researchers at the Fort Detrick laboratory conducted pioneering studies of potential germ weapons, identifying about fifty pathogens and toxins that were considered good candidates for germ warfare. Biological weapons researchers selected bacteria and toxins that could kill or incapacitate people and livestock (anthrax, encephalitis, yellow fever, botulinum toxin) as well as fungi or blights that could destroy food crops such as potatoes, wheat, and rice. Military officials argued that the work was primarily defensive because it could lead to the development of vaccines that would protect troops against biological weapons developed by America's enemies. However, the development of strategic biological weapons that could be used as bombs was also of interest. By 1970, the U.S. Army had a biological weapons arsenal that included pathogens classified as deadly or incapacitating microbes (anthrax, tularemia, brucellosis, Q fever, and Venezuelan equine encephalitis) and lethal or incapacitating toxins (botulinum and *Staphylococcus* enterotoxin B). Such agents were stored at Pine Bluff Arsenal in refrigerated bunkers and vans. Ideally, weaponized pathogens would be stored as inert powders, but the drying process is generally quite difficult and dangerous. Moreover, most microbes need refrigerated storage because they could not survive the drying process. Therefore, during the search for biological weapons, inspectors are particularly interested in refrigerated munitions bunkers.

In addition to collecting pathogens and toxins, bioweapons researchers were interested in the most effective means of exposing large numbers of people to biological agents. As part of an experimental program that lasted from 1949 to 1969, biological weapons researchers conducted hundreds of tests in populated areas throughout the United States. Generally, *Bacillus subtilis* or *Serratia marcescens*, which were thought to be harmless, were used in place of pathological agents in these experiments. Later studies revealed that *Serratia marcescens* can cause life-threatening infections in susceptible people. *Bacillus subtilis* or *Serratia marcescens* were dispersed from automobiles, boats, and airplanes; pumped into the ventilation ducts of selected buildings; or released in subway stations. Experiments conducted in San Francisco, California, in 1950 were followed by reports that people were suffering from unusual infections caused by *Serratia marcescens*. Information about these experiments did not reach the public until the 1970s, when investigative journalists raised questions about people who might have been harmed by the release of test bacteria in the 1950s.

American biowarfare researchers also collected information about the development and use of biological agents from Japanese scientists who directed the program established by the Imperial Japanese Army in the 1930s. The work of Sheldon H. Harris, American historian and author of *Factories of Death: Japanese Biological Warfare, 1932–45 and the American Cover-up* (1994), was important in revealing how leaders of Japan's bioweapons program conducted human experiments and deployed biological weapons against China. According to Chinese authorities, the use of biological weapons by the Imperial Japanese Army caused the deaths of more than 250,000 people in occupied China from 1932 until the end of World War II. The Japanese government essentially denied its involvement with biological weapons, until 2002, when a Japanese court acknowledged Japan's use of biological agents against civilians and prisoners, including the deliberate release of plague infected fleas and rats in China. Evidence also emerged about a facility known as Unit 731, the largest and most notorious center of Japanese biological weapons research.

The Japanese court ruled that Unit 731 had seriously harmed the Chinese plaintiffs but rejected a lawsuit seeking compensation on technical grounds. Unit 731, which had a staff of about three thousand scientists and technicians, was directed by Kitano Misaji and Shiro Ishii. Prisoners were used as guinea pigs in tests of the pathogens that cause anthrax, cholera, bubonic plague, glanders, dysentery, smallpox, typhoid, typhus, and other diseases. All of the research subjects, as many as ten thousand to twelve thousand prisoners, died or were killed in the course of these experiments. Ishii, Misaji, and other participants in this program were taken into American custody in 1946 and granted immunity from war crimes prosecution in exchange for information about their research. American scientists, who began their own biological warfare program in 1943 at Fort Detrick, Maryland, were very interested in the results of the experiments carried out by Ishii and other Japanese scientists.

Officially, the United States renounced the use of biological weapons intended to kill or incapacitate in 1969, when President Richard Nixon announced that the army's offensive biological weapons program would be terminated by executive order. Nixon's motives in making this decision were unclear and much debated. The president and his advisors might have been convinced that advances in conventional weaponry made chemical and biological weapons unnecessary as well as morally and ethically abhorrent. A more cynical explanation was that Nixon was trying to send other countries the misleading message that chemical and biological weapons were too unpredictable and unreliable to be militarily useful or effective. Renouncing offensive biological weapons did not actually involve terminating studies of such weapons because differences between studies of offensive and defensive aspects of biological warfare are minimal. Studies of potential bioweapons and the development of defensive medical measures were assigned to the U.S. Army Medical Research Institute of Infectious Diseases (USAMRIID). The Army Biological Laboratories at Fort Detrick, Maryland, were officially converted to defensive research in the 1970s.

Biological weapons have been called the poor man's atom bomb, but even countries with nuclear weapons established biological weapons programs after World War II. Despite extensive germ warfare research during and after World War II, most military experts were skeptical of their value in conventional warfare. Biological agents— bacteria, viruses, and toxins—are difficult to control, particularly in comparison to conventional weapons of mass destruction. Biological agents, incorporated into bombs, sprays, or aerosols, are capable of spreading in unpredictable ways without respecting national borders. Biological agents can have *backlash* and *blowback* effects that make them difficult to control and put those who are involved in the development and deployment of biological weapons at substantial risk. Although these problems may have been an obstacle to the use of bioweapons in conventional warfare, they would presumably not deter terrorists who accept the idea of suicide missions. A living weapon can be crude, unreliable, unpredictable, and uncontrollable but still perfectly suited to the goals of bioterrorists.

Experts on military planning generally assumed that major military powers would have no interest in using bioweapons once they had nuclear weapons. In contrast, stateless terrorists and rogue nations might consider biological weapons a viable, inexpensive alternative to conventional weapons. Even if bioweapons were useless in a military confrontation, an outbreak of a deadly, exotic disease would probably cause panic in civilian populations. Potential bioterrorists could pursue many ways of acquiring pathogens that could be used directly against people or to contaminate food and water supplies, damage the environment, and disrupt various industries. Many pathogens can be found in nature or easily obtained from academic laboratories and pharmaceutical or agricultural companies. Such microbes might cause diseases that are unfamiliar to modern physicians, which would delay the proper diagnosis of the first victims of the disease. As more cases appeared, the health care system would be overwhelmed with the tasks of isolating and caring for the sick; decontaminating areas where the biological agents had been released; administering vaccines, if possible; and dealing with panic, chaos, and misinformation. All of these factors could be applied to historical examples of the accidental and deliberate use of anthrax spores.

Experts on biowarfare have often called anthrax the ideal biological weapon. Before the crisis caused in the United States in 2001 by the simple expedient of sending envelopes containing anthrax spores, bioweapons were generally thought of in terms of aerosols, bombs, and other traditional forms of military hardware. Terrorist groups, unlike military planners, have attempted to exploit very simple methods of disseminating biological agents because their goal is to create panic, rather than win a military victory. For example, in 1984, members of the Rajneeshee cult used *Salmonella* bacteria to contaminate salad bars in Oregon restaurants. Allegedly, their goal was to influence local elections in Antelope, Oregon. About eight hundred people were sickened, some severely enough to require hospitalization, but there were no deaths. Later reports called this the first bioterrorism attack in the United States, but this episode was not widely publicized. In contrast, the anthrax letters created a media storm and panic that demonstrated the power of the threat of terrorism in the tense atmosphere following the September 11 attacks on the World Trade Center and the Pentagon. In terms of the study of emerging diseases, the anthrax attack of 2001 provided an example of what can be called *deliberately emerging diseases*, that is, disease outbreaks caused by pathogens used as biological weapons. This category could include well-known agents, such as anthrax, as well as previously unknown microbes or pathogens created in the laboratory by manipulating genetic factors responsible for virulence or drug resistance.

The first series of anthrax letters was sent out just one week after the September 11 terrorist attacks. As a result of letters sent to several newspapers, television reporters, and two U.S. senators, anthrax cases occurred in Florida, New York, Washington, D.C., and New Jersey. At least twenty-two people were infected; eleven people contracted deadly inhalation anthrax, and five people died. In addition to the danger to people who opened the letters containing the spores, the cross-contamination of other letters, post office equipment, mailboxes, and so forth created unpredictable patterns of spore dispersal. The sorting machines in the post office helped express the spores, allowing them to cross-contaminate other letters, and air currents dispersed them in unpredictable ways.

After struggling to cope with the anthrax attacks of 2001, the Centers for Disease Control and Prevention recommended strengthening the public health infrastructure at the federal, state, and local levels to improve surveillance and communication about unusual disease outbreaks. These policies would strengthen the nation's ability to deal with naturally transmitted diseases, such as influenza and SARS, as well as potential bioterrorist attacks. Nevertheless, epidemiologists find it very difficult to convince government officials to think of bioterrorism as a public health problem, rather than a disaster analogous to an explosion or fire.

At the time of the anthrax letter crisis, the American medical community had very little experience with anthrax, especially inhalation anthrax, which was generally thought to be fatal. Many people thought to be at risk were given ciprofloxacin (Cipro), a broad-spectrum oral fluoroquinolone, or doxycycline, a member of the tetracycline group. Infectious disease experts, however, worried that the decision to treat large numbers of people who were very unlikely to contract anthrax would increase the development of ciprofloxacin-resistant bacteria. The panic triggered by the anthrax attacks crippled the U.S. postal system for several months and launched an intensive search for the perpetrator.

At first, investigators speculated that the person who sent the anthrax letters might have stolen old laboratory samples of powdered anthrax. However, scientists quickly determined that the anthrax powder in the letters was probably made within the past two years. This indicated that the perpetrator was probably working in, or had access to, a modern microbiology laboratory. Unfortunately, this category included hundreds or even thousands of people, including the biodefense experts working with the Federal Bureau of Investigation (FBI). The anthrax used in the letters was identified as the Ames strain, which could be found in many U.S. biodefense research laboratories. Success in sequencing of the genome of *Bacillus anthracis*, and identifying genetically distinct subtypes, was critical to establishing the source of the material used in the anthrax letters. These studies also provided clues to the genetic factors that determine the virulence of different strains of the bacillus.

After ruling out foreign terrorists, FBI investigators turned their attention to scientists affiliated with biodefense facilities in the United States. Dr. Steven J. Hatfill, a researcher who worked at the U.S. biodefense program at Fort Detrick, Frederick, Maryland, became the focus of the FBI investigation, but despite four years of close scrutiny that Hatfill claimed rose to the level of harassment, he was not charged with any crimes. Although Hatfill insisted that he was not involved in the anthrax attacks, information about his background was widely reported by the media. Hatfill sued several reporters, including Nicholas D. Kristof (a columnist at the *New York Times*), the *New York Times*, and the Justice Department for defaming his reputation. In December 2006, the *New York Times* filed a motion with a federal judge to dismiss Hatfill's lawsuit, largely on the grounds that Hatfill had become a public figure through his public comments about the anthrax investigation. Therefore, Hatfill could not prove that he had been defamed by Kristof or that the columns demonstrated "actual malice," the legal standard that applies to defamation of public figures. Although Hatfill's suit against Kristof and the *New York Times* was dismissed, Kristof offered a public apology when a new suspect emerged. In 2008, Hatfill was cleared by the Justice Department and awarded a $4.6 million settlement for the lawsuit he had filed against the government.

On July 29, 2008, Bruce E. Ivins, a microbiologist who helped develop the controversial anthrax vaccine used to immunize American soldiers, killed himself after learning that federal prosecutors were preparing to indict him for the 2001 anthrax attacks. The Justice Department and the FBI announced that with the death of their chief suspect, they considered the case essentially closed. Ivins had been a researcher at the U.S. Army Medical Institute for Infectious Disease at Fort Detrick for more than twenty years. In particular, Ivins was considered an expert on anthrax, and the FBI had submitted samples of the 2001 anthrax preparations to him for analysis. Although FBI officials insisted that the evidence clearly indicated that Ivins was solely responsible for the anthrax attacks, skeptics considered the evidence circumstantial and asked for a more detailed and objective investigation. Friends and colleagues suggested that government agents, who were looking for a scapegoat in order to close their long, embarrassing, and fruitless investigation, had driven Ivins to suicide. Senator Patrick J. Leahy, chairman of the Senate Judiciary Committee and the target of one of the anthrax letters, was among skeptics who were not convinced that even if Ivins had been involved in the anthrax attacks, he had acted alone.

Thus, many questions about the identity and motives of the person (or persons) responsible for the anthrax attacks remained unresolved as of September 2008, when the FBI agreed to allow the National Academy of Sciences (NAS) to conduct an independent review of all available scientific evidence concerning the anthrax attacks. The prestigious NAS serves as the official adviser to the federal government on scientific and technical questions. According to NAS officials, a thorough investigation will be very expensive and time consuming.

The use of anthrax spores as an agent of bioterrorism led to renewed interest in the biology and pathology of *Bacillus anthracis* as well as laws that would limit access to deadly microbes. In 2003, scientists sequenced the genome of *Bacillus anthracis*. Although microbiologists hope that studies of the anthrax genome will lead to more effective therapeutic agents and preventive vaccines, such information could also be used to create more virulent, antibiotic-resistant, genetically modified forms of *Bacillus anthracis*.

Persistent contamination associated with sites where anthrax spores were analyzed, weaponized, or deliberately released underscores the difficulty of finding practical means of storing and securing biological weapons. The remarkable persistence of anthrax spores was demonstrated by bioweapons tests conducted on an island off the coast of Scotland during World War II. Allied tests of weaponized spores of *Bacillus anthracis* left Gruinard Island heavily contaminated. When testing ended, workers set the island on fire in an unsuccessful attempt to decontaminate it. In 1990, four years after contaminated areas were saturated with formaldehyde, Britain's "anthrax island" was declared safe. Another infamous test site for weaponized anthrax, Vozrozhdeniye Island in the Aral Sea, served as a bioweapons testing range for Biopreparat, the former Soviet Union's massive biowarfare research program.

Reports of accidents at germ warfare laboratories typically involve workers who were infected as a result of human error and carelessness, but biowarfare research facilities put the surrounding area at risk, as demonstrated by smallpox and anthrax outbreaks associated with biowarfare facilities that operated in the former Soviet

Union. Investigations of the worst outbreak of inhalation anthrax in history, an event that has been called a "biological Chernobyl" (a reference to the 1986 nuclear power plant accident in Ukraine), was ultimately attributed to the failure of maintenance workers to replace a critical air filter at the Biopreparat germ warfare facility that operated near Sverdlovsk, Russia. Attempting to conceal the source of the outbreak, Soviet authorities claimed that people had contracted anthrax by eating uninspected black market meat. Anthrax had been well known as a disease of livestock in the region since the early twentieth century. However, there was little doubt that the source of the Sverdlovsk anthrax outbreak of 1979 was a military facility conducting research on biological weapons. Although Soviet officials attempted to conceal the extent of the disaster, rumors about the deaths of hundreds or even thousands of people and animals appeared in newspapers outside the Soviet Union.

Detailed epidemiological investigations eventually revealed that at least sixty-six people had died, generally as the result of inhalation anthrax, and eleven survived. The survivors apparently had cutaneous anthrax. Hospital records indicate that anthrax patients were given antibiotics, supportive therapy, and artificial respiration. Fatalities usually occurred at home or within a few days of hospitalization, but survivors were generally in treatment for at least three weeks. Anthrax was also reported among sheep and cattle near Sverdlovsk, but many farmers in the area had recently vaccinated their sheep. A local emergency commission initially directed public health measures, including disinfection of homes, destruction of dogs and livestock, isolation of the sick, and a voluntary immunization program. According to local public health officials, about 80 percent of the people considered at risk were vaccinated.

In 1992, after the breakup of the Soviet Union, Russia's leaders admitted that the Sverdlovsk epidemic had been caused by the accidental release of weaponized anthrax spores. Studies of the Sverdlovsk outbreak by teams of Russian and American scientists were important in defining and differentiating the most deadly clinical forms of anthrax, that is, inhalation anthrax and gastrointestinal anthrax. In keeping with the general belief that human anthrax is not contagious, there was no evidence of person-to-person transmission during the outbreak. The information gained in studying the 1979 anthrax outbreak was useful to scientists during the 2001 anthrax crisis because there was very limited data for human anthrax, especially inhalation anthrax, in the medical literature. Physicians usually assumed that the incubation period for anthrax was two to six days; the data from Sverdlovsk indicated that the incubation period for fatal cases was usually nine to ten days, but might be as long as forty-three days. As indicated by experiments with nonhuman primates, anthrax spores can remain viable in the lung for many weeks. As the number of spores increases, the incubation period decreases.

Several factors in the 1990s called attention to the potential threat of biological weapons and bioterrorism. For the general public, popular books, such as Ken Alibek's autobiographical *Biohazard* (1999) and Richard Preston's novel *The Cobra Event* (1997), were important in raising awareness of biological weapons, especially the potential for creating more deadly agents with the tools of molecular biology. In 1992, Ken Alibek (Kanatjan Alibekov), first deputy director of Biopreparat, the Soviet bioweapons program, defected to the United States. Alibek, a physician and microbiologist, provided insights into the massive bioweapons programs of the former Soviet Union.

For U.S. military and political leaders, intelligence reports about Iraq's biological weapons program were a major concern in preparing for the first Persian Gulf War (1990–1991). Investigators suspected that the Iraqi government had sponsored studies of potential biowarfare agents, including *Bacillus anthracis*, *Salmonella typhi*, and botulinum toxin. After the war, investigators determined that the pathogens found in Iraqi laboratories had been obtained from the American Type Culture Collection (ATCC) in Virginia and the Pasteur Institute in Paris. Spokesmen for the ATCC and the Pasteur Institute said that all of their shipments had been legal because buyers claimed that the agents would be used for research and medical purposes. After the war, the United States, France, and other Western countries placed strict restrictions on the shipment of biological materials, and governments throughout the world attempted to control the use of all *select agents*, that is, microbes or toxins considered a threat to humans, food crops, and domesticated animals. A deep philosophical divide has emerged between scientists and intelligence officials over whether to withhold scientific information in the name of national security. Scientists argue that excessive restrictions would inhibit research, but would not necessarily keep bioterrorists from obtaining dangerous pathogens. Deadly agents, such as Ebola viruses, anthrax spores, and *Yersinia pestis*, exist in natural reservoirs.

A conference held in 1999, sponsored by the Johns Hopkins Center for Civilian Biodefense, the U.S. Department of Health and Human Services (HHS), the Infectious Diseases Society of American, and the American Society for Microbiology, urged preparedness for possible bioterrorism. Scientists acknowledged that advances in molecular biology and biotechnology increased the potential for creating more dangerous pathogens because the methods used to study the genes for virulence and antibiotic resistance could be used to create more lethal microbes. Such methods are becoming increasingly powerful. For example, the synthesis of the poliovirus, which was completed in 2002, had taken three years; one year later, scientists were able to assemble a comparable virus in only three weeks. Scientists are increasingly able to identify, isolate, and synthesize the virulence factors found in some of the most deadly microbes, as demonstrated by the sequencing and reconstruction of the genome of the influenza virus that caused the 1918 pandemic. Genetic maps of many pathogenic viruses and bacteria are widely available via the Internet and in scientific journals. As the case of the 2001 anthrax letters demonstrated, a scientist working in a program allegedly dedicated to biodefense research could use simple, even crude, means of dispersing deadly pathogens. Should such a scientist join a network of terrorists, pathogenic agents could presumably be transformed into weapons of mass destruction. Bioterrorists with access to modern laboratories might be able use information about the molecular biology of viruses and bacteria to create new pathogens by adding drug-resistance genes, virulence factors, and genes for toxins to existing microbes. Of course, the results of genetic manipulations are not always predictable. For example, the scientists who modified a mousepox virus in 2001 were investigating the possible use of infectious organisms for pest control, but the modified virus caused complete failure of the mouse immune system.

Predictions about the future development of biological weapons are also complicated by the growing realization that known disease-causing agents are only a very small component of the complex microbial world. Studies of emerging diseases suggest that disrupting natural ecosystems can result in transforming obscure agents, such as simian immunodeficiency viruses and the prions that cause scrapie in sheep, into deadly human pathogens.

NINE

❧∾∽❧

INFECTIOUS AGENTS AND NEW CONCEPTS: FROM CHRONIC DISEASES TO THE MICROBIOME

MICROBES AND CHRONIC DISEASES

Nineteenth-century scientists established the relationship between pathogenic microorganisms and contagious diseases by satisfying Koch's postulates, but providing proof of causality was difficult if scientists could not find an experimental animal or if the onset of disease symptoms involved multiple factors interacting over a long period of time. In the case of diseases that take many years to develop, complicating genetic, dietary, and environmental factors might be as critical as the initial infection. Therefore, scientists who suspected a relationship between microbes and chronic diseases generally found it difficult or impossible to provide rigorous proof.

The microbes associated with the development of a chronic disease might be eliminated after the patient recovers from the acute phase of the illness, but the initial infection might trigger a sequence of events that leads to permanent damage such as rheumatic heart disease after streptococcal infections. Some researchers suspect an association between some mental disorders—schizophrenia, bipolar disorder, obsessive-compulsive disorder—and infectious agents. Obsessive-compulsive disorder sometimes appears quite suddenly in children who have suffered from a streptococcal infection such as strep throat. If microbes are still in the body, but in a latent state, they might escape detection. Identifying and confirming an infectious cause of a chronic disease is complicated by several factors, such as environmental conditions and genetic differences in susceptibility and survival, and by complications that are due to multiple infections.

Epidemiological studies suggest that chronic conditions might occur in people suffering from several different infections, such as malaria and HIV, or hepatitis C and schistosomiasis, at the same time. Recent medical research suggests subtle and complex relationships between microbial infection and human health that could not be explored with the techniques previously available. The possibility that chronic diseases were linked to microbes was generally greeted with skepticism, but evidence of such relationships continues to accumulate. Advances in detection and diagnostic techniques have revealed that even conditions not typically associated with microorganisms may involve infectious agents. Evidence of the role of infectious agents in the development of ulcers, cancers, and other chronic conditions that were previously attributed to lifestyle factors, aging, or genetics has created another category of emerging diseases that could be thought of as *newly appreciated infections*. However, the broader implications of these findings must be interpreted with caution because microbes are so ubiquitous that finding them in association with various chronic conditions may be merely coincidental. For example, the common Epstein-Barr virus (EBV) seems to cause chronic disease in some people but produces no obvious symptoms of acute or chronic disease in others. Such observations could mean that the virus does not cause the diseases in question and that the alleged association is coincidental, or that genetic factors, environmental factors, or age at infection determine the course of disease.

Since Louis Pasteur and Robert Koch established the modern germ theory of disease, scientists have provided rigorous proof that microbial agents cause acute illnesses, epidemic diseases, and wound infections, but infectious organisms have now been clearly linked to certain chronic conditions such as gastrointestinal ulcers and various cancers. Some pathogens may trigger an immune response that eventually leads to chronic inflammation or autoimmune disorders. In other cases, acute, chronic, latent, or recurrent infections or coinfections may lead to serious chronic diseases. Many claims of a linkage between an infectious agent and chronic disorders remain purely speculative or highly controversial, but microbes are now suspects in conditions previously blamed on lifestyle, genes, and environmental factors. Microorganisms have been implicated, if not convicted, of playing a role in the development of some chronic and autoimmune diseases such as asthma, ulcers, kidney stones, type 1 diabetes, multiple sclerosis, inflammatory bowel disease, atherosclerosis, and cardiovascular disease. Some researchers have suggested that antigens on certain viruses might resemble normal components of the cells of the host. This so-called molecular mimicry could cause the immune system to attack its own tissues, leading to chronic and autoimmune disorders.

Proof that microbes act as triggers for the development of chronic diseases would have major clinical and public health implications. Chronic diseases, such as heart disease, cancer, stroke, chronic obstructive pulmonary disease, diabetes, and Alzheimer's disease, are the leading causes of illness and death in the United States today. If microbes cause or contribute to some of these conditions, the discovery of a means to prevent or block the disease process would have profound effects; previously intractable chronic conditions might respond to antibiotics, antiviral drugs, or vaccines. Traditional methods of detecting and isolating microbes may be inadequate if microbes exist in a latent state or if a disease is caused by novel or rare pathogens.

New techniques make it possible for scientists to investigate aspects of the relationship between infectious agents and human disease that were previously impossible. Where traditional medical microbiology cannot establish the relationship between microbes and chronic diseases, evidence may depend on new analytical tools and approaches generated by molecular biology, genomics, and biotechnology. New methodologies—genomics, proteomics, and DNA microarray technology—allow scientists to classify bacteria in terms of ribosomal RNA sequences and other molecular characteristics. Such studies have revealed previously unsuspected microbial diversity, including agents that cannot be grown or isolated using traditional culture-based methods. Instead of diagnosing a disease-causing agent by culturing a microbe, scientists look for *molecular signatures*, that is, sequence-based molecular methods that can detect evidence of the pathogen or the immunological response of the victim.

Since the 1980s, rigorous proof of the relationship between infectious agents and specific chronic diseases has emerged for *Helicobacter pylori* and peptic ulcers, human papillomaviruses and cervical cancer, hepatitis viruses and liver cancer, and so forth. The bacterium *Helicobacter pylori* has been linked to a number of disorders, including gastritis, peptic ulcers, stomach and duodenal cancers (gastric adenocarcinoma), and certain types of lymphoma. Other connections between infections and chronic diseases are suspected, but not proven. The age at which people are exposed to an infectious agent may be critical in determining the interval between infection and the onset and severity of disease, as in the case of hepatitis B virus and chronic complications. Finding evidence that a specific microbe could cause a chronic condition should eliminate many ineffective treatments and encourage the use of appropriate antibiotics or preventive vaccines. However, if fear of chronic disease leads to the widespread abuse of antibiotics and other drugs, the risks of developing drug-resistant strains of microbes could outweigh the still uncertain benefits of prevention.

INFECTIOUS AGENTS, CHRONIC DISEASES, AND CANCER

Researchers suspect that some viruses may be linked to subtle changes in human cells that lead to chronic conditions. Herpesviruses, members of the notorious *Herpesviridae* family, are especially known for causing both acute and latent infections. Various members of this group cause cold sores, genital herpes, roseola, and other diseases. During the 1970s, shortly before the discovery of AIDS, genital herpes raised public awareness of persistent, recurrent viral infections. Human herpes 6 and 7 have been implicated in various chronic conditions, including Hodgkin's lymphoma, leukemia, and chronic fatigue syndrome. Throughout history, there have been reports of clusters of a condition physicians referred to as *asthenia*, a combination of weakness and a host of vague, nonspecific symptoms. Asthenia-like cases have been called hypochondria, malingering, epidemic neuromyasthenia, chronic EBV syndrome, mass hysteria, postviral asthenia syndrome, or chronic fatigue syndrome. Clinicians who encountered clusters of patients with this condition speculated about the possibility that the chronic fatigue was the result of an undiagnosed viral infection that led to inflammation or an autoimmune reaction. Reactivation of latent herpes viruses has been found in patients whose immune systems were compromised by HIV/AIDS, chemotherapy for cancer, or the immunosuppressive drugs taken by bone marrow and organ transplantation patients.

In 1926, the Nobel Prize in Physiology or Medicine was awarded to Danish physician Johannes Andreas Grib Fibiger for his discovery that a parasitic worm he called *Spiroptera neoplastica* caused gastric cancer in rats. His findings and conclusions were later refuted, his experimental work dismissed as primitive, and this award became a source of embarrassment to the Nobel Assembly of the prestigious Karolinska Institute. No other Nobel Prize was awarded for cancer research until 1966, when eighty-seven-year-old Francis Peyton Rous won the Nobel Prize in Physiology or Medicine for his 1911 discovery of a filterable virus that caused cancer in chickens. When other researchers refuted Fibiger's work, his ideas about the relationship between parasites and cancer were ridiculed or ignored, but eventually, he was credited with stimulating important experimental work on the induction of cancer. Originally trained as a microbiologist, Fibiger also carried out valuable studies of diphtheria and tuberculosis, including demonstrations that, contrary to Koch's assessment, the milk of cows with bovine tuberculosis could transmit the disease to humans.

In his Nobel Prize Lecture, "Investigations on *Spiroptera carcinoma* and the Experimental Induction of Cancer," Fibiger reviewed the experiments he had carried out since 1907, when he first observed large tumors in the stomachs of three wild rats that had been captured for use in tuberculosis research. Citing previous reports that parasites had been found in association with tumors in rats and mice, Fibiger did not claim that his study was totally original. Nevertheless, he emphasized the point that his experiments were conducted on a much larger scale than those of his predecessors. Fibiger's search for the causative agent of cancer began when he examined samples of the tumors under the microscope and discovered traces of parasitic nematode worms and their eggs. He concluded that the parasites, which he called *Spiroptera neoplastica*, had caused the tumors. However, he was unable to find similar stomach cancers when he examined hundreds of other wild rats. Suspecting that the worms were transmitted by an intermediate host, Fibiger sought out rats that could have acquired the parasites from cockroaches. Biologists knew that parasitic worms typically spent part of their life cycles in roaches. In nature, nematode eggs develop into larvae when they are consumed by roaches. The larvae make their way from the intestines of their intermediate host to its muscles, where they form cysts. Rats become infested when they eat infected roaches. The encysted worms are released in the rat's stomach and develop into sexually mature worms. When Fibiger examined rats living in a sugar refinery that regularly feasted on roaches, he found that more than half of these rodents had worms in their stomachs, and several had stomach tumors. In a new series of experiments, Fibiger found that captive rats given a diet of roaches infested with nematode larvae developed tumors of the stomach, but rats that consumed adult nematodes or their eggs did not.

Despite the Nobel Prize awarded to Fibiger for his *Spiroptera carcinoma* theory, skeptics argued that he had not provided unequivocal evidence that the worms were the direct cause of the tumors; that is, the alleged association between parasites and tumors could have been merely coincidental, or the parasites might have been a secondary development in animals weakened by tumors. Other researchers suggested that the tumors were the result of irritation caused by parasites in animals weakened by a vitamin A deficiency or that cancerous growths had been induced by a virus carried by the worms or roaches.

Fibiger's major claims for his infamous cancer-causing nematode *Spiroptera carcinoma* studies were thoroughly rejected, but his reputation has been somewhat rehabilitated because of the role he played in establishing the experimental study of cancer in laboratory animals. Other researchers succeeded in establishing experimental systems in which cancers, especially skin cancers, were induced by means of chronic irritation—chemical or mechanical—of susceptible tissues. Although Fibiger's work did not prove that *Spiroptera neoplastica* caused cancer, it did raise the question of whether infectious agents might trigger the development of some cancers. Peyton Rous's experiments on Rous sarcoma, epidemiological studies of the relationship between certain chronic parasitic infections and cancers, the development of vaccines that prevent cancers induced by human papilloma viruses, and the demonstration of the role of *Helicobacter pylori* in the induction of stomach cancers provide a demonstration of the power of the idea encapsulated in Fibiger's 1926 Nobel Prize. Today, scientists are actively investigating the relationship between viruses and cancers, and many are convinced that infectious agents cause a significant fraction of the global burden of human cancer.

HELICOBACTER PYLORI AND PEPTIC ULCERS

One of the most surprising but well-authenticated examples of a previously unsuspected relationship between a chronic condition and an infectious agent was the demonstration that *Helicobacter pylori* causes peptic ulcers. Chronic *Helicobacter pylori* infections have also been linked to cancer of the stomach and certain types of lymphomas. In 2005, Barry J. Marshall and J. Robin Warren shared the Nobel Prize in Medicine or Physiology for their work on *Helicobacter pylori*. Peptic ulcers, caused by the erosion of the lining of the stomach or the duodenum (the portion of the small intestine that is connected to the stomach), produce severe abdominal pain and gastrointestinal bleeding. When chronic peptic ulcers perforate the intestinal wall, microbes from the gastrointestinal tract can enter the abdominal cavity, which can result in peritonitis and death. For many years, physicians assumed that peptic ulcers were caused by stress and dietary factors. Conventional therapy included bland diets, stress management, the administration of various forms of bismuth, or surgery to remove severely damaged sections of the stomach. Claims that gastric and duodenal ulcers were caused by bacterial infections were generally dismissed as impossible, despite several reports that unusual bacteria had been found in the stomach of patients with ulcers. In 1940, A. Stone Freedberg identified the curved bacteria, now known as *H. pylori*, in mucosal tissue removed from the stomachs of patients undergoing operations for ulcers and other illnesses. Although Freedberg published an account of his findings, he was not able to grow the bacteria in laboratory cultures. Several other researchers reported similar findings and suggested that ulcers might be caused by infection, but studies conducted in the 1950s found no bacteria in more than one thousand stomach specimens. The issue seemed to be settled until the 1980s, when Marshall and Warren identified *H. pylori* in ulcer patients. To substantiate the theory he and Robin Wright had about gastric ulcers, Marshall, who was certified free of *H. pylori* and stomach ulcers, drank a culture of *H. pylori*. When Marshall was diagnosed with gastritis, the first stage of an ulcer, *H. pylori* was isolated from his stomach. He was restored to health after treatment with antibiotics.

Unfortunately, Marshall's demonstration did not provoke an immediate change in the treatment of ulcers. Skeptics found it difficult to believe that allegedly pathogenic bacteria could establish chronic infections in the acidic atmosphere of the stomach, and bacteriologists noted that *H. pylori* cultures prefer to grow at a neutral pH. These objections were resolved by evidence that *H. pylori* were able to live in the gastric mucosa because the mucous that coats the lining of the stomach protects them from stomach acid. White blood cells, unable to reach the niche occupied by *H. pylori*, generally die and release their contents into the stomach lining. The chronic, ineffective inflammatory response is a major factor in the development of chronic gastritis and peptic ulcers. In some patients, bacterial infection apparently leads to chronic inflammation, increased cell proliferation, and stomach cancer.

As the medical community gradually accepted the idea that *Helicobacter pylori* infection was associated with gastritis and peptic ulcers, a revolution in treatment followed. Many questions about the origin and dissemination of *H. pylori* infections remain unanswered, although it is clear that *H. pylori* can be transmitted by contaminated food and water. In third world countries, *H. pylori* is found in about 80 percent of the adult population. In the United States, the rate of *H. pylori* infection is about 50 percent, but many factors affect the prevalence of infection. Some scientists think that *H. pylori* infection was already established in ancient hominids. Therefore, studies of *H. pylori* variations in different parts of the world could provide evidence of human evolution and patterns of migration out of Africa. The identification of genes that appear to predispose people to the chronic disorders associated with *H. pylori* infections might also be related to the antiquity of interactions between humans and these bacteria. However, some studies suggest that *H. pylori* was acquired from other animals in the more recent past. Similar bacteria have been found in dogs, sheep, cats, horses, cows, pigs, and some primates. New species are likely to be recognized when the stomach and gastrointestinal tracts of other animals are screened for similar bacteria.

Despite the high prevalence of *H. pylori* infections throughout the world, the incidence of ulcers is generally very low. Searching for the factors involved in the development of ulcers, researchers hope that human genomics will explain why so many people are chronically infected with *H. pylori*, but only a small minority develop ulcers and cancer. Understanding the factors involved might lead to the identification of susceptible individuals and the development of methods of prevention and treatment. In accordance with the rule that every silver lining must have a cloud, some researchers suggest that eliminating *H. pylori* infections might have negative consequences. When *H. pylori* infections are cured by antibiotics, the environment of the stomach might become more acidic, which could produce other problems such as gastric reflux and adenocarcinoma of the esophagus.

THE HYGIENE HYPOTHESIS

In industrialized countries the prevalence of *H. pylori* infections has been diminishing at least since the 1950s, but in the not so distant past, essentially all people were probably colonized by *Helicobacter*. Some researchers suggest that there might be a relationship between the decrease in the prevalence of *Helicobacter pylori* infections and the rise in childhood asthma and allergies. The idea that a general decrease in the prevalence of infectious diseases, especially during infancy and early childhood, is related to increases in asthma, allergies, autoimmune diseases, and chronic inflammatory disorders has been called the *hygiene hypothesis*.

One of the first versions of the hygiene hypothesis was published by David P. Strachan in the *British Medical Journal* in 1989 as a possible explanation for the observation that asthma and allergic diseases, such as hay fever and eczema, were less common in children from larger families than among only children. Similarly, children who attended day care and children who grew up on a farm or in areas with relatively poor sanitation were supposedly less likely to develop allergies and asthma. Some researchers concluded that exposure to many childhood illnesses provided protection from allergies and asthma. Accounts of the hygiene hypothesis were widely circulated in the popular press, the news media, and some medical journals. It was not uncommon for commentators to conclude that the hygiene hypothesis indicated that "dirt" might be good for children. Studies that questioned the alleged relationship between childhood diseases and protection from asthma, allergies, and inflammatory disorders received very little publicity.

According to advocates of the hygiene hypothesis, as infectious diseases decreased, the prevalence of allergies, asthma, and autoimmune diseases increased in wealthy, industrialized countries because improvements in sanitation, domestic cleanliness, and personal hygiene protected infants and children from exposure to once universal parasites and microbial agents. Early proponents of the hygiene hypothesis generally assumed that experiencing a series of minor illnesses during early childhood was necessary for the normal development of the immune system. Presumably, through encounters with a wide array of challenges, the immature immune system would learn how to distinguish between harmless materials and real threats. Throughout human evolution, infants and children had been exposed to, and adapted to, a series of infections caused by parasites, bacteria, and other noxious entities. Children growing up without the burden of infections faced by generations of human ancestors might develop a tendency to overreact to minor, normally harmless entities, which could lead to allergies, asthma, and autoimmune diseases. Later versions of the hygiene hypothesis proposed that a child does not need to experience infections and diseases but does need to achieve normal colonization of the body by common microbes for the development of a balanced, functional immune system. Thus, in addition to the problems caused by unnatural, modern cleanliness, the universal use of antibiotics to treat minor illnesses during early childhood could disrupt the establishment of the body's normal microflora by killing microbes that would have been part of the proper education of the developing immune system.

Today, residents of wealthy, industrialized nations have little or no knowledge of diseases caused by parasitic worms, but when Norman R. Stoll presented his famous presidential address, "This Wormy World," to the American Society of Parasitologists in 1946, parasitic worms were still considered ubiquitous and persistent enemies of the human race. In Princeton, New Jersey, where Stoll lived, 23 percent of the children were infested with some kind of worm. Much of Stoll's lecture was devoted to the problem of trichinosis, which affected about one in six Americans at the time. The parasite *Trichina spiralis* was first described in 1835 by British pathologist James Paget. It was later associated with trichinosis, a potentially deadly disease caused by parasitic worms found in many wild and domesticated animals. Parasitic worms do not kill well-nourished people, but they remain a great burden in many impoverished parts of the world.

Advocates of this version of the hygiene hypothesis, sometimes referred to as the "Old Friends Hypothesis," argue that eliminating common intestinal parasites was a significant factor in the increased prevalence of asthma and allergies as well as a group of conditions collectively known as irritable bowel diseases such as Crohn's disease and ulcerative colitis. Irritable bowel diseases appear to occur when the immune system attacks the intestines, causing chronic inflammation. Ulcerative colitis is usually restricted to the large intestine and involves inflammation of the superficial layers of the bowel lining. In some cases, however, more extensive damage to the intestinal wall can occur. Crohn's disease causes extensive damage to the lining of the small and large intestines, resulting in cramps, diarrhea, and rectal bleeding. In addition to intestinal problems, Crohn's disease is associated with painful skin ulcers, eye disorders, inflammation of the liver, arthritis, and other complications. In the 1930s, gastroenterologist Burrill Bernard Crohn described a condition he called terminal or regional ileitis, which is now known as Crohn's disease. Crohn suggested that the disease was caused by *Mycobacterium paratuberculosis*, a pathogen that causes an intestinal disease in sheep and cattle known as Johne's disease. Various causes for Crohn's have been proposed, including bacterial pathogens, diet, environmental factors, immune system disorders, or a combination of genetic and environmental factors.

Irritable bowel diseases were apparently quite rare before the 1930s, but by the 1970s, they were fairly common in wealthy countries. Instead of resorting to explanations based on genetics or the possibility that unknown toxic factors found in wealthy, industrialized countries had caused a sharp increase in irritable bowel diseases, advocates of the hygiene hypothesis suggest that some factor or factors that had previously inhibited the development of chronic bowel diseases had essentially disappeared as a consequence of modern lifestyles. Several lines of evidence suggested that inflammatory bowel conditions have become more prevalent in countries where children are no longer routinely exposed to parasitic worms. Theoretically, the parasitic worms that were so common among our ancestors and are still highly prevalent among people living in underdeveloped tropical countries might provide chemicals that suppress certain harmful immune system responses. Successful parasites have mastered the art of life as "slow predators" that take up long-term residence in their prey. Instead of killing their host, parasitic worms have evolved strategies that allow them to evade or modulate the host's immune responses so that they can continuously consume nutrients supplied by their living, if somewhat debilitated, host. Small, clinical tests of this concept, performed in 2005, were widely reported in the popular media. Volunteers suffering from ulcerative colitis or Crohn's disease were given a placebo or the eggs of the pig whipworm, *Trichuris suis*, a harmless intestinal worm that does not cause disease in humans. Pig whipworms live only a short time in humans and cannot be transmitted to another person. Although the number of people involved in the experiment was small, the results were encouraging. Many of the patients given *Trichuris suis* eggs reported significant improvement. Scientists have also investigated the possibility that hookworm infestations and schistosomiasis suppress or prevent allergies and autoimmune disorders.

Critics of the hygiene hypothesis have questions about its validity as well as ethical concerns about the way the popular media have portrayed the parasites that are responsible for so much human suffering throughout the world as harmless, even benevolent, therapeutic agents. Major campaigns were conducted in the United States during the twentieth century to eliminate hookworm infections, but in poor tropical countries, these parasites still kill sixty-five thousand people a year and cause debilitating anemia in hundreds of thousands of people. Nevertheless, preliminary human tests of hookworm therapy for irritable bowel diseases have been widely reported as demonstrations of proof of concept. If further studies demonstrate the efficacy of worm therapy, the specific chemical signals that parasites produce to suppress the immune system might be identified, isolated, and modified. Derivatives of the chemical signals produced by parasites might prevent or control allergies and autoimmune conditions without the threat of hookworm disease or a dangerous suppression of the immune system.

Not surprisingly, the hygiene hypothesis has become one of the many reasons that parents give for rejecting preventive immunizations for their children. Leaders of the antivaccination movement claim that infectious diseases, such as colds, influenza, measles, and chicken pox, are a normal part of childhood and that natural exposure to such diseases is essential for proper maturation of the immune system. However, many studies show that high levels of illness during childhood are associated with poor health throughout life and a greater chance of premature death. Medical experts warn that the idea that contracting childhood infections and maintaining a permanent population of parasitic worms are good for the immune system is very dangerous. Moreover, the childhood diseases that are typically the target of preventive vaccines are the diseases that humans have experienced for only a tiny fraction of human evolution. Highly contagious diseases, such as measles and smallpox, were not part of the long evolutionary history that shaped the human immune system. Such diseases could only become the inevitable diseases of childhood in large, densely populated human societies. Human beings lived as hunter-gatherers until about eight to ten thousand years ago, when they began to cultivate crops and domesticate animals. Most of the contagious diseases targeted by vaccines did not play a significant role in the lives of our ancestors until they domesticated animals and began crowding together in large settlements about five thousand years ago. Cities with populations large enough to sustain most epidemic diseases first appeared about four thousand years ago. So it is reasonable to say that human beings have survived *despite* epidemic diseases, but it is not reasonable to assume that smallpox and measles were significant forces in human evolution.

Advocates of the hygiene hypothesis who suggest that a bit of dirt is good for infants might want to think about the relationship between infant botulism, a potentially fatal disease first recognized in the 1970s, and the distribution of *Clostridium botulinum* spores. *Clostridium* spores have been found in honey, but they are also widely present in the environment, especially in soil. Infant botulism is caused by the germination of *Clostridium* spores in the infant's immature gastrointestinal tract. Moreover, even in a very clean, modern environment, it is unlikely that any human being can actually escape the world of germs. Perhaps the most logical explanation for the relative absence of asthma, allergies, and autoimmune disorders in impoverished, developing countries is the fact that so many infants and children die of diarrheas, fevers, and other infectious diseases that rich children almost never experience.

THE HUMAN MICROBIOME PROJECT

Since the establishment of the germ theory of disease, microorganisms have generally been thought of as disease-causing entities. Medical microbiology generally encouraged ways of thinking about microbes as alien agents that invaded the human body to cause disease. However, the microbial world is incredibly complex, and its inhabitants play many roles essential to the survival of life on earth and the health of the planet. Indeed, human life depends on the balance between our own cells and the microorganisms that inhabit our bodies as well as our interactions with environmental microbes. Germs are unavoidable and, except for specific pathogens, usually innocuous for people with a normal immune system and, perhaps, a full complement of commensal microbes. Hundreds of previously unrecognized species of bacteria normally live on and within the human body, especially in the intestines, and even in tissues previously thought to be free of microbes. Gut microbes perform many essential functions, including the digestion of complex plant materials, the synthesis of vitamins, and the production of enzymes needed to metabolize cholesterol and bile acids. When broad-spectrum antibiotics are used to kill a specific pathogen, the entire microbial community can be seriously disrupted, which may create a niche for dangerous pathogens.

Elie Metchnikoff, a pioneer immunologist best known for his discovery of phagocytes (the white blood cells that engulf microbial invaders), was convinced that the putrefaction caused by bacteria inside the gastrointestinal tract caused senility, atherosclerosis, gray hair, and premature death. In a prediction that seems particularly misguided today, Metchnikoff asserted that eventually, specialized surgeons would routinely remove the entire human colon to prevent chronic poisoning by the intestinal flora. Other scientists have argued that we should try to think of the human body as a complex, interdependent community comprised of human and microbial cells. Specifically, human cells make up only about 10 percent of this community. The vast majority of the microbial cells that make up the other 90 percent of the body constitute a complex bacterial ecosystem residing in the gastrointestinal tract.

In 2005, scientists representing the National Human Genome Research Institute and an international consortium of researchers launched the Human Gut Microbiome Initiative. The term *microbiome* generally refers to all the microbes that live in and on a normal, healthy human being. Often referred to as the second, and more challenging human genome project, the Human Gut Microbiome Initiative was dedicated to establishing a census or community profile of the bacteria that live in the normal human gastrointestinal system. Techniques developed during the Human Genome Project are being used to begin the immense task of identifying and sequencing all the genes of the human gut microflora. The Human Gut Microbiome Project, however, is just part of the Human Microbiome Project, which will eventually create a catalog of all the microbial species that live in and on every niche of the human body. The goal of the Human Microbiome Project is to characterize the entire human microbiota and study the effect of these microbial communities on human development, physiology, immunity, nutrition, and health. As in the case of the Human Genome Project, researchers expect the Human Microbiome Project to generate new techniques as well as new ideas. The Human Microbiome Project has become part of the National Institutes of Health's New Pathways to Discovery and its Roadmap for Medical Research. The goals and methods encapsulated in the Human Microbiome Project reflect a fundamental shift in microbiology that is likely to have a profound impact on the way we envision human health and physiology.

According to microbiome researchers, the collection of human and microbial genes within the body should be thought of as a complex *metagenome*, in which the total number of microbial genes probably exceeds the number of genes in the human genome by orders of magnitude. Human beings might then be represented as *superorganisms*, whose metabolic processes represent the totality of microbial and human cell biology. Our physiological status is thus the product of the interactions between our human and microbial genomes. Ultimately, scientists would like to isolate, sequence, and analyze the genomes of all members of the microbial community, but the first phase of the Human Microbiome Project plan calls for the study of about one hundred representative microbial species. Although the task of characterizing the trillions of microbial cells in the gut has just begun, scientists suspect that the microbial population as a whole can probably be resolved into hundreds or thousands of individual species.

Microbiology, as established by Louis Pasteur, Robert Koch, and other nineteenth-century pioneers, focused on the study of individual species as isolated units. To prove that a specific microbe caused a specific disease, classical microbiologists had to grow pure cultures of the alleged pathogen. Classical methods could not, however, produce laboratory cultures of many microbial species or explore the relationships among the individual microbial species in complex communities. New techniques that analyze the total DNA in a microbial community eliminate the need to culture each member of natural microbial communities. The advances in DNA sequencing methods that make it possible to analyze the genetic material derived from an entire microbial community have created a new field of study known as *metagenomics*. The total genomic material of the microbial communities that live in and on human beings constitutes the human metagenome. Using this approach, scientists are attempting to analyze representative genes of all bacterial species in the microbiome and characterize possible relationships between changes in microbial communities and human health. Understanding the ways in which complex microbial ecosystems function may eventually reveal the factors that transform normally harmless microbes into deadly pathogens.

BIBLIOGRAPHY

Abraham, T. (2005). *Twenty-first Century Plague: The Story of SARS*. Baltimore: Johns Hopkins University Press.

Alibek, K., with Handelman, S. (1999). *Biohazard: The Chilling True Story of the Largest Covert Biological Weapons Program in the World—Told from Inside by the Man Who Ran It*. New York: Random House.

Allen, A. (2007). *Vaccine: The Controversial Story of Medicine's Greatest Lifesaver*. New York: W. W. Norton.

Armus, D., ed. (2003). *Disease in the History of Modern Latin America: From Malaria to AIDS*. Durham, NC: Duke University Press.

Barnes, D. S. (2006). *The Great Stink of Paris and the Nineteenth-Century Struggle against Filth and Germs*. Baltimore: John Hopkins University Press.

Barry, J. M. (2004). *The Great Influenza: The Epic Story of the Deadliest Plague in History*. New York: Viking Press.

Bashford, A., ed. (2007). *Medicine at the Border: Disease, Globalization, and Security, 1850 to the Present*. New York: Palgrave.

Baxby, D. (2001). *Smallpox Vaccine, Ahead of Its Time: How the Late Development of Laboratory Methods and Other Vaccines Affected the Acceptance of Smallpox Vaccine*. Berkeley, England: Jenner Museum.

Bazin, H. (2000). *The Eradication of Smallpox: Edward Jenner and the First and Only Eradication of a Human Infectious Disease*. San Diego, CA: Academic Press.

Becker, U. (2007). *Light at the End of the Tunnel? The Sixth Review Conference of the Biological Weapons Convention*. Frankfurt, Germany: Peace Research Institute Frankfurt.

Behrman, G. (2004). *The Invisible People: How the U.S. Has Slept through the Global AIDS Pandemic, the Greatest Humanitarian Catastrophe of Our Time.* New York: Free Press.

Beveridge, W. I. B. (1978). *Influenza, the Last Great Plague: An Unfinished Story of Discovery.* New York: Prodist.

Black, J. G. (2008). *Microbiology: Principles and Explorations.* 7th ed. Hoboken, NJ: Wiley.

Bourdelais, P. (2006). *Epidemics Laid Low: A History of What Happened in Rich Countries.* Translated by Bart K. Holland. Baltimore: Johns Hopkins University Press.

Brandt, A. M. (1987). *No Magic Bullet: A Social History of Venereal Disease in the United States since 1880.* New York: Oxford University Press.

Brock, T. D. (1999). *Milestones in Microbiology 1546 to 1940.* Washington, DC: ASM Press.

———. (1999). *Robert Koch: A Life in Medicine and Bacteriology.* Washington, DC: ASM Press.

Brody, S. N. (1974). *The Disease of the Soul: Leprosy in Medieval Literature.* Ithaca, NY: Cornell University Press.

Burroughs, T., Knobler, S., and Lederberg, J., eds. (2002). *The Emergence of Zoonotic Diseases: Understanding the Impact on Animal and Human Health.* Washington, DC: National Academies Press.

Cairns, J., Stent, G. S., and Watson, J. D., eds. (2007). *Phage and the Origins of Molecular Biology.* 2nd ed. New York: Cold Spring Harbor Laboratory of Quantitative Biology.

Calendar, R., and Abedon, S. T., eds. (2006). *The Bacteriophages.* New York: Oxford University Press.

Campkin, B., and Cox, R., eds. (2007). *Dirt: New Geographies of Cleanliness and Contamination.* London: I. B. Tauris.

Carlin, C. L., ed. (2005). *Imagining Contagion in Early Modern Europe.* New York: Palgrave Macmillan.

Carmichael, A. G. (1986). *Plague and the Poor in Renaissance Florence.* New York: Cambridge University Press.

Carter, K. C., ed. (1987). *Essays of Robert Koch.* Translated by K. C. Carter. New York: Greenwood Press.

———. (2003). *The Rise of Causal Concepts of Disease: Case Histories.* Burlington, VT: Ashgate.

Chase, A. (1982). *Magic Shots: A Human and Scientific Account of the Long and Continuing Struggle to Eradicate Infectious Diseases by Vaccination.* New York: William Morrow.

Cipolla, C. M. (1992). *Miasmas and Disease: Public Health and the Environment in the Pre-industrial Age.* Translated by Elizabeth Potter. New Haven, CT: Yale University Press.

Cliff, A., Haggett, P., and Smallman-Raynor, M. (1993). *Measles: An Historical Geography of a Major Human Viral Disease, from Global Expansion to Local Retreat, 1840–1990.* Oxford: Blackwell.

Cohen, M. (1989). *Health and the Rise of Civilization.* New Haven, CT: Yale University Press.

Cole, L. A. (1990). *Clouds of Secrecy: The Army's Germ Warfare Tests over Populated Areas.* Savage, MD: Rowman and Littlefield.

———. (2003). *The Anthrax Letters: A Medical Detective Story.* Washington, DC: Joseph Henry Press.

Colgrove, J. (2006). *State of Immunity: The Politics of Vaccination in Twentieth-Century America.* Berkeley: University of California Press.

Conrad, L. I., and Wujastyk, D., eds. (2000). *Contagion: Perspectives from Pre-Modern Societies.* Brookfield, VT: Ashgate.

Crosby, A. W. (1986). *Ecological Imperialism: The Biological Expansion of Europe, 900–1900.* New York: Cambridge University Press.

———. (2003). *America's Forgotten Pandemic: The Influenza of 1918.* New York: Cambridge University Press.

Cueto, M. (2001). *The Return of Epidemics: Health and Society in Peru during the Twentieth Century.* Burlington, VT: Ashgate.

Daniel, T. M. (2000). *Pioneers in Medicine and Their Impact on Tuberculosis.* Rochester, NY: University of Rochester Press.

Daniel, T. M., and Robbins, F. C., eds. (1997). *Polio.* Rochester, NY: University of Rochester Press.

Debré, P. (2000). *Louis Pasteur.* Baltimore: Johns Hopkins University Press.

Demaitre, L. E. (2007). *Leprosy in Premodern Medicine: A Malady of the Whole Body.* Baltimore: Johns Hopkins University Press.

De Palo, G., Rilke, F., and Zur Hausen, H., eds. (1986). *Herpes and Papilloma Viruses.* New York: Raven Press.

Diener, T. O. (1979). *Viroids and Viroid Diseases.* New York: Wiley.

Dormandy, T. (2000). *White Death: A History of Tuberculosis.* New York: New York University Press.

Doupher, B. V., ed. (2006). *Prions: New Research.* New York: Nova Science.

Dubos, R. J. (1988). *Pasteur and Modern Science.* Edited by Thomas D. Brock. Madison, WI: Science Tech.

Duesberg, P. (1996). *Inventing the AIDS Virus.* Washington, DC: Regnery.

Durbach, N. (2005). *Bodily Matters: The Anti-Vaccination Movement in England, 1853–1907.* Durham, NC: Duke University Press.

Edmond, R. (2007). *Leprosy and Empire: A Medical and Cultural History.* New York: Cambridge University Press.

Endicott, S., and Hagerman, E. (1999). *The United States and Biological Warfare: Secrets from the Early Cold War and Korea.* Bloomington: Indiana University Press.

Essex, M., Todaro, G., and Zur Hausen, H., eds. (1980). *Viruses in Naturally Occurring Cancers.* Cold Spring Harbor, NY: Cold Spring Harbor Laboratory.

Estes, J. W., and Smith, B. G., eds. (1997). *A Melancholy Scene of Devastation: The Public Response to the 1793 Philadelphia Yellow Fever Epidemic.* Canton, MA: Science History.

Farley, J. (1997). *The Spontaneous Generation Controversy from Descartes to Oparin.* Baltimore: Johns Hopkins University Press.

Farmer, P., ed. (1999). *The Global Impact of Drug-Resistant Tuberculosis.* Boston, MA: Harvard Medical Schools.

Fauci, A. S. (2003). *Bioterrorism: A Clear and Present Danger.* Santa Monica, CA: RAND Corporation.

Fee, E., and Acheson, R. M. (1991). *A History of Education in Public Health: Health That Mocks the Doctors' Rules.* New York: Oxford University Press.

Feldman, E. A., and Bayer, R., eds. (1999). *Blood Feuds: AIDS, Blood, and the Politics of Medical Disaster.* New York: Oxford University Press.

Fenner, F. (1988). *Smallpox and Its Eradication.* Geneva, Switzerland: World Health Organization.

Fenner, F., and Gibbs, A., eds. (1988). *Portraits of Viruses. A History of Virology.* New York: Karger.

Fracastoro, G. (1984). *Fracastoro's "Syphilis": Introduction, Text, Translations, and Notes with a Computer-Generated Word Index by Geoffrey Eatough.* Liverpool, England: Francis Cairns.

Gandy, M., and Zumla, A., eds. (2003). *The Return of the White Plague: Global Poverty and the "New" Tuberculosis.* London: Verso.

Garrett, L. (1994). *The Coming Plague: Newly Emerging Disease in a World out of Balance.* New York: Farrar, Straus and Giroux.

————. (2000). *Betrayal of Trust: The Collapse of Global Public Health.* New York: Hyperion.

Garrett, R., and Klenk, H.-P., eds. (2007). *Archaea: Evolution, Physiology, and Molecular Biology.* Malden, MA: Blackwell.

Geison, G. L. (1995). *The Private Science of Louis Pasteur.* Princeton, NJ: Princeton University Press.

Geiter, L., ed. (2000). *Ending Neglect: The Elimination of Tuberculosis in the United States.* Washington, DC: National Academies Press.

Glynn, I., and Glynn, J. (2004). *The Life and Death of Smallpox.* Cambridge: Cambridge University Press.

Goudsmit, J. (2004). *Viral Fitness: The Next SARS and West Nile in the Making.* New York: Oxford University Press.

Gould, T. (1995). *A Summer Plague: Polio and Its Survivors.* New Haven, CT: Yale University Press.

————. (2005). *A Disease Apart: Leprosy in the Modern World.* New York: St. Martin's Press.

Grmek, M. D. (1990). *History of AIDS: Emergence and Origin of a Modern Pandemic.* Translated by R. C. Maulitz and J. Duffin. Princeton, NJ: Princeton University Press.

Guillemin, J. (1999). *Anthrax: The Investigation of a Deadly Outbreak.* Berkeley: University of California Press.

Gussow, Z. (1989). *Leprosy, Racism and Public Health: Social Policy in Chronic Disease Control.* Boulder, CO: Westview Press.

Hadidi, A., ed. (2003). *Viroids.* Enfield, NH: Science.

Hamlin, C. R. (1998). *Public Health and Social Justice in the Age of Chadwick.* New York: Cambridge University Press.

Hammonds, E. M. (1999). *Childhood's Deadly Scourge: The Campaign to Control Diphtheria in New York City, 1880–1930.* Baltimore: Johns Hopkins University Press.

Harden, V. A. (1990). *Rocky Mountain Spotted Fever: History of a Twentieth-Century Disease.* Baltimore: Johns Hopkins University Press.

Harris, S. H. (2002). *Factories of Death: Japanese Biological Warfare, 1932–45 and the American Cover-Up.* Rev. ed. New York: Routledge.

Häusler; T. (2006). *Viruses vs. Superbugs: A Solution to the Antibiotics Crisis?* Translated by K. Leube. New York: Macmillan.

Hays, J. N. (1997). *The Burdens of Disease: Epidemics and Human Response in Western History.* New Brunswick, NJ: Rutgers University Press.

Headrick, D. R. (1981). *The Tools of Empire: Technology and European Imperialism in the Nineteenth Century.* New York: Oxford University Press.

Hooper, E. (1999). *The River: A Journey to the Source of HIV and AIDS.* Boston, MA: Little, Brown.

Hopkins, D. R. (2002). *The Greatest Killer: Smallpox in History.* Chicago: University of Chicago Press.

Hughes, S. S. (1977). *The Virus: A History of the Concept.* New York: Science History.

Humphreys, M. (2001). *Malaria: Poverty, Race and Public Health in the United States.* Baltimore: Johns Hopkins University Press.

Institute of Medicine, National Academy of Sciences (1986). *Confronting AIDS: Directions for Public Health, Health Care, and Research.* Report prepared by the Committee on a National Strategy for AIDS of the Institute of Medicine. Washington, DC: National Academies Press.

Jarcho, S. (2000). *The Concept of Contagion in Medicine, Literature and Religion.* Malabar, FL: Krieger.

Johnson, S. (2006). *The Ghost Map: The Story of London's Most Terrifying Epidemic—and How It Changed Science, Cities, and the Modern World.* New York: Riverhead Books / Penguin Group.

Kiple, K. F., ed. (1993). *The Cambridge World History of Human Disease.* New York: Cambridge University Press.

Kiple, K. F., and Beck, S. V., eds. (1997). *Biological Consequences of the European Expansion, 1450–1800.* Brookfield, VT: Ashgate.

Knobler, S. L., ed. (2003). *The Resistance Phenomenon in Microbes and Infectious Disease Vectors: Implications for Human Health and Strategies for Containment.* Washington, DC: National Academies Press.

———, ed. (2004). *The Infectious Etiology of Chronic Diseases: Defining the Relationship, Enhancing the Research, and Mitigating the Effects.* Washington, DC: National Academies Press.

———, ed. (2004). *Learning from SARS: Preparing for the Next Disease Outbreak. Workshop Summary.* Washington, DC: National Academies Press.

Knobler, S., Lederberg, J., and Pray, L. A., eds. (2002). *Considerations for Viral Disease Eradication: Lessons Learned and Future Strategies.* Washington, DC: National Academies Press.

Knobler, S., Mahmoud, A., and Lemon, S., eds. (2006). *The Impact of Globalization on Infectious Disease Emergence and Control: Exploring the Consequences and Opportunities. Forum on Microbial Threats.* Washington, DC: National Academies Press.

Kolata, G. B. (2000). *Flu: The Story of the Great Influenza Pandemic of 1918 and the Search for the Virus That Caused It.* London: Macmillan.

Krause, R. M. (1981). *The Restless Tide: The Persistent Challenge of the Microbial World.* Washington, DC: National Foundation for Infectious Diseases.

Kunitz, S. J. (1994). *Disease and Social Diversity: The European Impact on the Health of Non-Europeans.* Oxford: Oxford University Press.

Kutter, E., and Sulakvelidze, A. (2005). *Bacteriophages: Biology and Applications.* Boca Raton, FL: CRC Press.

Lal, S. K., ed. (2006). *Emerging Viral Diseases of Southeast Asia.* New York: Karger.

Leavitt, J. W. (1996). *Typhoid Mary: Captive to the Public's Health.* Boston, MA: Beacon Press.

Lechevalier, H. A., and Solotorovsky, M. (1974). *Three Centuries of Microbiology.* New York: Dover.

Lederberg, J., ed. (1999). *Biological Weapons: Limiting the Threat.* Cambridge, MA: MIT Press.

Lederberg, J., Shope, R. E., & Oaks, S. C., eds. (1992). *Emerging Infections: Microbial Threats to Health in the United States.* Washington, DC: National Academies Press.

Lee, R. A. (2007). *From Snake Oil to Medicine: Pioneering Public Health.* Westport, CT: Praeger.

Lesch, J. E. (2007). *The First Miracle Drugs: How the Sulfa Drugs Transformed Medicine.* New York: Oxford University Press.

Levy, B. S., and Sidel, V. W., eds. (2007). *War and Public Health.* 2nd ed. New York: Oxford University Press.

Loudon, I. (2000). *The Tragedy of Childbed Fever.* New York: Oxford University Press.

Magner, L. N. (2002). *A History of the Life Sciences.* New York: Marcel Dekker.

———. (2005). *A History of Medicine.* New York: Taylor and Francis.

Markel, H. (2004). *When Germs Travel: Six Major Epidemics That Have Invaded America since 1900 and the Fears They Have Unleashed.* New York: Pantheon Books.

McCarthy, M. P. (1987). *Typhoid and the Politics of Public Health in Nineteenth-Century Philadelphia.* Philadelphia: American Philosophical Society.

McLean, A., May, R. M., Pattison, J., and Weiss, R. A., eds. (2005). *SARS: A Case Study in Emerging Infections.* Oxford: Oxford University Press.

McMichael, T. (2001). *Human Frontiers, Environments and Disease: Past Patterns, Uncertain Futures.* Cambridge: Cambridge University Press.

McNeill, W. H. (1998). *Plagues and Peoples.* New York: Anchor Books.

Miller, J., Engelberg, S., and Broad, W. (2002). *Germs: Biological Weapons and America's Secret War.* New York: Simon and Schuster.

Moberg, C. L., and Cohn, Z. A., eds. (1990). *Launching the Antibiotic Era: Personal Accounts of the Discovery and Use of the First Antibiotics.* New York: Rockefeller University Press.

Money, N. P. (2007). *The Triumph of the Fungi: A Rotten History.* New York: Oxford University Press.

Moore, J. (2002). *Parasites and the Behavior of Animals.* New York: Oxford University Press.

Morris, R. D. (2007). *The Blue Death: Disease, Disaster, and the Water We Drink.* New York: HarperCollins.

Morse, S. S., ed. (1993). *Emerging Viruses.* Oxford: Oxford University Press.

Muraskin, W. (1995). *The War against Hepatitis B: A History of the International Task Force on Hepatitis B Immunization.* Philadelphia: University of Pennsylvania Press.

———. (1998). *The Politics of International Health: The Children's Vaccine Initiative and the Struggle to Develop Vaccines for the Third World.* Albany, NY: SUNY Press.

Murray, C. J. L., and Lopez, A. D. (1996). *Global Health Statistics: A Compendium of Incidence, Prevalence, and Mortality Estimates for Over 200 Conditions.* Cambridge, MA: Harvard University Press.

Neustadt, R. E., and Fineberg, H. V. (1983). *The Epidemic That Never Was: Policy-making and the Swine Flu Scare.* New York: Vintage Books.

Nuland, S. B. (2003). *The Doctors' Plague: Germs, Childbed Fever and the Strange Story of Ignac Semmelweis.* New York: W. W. Norton.

Nunnally, B. K., and Krull, I. S., eds. (2004). *Prions and Mad Cow Disease.* New York: Marcel Dekker.

Offit, P. A. (2005). *The Cutter Incident: How America's First Polio Vaccine Led to the Growing Vaccine Crisis.* New Haven, CT: Yale University Press.

———. (2008). *Autism's False Prophets: Bad Science, Risky Medicine, and the Search for a Cure.* New York: Columbia University Press.

Oshinsky, D. M. (2005). *Polio: An American Story.* New York: Oxford University Press.

Packard, R. M. (2007). *The Making of a Tropical Disease: A Short History of Malaria.* Baltimore: Johns Hopkins University Press.

Parascandola, J., ed. (1980). *The History of Antibiotics: A Symposium.* Madison, WI: American Institute for the History of Pharmacy.

———. (2008). *Sex, Sin, and Science: A History of Syphilis in America.* Westport, CT: Praeger.

Parry, H. B. (1983). *Scrapie Disease in Sheep: Historical, Clinical, Epidemiological, Pathological, and Practical Aspects of the Natural Disease.* New York: Academic Press.

Perleth, M. (1997). *Historical Aspects of American Trypanosomiasis (Chagas' Disease).* Frankfurt am Main, Germany: Peter Lang.

Peters, C. J., and Calisher, C. H., eds. (2005). *Infectious Diseases from Nature: Mechanisms of Viral Emergence and Persistence.* New York: Springer.

Peto, R., and Zur Hausen, H., eds. (1986). *Viral Etiology of Cervical Cancer.* Cold Spring Harbor, NY: Cold Spring Harbor Laboratory.

Pilch, R. F., and Zilinskas, R. A., eds. (2005). *Encyclopedia of Bioterrorism Defense.* Hoboken, NJ: Wiley–Liss.

Plotkin, S., and Fantini, B., eds. (1996). *Vaccinia, Vaccination and Vaccinology: Jenner, Pasteur, and Their Successors.* Paris: Elsevier.

Poser, C. M., and Bruyn, G. W. (2000). *An Illustrated History of Malaria.* Boca Raton, FL: CRC Press.

Preston, R. (2002). *The Demon in the Freezer: A True Story.* New York: Random House.

Prusiner, S. B., ed. (2004). *Prion Biology and Diseases.* 2nd ed. Cold Spring Harbor, NY: Cold Spring Harbor Laboratory.

Rabenau, H. F., Cinatl, J., and Doerr, H. W., eds. (2004). *Prions: A Challenge for Science, Medicine and the Public Health System.* New York: Karger.

Razzell, P. (1977). *Edward Jenner's Cowpox Vaccine: The History of a Medical Myth.* Sussex, England: Caliban Books.

Regis, E. (1999). *The Biology of Doom: The History of America's Secret Germ Warfare Project.* New York: Henry Holt.

Reynolds, L. A., and Tansey, E. M., eds. (2003). *Foot and Mouth Disease: The 1967 Outbreak and Its Aftermath.* London: Wellcome Trust Centre for the History of Medicine.

Rhodes, R. (1998). *Deadly Feasts: The "Prion" Controversy and the Public's Health.* New York: Simon and Schuster.

Rifkind, D., and Freeman, G. L. (2005). *The Nobel Prize Winning Discoveries in Infectious Diseases.* London: Elsevier / Academic.

Riley, J. C. (2001). *Rising Life Expectancy: A Global History.* New York: Cambridge University Press.

Rosen, G. (1993). *A History of Public Health.* Introduction by Elizabeth Fee. Biographical essay and new bibliography by Edward T. Morman. Baltimore: Johns Hopkins University Press.

Rosenberg, C. E. (1987). *The Cholera Years: The United States in 1832, 1849, and 1866.* Chicago, IL: University of Chicago Press.

Rosner, D., ed. (1995). *Hives of Sickness: Public Health and Epidemics in New York City.* New Brunswick, NJ: Rutgers University Press.

Ryan, F. (1993). *The Forgotten Plague: How the Battle against Tuberculosis Was Won—and Lost.* Boston, MA: Little, Brown.

Sachs, J. S. (2007). *Good Germs, Bad Germs: Health and Survival in a Bacterial World.* New York: Hill and Wang.

Sagan, D., and Margulis, L. (1993). *Garden of Microbial Delights: A Practical Guide to the Subvisible World.* Dubuque, IA: Kendall Hunt.

Salyers, A. A., and Whitt, D. D. (2005). *Revenge of the Microbes: How Bacterial Resistance Is Undermining the Antibiotic Miracle.* Washington, DC: ASM Press.

Scott, S., and Duncan, C. J. (2001). *Biology of Plagues: Evidence from Historical Populations.* New York: Cambridge University Press.

Semancik, J. S., ed. (1987). *Viroids and Viroid-like Pathogens.* Boca Raton, FL: CRC Press.

Seytre, B., and Shaffer, M. (2005). *The Death of a Disease: A History of the Eradication of Poliomyelitis.* New Brunswick, NJ: Rutgers University Press.

Silverstein, A. M. (1981). *Pure Politics and Impure Science: The Swine Flu Affair.* Baltimore: Johns Hopkins University Press.

Smith, J. S. (1990). *Patenting the Sun: Polio and the Salk Vaccine.* New York: William Morrow.

Smith, V. (2007). *Clean: A History of Personal Hygiene and Purity.* New York: Oxford University Press.

Smolinski, M. S., Hamburg, M. A., and Lederberg, J., eds. (200). *Microbial Threats to Health: Emergence, Detection, and Response.* Washington, DC: National Academies Press.

Snodgrass, M. E. (2003). *World Epidemics: A Cultural Chronology of Disease from Prehistory to the Era of SARS.* Jefferson, NC: McFarland.

Snow, J. (1965). *Snow on Cholera: Being a Reprint of Two Papers.* New York: Hafner.

Spencer, C. (2004). *Mad Cows and Cannibals: A Guide to the Transmissible Spongiform Encephalopathies.* Upper Saddle River, NJ: Pearson / Prentice Hall.

Staley, J. T., and Reysenbach, A.-L. (2002). *Biodiversity of Microbial Life.* New York: Wiley–Liss.

Summers, W. C. (1999). *Félix d'Hérelle and the Origins of Molecular Biology.* New Haven, CT: Yale University Press.

Thomas, A. (2005). *Twenty-first Century Plague: The Story of SARS.* Baltimore: Johns Hopkins University Press.

Tierno, P. M., Jr. (2001). *The Secret Life of Germs: Observations and Lessons from a Microbe Hunter.* New York: Pocket Books.

Tomes, N. (1998). *The Gospel of Germs: Men, Women, and the Microbe in American Life.* Cambridge, MA: Harvard University Press, 1998.

Torrey, E. F., and Yolken, R. H. (2005). *Beasts of the Earth: Animals, Humans, and Disease.* New Brunswick, NJ: Rutgers University Press.

Venter, J. C. (2007). *A Life Decoded. My Genome: My Life.* New York: Viking / Penguin.

Watts, S. (1998). *Epidemics and History: Disease, Power and Imperialism.* New Haven, CT: Yale University Press.

Wickner, R. B. (1997). *Prion Diseases of Mammals and Yeast: Molecular Mechanisms and Genetic Features.* New York: Springer.

Williams, P., and Wallace, D. (1989). *Unit 731: Japan's Secret Biological Warfare in World War II.* New York: Free Press.

Wilson, M. (2005). *Microbial Inhabitants of Humans: Their Ecology and Role in Health and Disease.* New York: Cambridge University Press.

Wilson, M. E., Levins, R., and Spielman, A., eds. (1994). *Disease in Evolution: Global Changes and Emergence of Infectious Diseases.* New York: New York Academy of Sciences.

Worboys, M. (2000). *Spreading Germs: Disease Theories and Medical Practice in Britain, 1865–1900.* New York: Cambridge University Press.

World Health Organization (1980). *The Global Eradication of Smallpox. Final Report of the Global Commission for the Certification of Smallpox Eradication, Geneva, December 1979.* Geneva, Switzerland: World Health Organization.

Ziporyn, T. (1988). *Disease in the Popular American Press: The Case of Diphtheria, Typhoid Fever, and Syphilis, 1870–1920.* New York: Greenwood Press.

Zubay, G., ed. (2005). *Agents of Bioterrorism: Pathogens and Their Weaponization.* New York: Columbia University Press.

Zuk, M. (2007). *Riddled with Life: Friendly Worms, Ladybug Sex, and the Parasites That Make Us Who We Are.* Orlando, FL: Harcourt.

Zur Hausen, H. (2006). *Infections Causing Human Cancer.* Chichester, England: Wiley.

INDEX

Acquired immune deficiency syndrome, see AIDS

AIDS (acquired immune deficiency syndrome), 89, 150, 154, 156–66, 198; AIDS denialists, 158–59, 163–66; antiretroviral drugs, 165–67; causative agent, discovery of, 158; emerging diseases, 151; leprosy, 14–15; *Pneumocystis carinii* pneumonia, xx, 157; reverse transcriptase, 86, 166; tuberculosis, 65–66; vaccine prospects, 88, 166–68

Alibek, Ken (Kanatjan Kalibekov), 119, 192–93

Anthrax, bioterrorism, 39, 132, 150–51, 188–91; causative agent, discovery of, 37–38; clinical patterns, 37, 39, 189, 192; genome of, 191; spore formation, 38–39, 191; Sverdlovsk anthrax outbreak, 191–93; vaccine, 39, 132. *See also* Anthrax letters

Anthrax letters, 150–51, 188–91. *See also* Bioterrorism

Antibiotics, 62–66, 79, 189–90

Antisepsis, 41, 50, 53–56, 61

Antivaccinationists (vaccine resisters), 128–32; Guardasil, opposition to, 134; hygiene hypothesis as rationale, 204; mandatory vaccination, opposition to, 114–15, 128–29; religious exemptions to mandatory vaccination, 129–30, 134

Archaeans, xv–xvi

Asepsis, 55–56

Asiatic cholera, 98–99. *See also* Cholera

Atmospheric-miasmatic theory of disease, 20

Autism, 129–31

Autoclave, 56

Avian flu, 181, 183–84. *See also* Influenza

Bacteria, drug resistant, 62, 65–67; MRSA, 69–70; phage therapy and, 79–81; tuberculosis and, 66–70

Bacterial virus. *See* Bacteriophage
Bacteriophage (bacterial virus), 70–71;
    discovery of, 77–81; lysogenic, 84; lytic,
    84. *See also* Phage and Phage therapy
Baltimore, David, 86–87, 166–68
Barr, Yvonne, 87–88
Bassi, Agostino, 27–28
Bdellovibrio, 70–71
Behring, Emil von, 58–59
Beijerinck, Willem, 75
Bejel, *See* Syphilis
Biological weapons, 185–194; select agents
    (microbes and toxins) as potential
    biological weapons, 186–87, 193;
    dispersal, potential methods of, 186, 189.
    See also Bioterrorism
Bioterrorism, anthrax, as biological weapon,
    39, 150, 188–91, 193; smallpox, as
    biological weapon, 118–19, 185–94
Black Death, 9, 12. *See also* Bubonic plague
Bonomo, Giovanni Cosimo, 27
Botox, 155
Botulism, 155, 205
BSE (bovine spongiform encephalopathy),
    93–94. *See also* Mad cow disease. *See also*
    Prions
Boylston, Zabdiel, 113
Bruce, David, 147
Bubonic plague, 9–12
Budd, William, 43, 104–5
Bugie, Elizabeth, 64
Burkitt, Denis Parsons, 87
Burkitt's lymphoma, 87–88
Burnet, Macfarlane, 149

Calmette, Albert, 45
Carbolic acid (phenol), 55–56, 61
Carrión, Daniel Alcides, 146
Carrión's disease (bartonellosis, verruga
    peruana, Oroya fever), 146
Carson, Rachel, 140
Central dogma of molecular biology, 85–86
Cervical cancer, 133–34

Chadwick, Edwin, 97–98, 103
Chagas, Carlos, 146
Chagas' disease, xxi, 68, 144–45
Chain, Ernst Boris, 63
Chamberland, Charles, 39, 55–56, 74;
    Chamberland filter, 74–76
Chase, Martha, 85
Chemical warfare, 185
Chikungunya virus, 172–74
Childbed fever (puerperal fever), 49–53
Cholera, 79, 98–104, 144; Broad Street
    outbreak, 99–100; cholera vibrio,
    discovery of, 101–2
Chronic diseases, epidemiological transition
    and, 149–50, 195–201; infectious agents
    as causative factors, 88, 195–210. *See also*
    Human Microbiome Project and Hygiene
    hypothesis
Cohn, Ferdinand, 26–27, 38
Columbus, Christopher, 22, 25
Commensalism, 2, 205–7
Communication, bacterial (quorum sensing),
    xviii–xix, 70. *See also* Microbial ecology
Conquest of the Americas, demographic
    catastrophe and role of European diseases,
    16–17
Contagion, theory of disease, 20–25, 27–28
Cowpox, 113, 117. *See also* Smallpox
Creutzfeldt-Jakob disease (CJD), 91–92
Crick, Frances, 85
Crohn's disease, 203–4
Curtis, Tom, 159
Cutter Incident, 122, 125–27

DDT (dichlorodiphenyltrichloroethane),
    140–41
Delbrück, Max, 85
Dengue fever, 141–42, 144, 173
D'Hérelle, Felix, 77–79, 80, 83
Diener, Theodor O., 90
Diphtheria, 57–59, 128–29
Disinfectants, 40–41, 54–56, 61
Domagk, Gerhard, 61–62

DPT (diphtheria, pertussis, tetanus vaccine), 59, 128–29
Dracunculiasis (guinea worm disease), 145–47
Drug resistant bacteria. See Bacteria, drug resistant
Duesberg, Peter, 163–66
Dulbecco, Renato, 86

Eberth, Carl Joseph, 105
Ebola fever, 59, 152, 156, 169–71; amplifiers, hospitals as, 170
Ehrenberg, Christian Gottfried, 26
Ehrlich, Paul, 25, 60–61, 62
Elephantiasis (filariasis), 134, 142, 145
Eliava, George, 79
Emerging diseases, 25, 150–54, 189
Enders, John, 121–22
Epidemiological transition, 149–50
Epstein, Michael Anthony, 87–88
Epstein-Barr virus (EBV), 87–88, 196, 198
Escherich, Theodor, 155
Escherichia coli O157:H7, 155–56
Etiological principle, 30–31
Eukaryotes, xvi
Extremophiles, xv–xvii

Farr, William, 100
Fauci, Anthony, 168
Feldman, William H., 64
Fibiger, Johannes Andreas, 198–99
Filariasis (elephantiasis), 134, 142, 145
Filoviruses, 169
Fleming, Alexander, 62–63
Florey, Howard Walter, 63–64
FMD (foot-and-mouth disease), 74, 76–77
Fomites, 21
Food-borne diseases (food poisoning), 154–56
Fracastoro, Girolamo, 20–22, 25, 28–29, 33
Frank, Johann Peter, 96
Franklin, Benjamin, 130
Frosch, Paul, 76

Gaffky, George, 105
Gajdusek, Carleton, 91–92
Galen, 8
Gallo, Robert, 158
Genital herpes, 133–34. *See also* Human papilloma virus
Germ theory of disease, modern, 28–31; popularization of, 45–47
Global Network for Neglected Tropical Diseases, 144
Global warming, 148
Gonorrhea, 25, 62, 64
Gram stain, xvii
Gram, Hans Christian, xvii
Graunt, John, 96
Great Stink of London, 98
Gregg, Norman, 127
Guérin, Jean-Marie Camille, 45
Guillain-Barré syndrome, 129, 182
Guinea worm disease (dracunculiasis), 145–47

Hamilton, Alice, 105–6
Hand washing, 52–53, 67–68
Hankin, Ernest Hanbury, 79
Hansen, Gerhard, 13
Hansen's disease (leprosy), 13–15
Hantavirus fever, 152, 171–72
Hata, Sahachiro, 61
Hatfill, Steven J., 190
Hausen, Harald zur (Zur Hausen, Harald), 133–34
Healthy carrier, 2, 106–9
Helicobacter pylori, 163, 197, 199–210; cancers and, 200–201; peptic ulcers and, 199–200; prevalence of, 200–201
Hemorrhagic fevers, 59–60, 168–73
Henle, Jacob, 28–30
Hepatitis viruses, 89, 90, 132
Herpesviruses, 197–98. *See also* Human papilloma virus
Hershey, Alfred, 85
Hershey-Chase experiment, 85

Hilleman, Maurice R., 132, 179

Hinshaw, Horton Corwin, 64

Hippocratic medicine, 7, 8, 20

HIV (human immunodeficiency virus). *See* AIDS

HIV/AIDS. *See* AIDS

Hoffman, Paul Erich, 25

Holmes, Oliver Wendell, 50–51

Hooper, Edward, 159

HPV, *See* Human papilloma virus

Hultin, Johan, 180

Human Genome Project, 206

Human Gut Microbiome Initiative, 206–7

Human immunodeficiency virus (HIV). *See* AIDS

Human Microbiome Project, 205–7

Human papilloma virus (HPV), 89, 132–34

Hygiene hypothesis, 121, 201–5

Immune response, 56–57, 59–60, 112, 202–5

Influenza, 88, 175–84; pandemic influenza, 176–80

Invisible-filterable viruses. *See* Viruses

Irritable bowel syndromes, 203–5. *See also* Hygiene hypothesis

Ishii, Shiro, 187

Ivanovski, Dimitri, 75

Ivins, Bruce E., 190–91

Jenner, Edward, 35, 58, 113–18

Kaposi's sarcoma, 89, 157. *See also* AIDS

Kellogg, John Harvey, 46

Kilbourne, Edwin D., 182

Kitasato, Shibasaburo, 10, 58–59

Klebs, Theodor, 57

Koch, Robert, 30, 37–44, 196; cholera, 101, 105–6; tuberculin, 44–45, 54, 58, 64, 74

Koch's postulates, 43, 74, 129, 195

Koprowski, Hilary, 159–60

Kuru, 91–92. *See also* Prions

Landsteiner, Karl, 121

Lassa fever, 59, 156, 171

Laveran, Charles-Louis-Alphonse, 134

Lederberg, Joshua, 85

Leeuwenhoek, Antoni van, 26

Legionnaires' disease (legionellosis, Pontiac fever), 151–52

Leishmaniasis (black fever or kala-azar), 142–43, 145, 147

Leper, 12, 14. *See also* Hansen's disease and Leprosy

Leprosy (Hansen's disease), 12–15, 20

Lice, 16, 143–44

Liebig, Justus von, 30, 33

Linnaeus, Carl von, 26

Lister, Joseph, 53–55, 67, 68

Listeriosis, 155

Loeffler, Friedrich, 57, 76

Louis, Pierre Charles Alexandre, 104

Lucretius, 8

Luria, Salvador, 84, 85

Lwoff, André, 84–85

Lyme disease, 144

Lymerix vaccine, 144

Maalin, Ali Maow, 115

Mad cow disease (BSE), 93–94, 152

Magic bullets, 60–61, 70

Malaria, 6, 8–9, 134–42; clinical forms, 8–9

Mallon, Mary, 106–8. *See also* Typhoid Mary

Manson, Patrick, 134

Marburg fever, 169

Marek's disease (range paralysis), 132

Mather, Cotton, 113

Mayer, Adolf Eduard, 75

Mbeki, Thabo, 165–66

MDR-TB (multidrug-resistant tuberculosis), 66–67

Measles, 111, 119–20, 204–5. *See also* MMR

Metagenome, 206

Metchnikoff, Elie, 71, 205

Miasma (poisonous vapor, noxious air), 19.
  See also Miasmatic theory of disease
Miasmatic theory of disease, 19, 20, 22,
  95–98
Microbial ecology, xxi, 94, 206–7; quorum
  sensing (bacterial communication),
  xviii–xix, 70
Misaji, Kitano, 187
Mizutani, Satoshi, 86–87
MMR (measles, mumps, rubella vaccine),
  127, 130–32
Molecular mimicry, 196
Molecular phylogenetics, xv
Molecular signatures, 197
Monkeypox, 117
Montagnier, Luc, 158
Montagu, Mary Wortley, 112–13
Mr. N, 107–8
MRSA (methicillin-resistant *Staphylococcus
  aureus*), 68–70
Murray, Polly, 144
Mycobacterium tuberculosis, 41, 64. *See also*
  Tuberculosis
Mycology, xix–xx

Native Americans, impact of European
  diseases on, 16–17
Neglected tropical diseases, 144–48
Neolithic Revolution, 3–4
Nicolle, Charles, 143
Nightingale, Florence, 54
Nipah virus, 172–73
Nixon, Richard, 187–88
Nosocomial infections, 67–69

O'Brien, Muriel, 89
Oral rehydration, 102–3
Oroya fever, 146

Pacini, Filippo, 101
Paget, James, 202
Paleolithic era (Old Stone Age), 3
Paleopathology, 2–3, 24–25

Pap smear, 133
Papanicolaou, George N., 133
Parasites, xx-xxi, 134, 145, 203
Parker, Janet, 116–17
Pasteur, Louis, 30, 31–37, 54–56, 74, 196;
  anthrax, 38–39; childbed fever, 53;
  fermentation, 32–33, 34; pasteurization,
  34; rabies vaccine, 35–37, 58; silkworm
  diseases, 34; spontaneous generation,
  33–34
Pasteurella pestis, 11. *See Yersinia pestis*
Pasteurization, 34, 42, 46
Penicillin, 62–64
Penicillium notatum, 62–64
Pertussis (whooping cough), 128–29, 154
Petri, Richard Julius, 40
Pettenkofer, Max von, 97, 101
Peyer, Johann, 104–5
Phage (bacteriophage), 70–71, 77–81, 84,
  84. *See also* Phage therapy
Phage therapy, 70–71, 78–83, 85
Pinta, 23–24. *See also* Syphilis
Plague, bubonic. *See* Bubonic plague
Pneumocystis carinii pneumonia. *See* AIDS
Poliomyelitis (infantile paralysis, polio),
  121–25; eradication programs, 123–25;
  genome of poliovirus, 125; *Gottsdanker v.
  Cutter Laboratories*, 126; resurgence,
  123–25; Sabin vaccine, 122–24; Salk
  vaccine, 122–27; speculations about
  vaccine trials in Africa and AIDS
  epidemic, 159–60; synthesis of poliovirus
Pontiac fever. *See* Legionnaires' disease
Poor Law Commission, 97–98
Population density and disease, 1–2, 153–54,
  204–5
Post hoc ergo propter hoc (logical fallacy), 129
Potato spindle tuber disease, 89–90. *See also*
  Viroids
Poxviruses, 111, 117. *See also* Smallpox and
  Monkeypox
Preston, Richard, 171, 193
Prions, 89, 91–94, 194

Probiotic therapy, 71
Prokaryotes, xv
Prontosil, 62. *See also* Sulfanilamide and Sulfa drugs
Prophage, 85
Provirus hypothesis, 86
Prowazek, Stanislaus, 143
Prusiner, Stanley, 92
Puerperal fever (childbed fever), 49–53
Pylarini, Jacob, 113

Quarantine regulations, 9, 21
Quorum sensing (bacterial communication), xviii–xix

Rabies, 35–37, 74
Rajneeshee cult, 189. *See* Bioterrorism
Raymer, William B., 89–90
Redi, Francesco, 33
Reed, Walter, 136
Retroviruses, 86–87
Reverse transcriptase, 86–87, 166
Rhazes, 111–12
Rickets, Howard Taylor, 73, 143
Rickettsia, 143–44, 173
Rift Valley fever, 172–73
Rigoni-Stern, Domenico Antonio, 133
Rinderpest, 5, 120, 154
Robbins, Frederick, 121–22
Rocha-Lima, Henrique da, 143
Rocky Mountain spotted fever, 143, 173
Ross, Ronald, 134
Rotavirus vaccine, 131
Rous sarcoma virus (RSV), 86–87
Rous, Francis Peyton, 86–87, 132, 198
Roux, Émile, 39, 57
Rubella (German measles), 127
Rush, Benjamin, 54, 135

Sabin, Albert, 122–23
Salk, Jonas, 122–23
Salvarsan, 25, 56, 60–61, 62
Sanitary reform, 20, 46–47, 96–98

SARS (severe acute respiratory syndrome), 152, 156, 175, 183, 189
Scabies, 27
Schatz, Albert, 64, 65
Schaudinn, Fritz Richard, 25
Schick test, 59
Schick, Béla, 59
Schistosomiasis, 6, 142, 145
Schwann, Theodor, 30
Scrapie, 91–92. *See also* Prions
Semmelweis, Ignaz Philipp, 50–53, 68
Serum therapy, 56–60
Severe acute respiratory syndrome (SARS), 152, 156, 175, 183, 189
Shattuck, Lemuel, 98
Shope, Richard, 133
Sick building syndrome, xx
Sickle cell anemia, 2, 139
Simond, Paul-Louis, 10
SIV (simian immunodeficiency virus), 159–60, 167, 194. *See also* AIDS
Slave trade and disease, 16–17
Sleeping sickness (trypanosomiasis), 5, 61, 145, 147–48
Slow virus. *See* Prions
Smallpox, 28, 58, 111–19, 128, 204–5
Smith, Theobald, 143
Snow, John, 99–100
Spontaneous generation, 27, 30, 33–34
Stanley, Wendell Meredith, 75–76
Staphylococcus aureus, 68–70
Steere, Allen C., 144
Stoll, Norman R., 202
Strachan, David P., 201
Streptomycin, 45, 64–65
Sulfa drugs (sulfanilamide), 56, 61–63
Sulfanilamide, 56, 61–63
Sverdlovsk. *See* Anthrax
Swine flu, 151, 181–83
Sydenham, Thomas, 111–12
Synthetic genomics, 83, 125, 193–94
Syphilis, 20, 22–25, 60–61, 68

Taubenberger, Jeffrey, 180–81
Temin, Howard, 86–87, 166
Tetanus, 58
Texas cattle fever, 143
Thalassemia, 139
Theiler, Max, 136
Thimerosal, 130
Thucydides, 7
Ticks (as vectors), 143–44
Timoni, Emanuel, 113
Tobacco mosaic disease, 74–76
Trachoma, 147
Transmissible spongiform encephalopathies. *See* Prions
Treponematoses, 23–25
Trichinosis, 202
Trypanosomiasis (sleeping sickness), 5, 61, 142, 145, 147–48
Tsetse fly, 145, 147
Tshabalala-Msimang, Manto, 165–66
Tuberculin, 44–45
Tuberculosis, 41–43, 64–65
Tumor viruses, 86–89, 132–34; anticancer vaccines, 132–34
Tumpey, Terrence, 180–81
Twort, Frederick, 77–79
Twort-d' Hérelle particles, 78. *See* Bacteriophage
Typhoid fever, 104–9, 154
Typhoid Mary (Mary Mallon), 106–8
Typhus fever, 73, 105, 143–44

Unpasteurized milk (raw milk) and disease, 34, 155

Vaccines, *Gottsdanker v. Cutter Laboratories*, 126; liability issues, 126–27, 130–32; Lymerix, 144; swine flu vaccine, 182
Varro, Marcus Terentius, 8, 25
Vectors (insects and arthropods), 73, 134–42; resurgence of diseases transmitted by, 141–42

Venereal disease (sexually transmitted disease), 22
Venter, J. Craig, 83
Villemin, Jean Antoine, 43
Virgin soil epidemics, 2, 120, 204–5
Viroids, 89–91
Virology, 74, 83–84
Viruses, antiviral drugs, 88, 183; changing definitions of, 73–74, 84; contagion and, 73–74; invisible-filterable virus, 27, 73–75; molecular biology and, 83–86; virology as new discipline, 74, 83–84
Vitruvius, 8

Wakefield, Andrew, 131
Waksman, Selman A., 45, 64–65
Waterborne diseases, 98–104. *See also* Cholera and Typhoid fever
Waterhouse, Benjamin, 114
Watson, James D., 85
Weller, Thomas, 121–22
West Nile fever, 68, 141, 152, 156, 174
White, Ellen G., 46
Whitehead, Henry, 100
Whooping cough (pertussis), 128–29
Woese, Carl R., xv
Wolbachia bacteria, 142

XDR-TB (extremely drug-resistant tuberculosis), 66–67
Xenophylla cheopsis, 11

Yaws, 23–24. *See also* Syphilis
Yellow fever, 135–37, 141
Yersin, Alexandre, 10–11, 57
Yersinia pestis, 10–12, 154
Yersinia pseudotuberculosis, 11

Zika virus, 173
Zinder, Norton, 85
Zoonoses, 4–5, 76, 154, 201
Zur Hausen, Harald, 133–34

About the Author

LOIS N. MAGNER is Professor Emerita at Purdue University. She is the author of *Doctors, Nurses, and Medical Practitioners: A Bio-Bibliographical Sourcebook* (Greenwood Press, 1998), *A History of Medicine: Second Edition, Revised and Expanded* (2005), and *A History of the Life Sciences: Third Edition, Revised and Expanded* (2002).